CALCIUM ENTRY BLOCKERS IN CARDIOVASCULAR AND CEREBRAL DYSFUNCTIONS

DEVELOPMENTS IN CARDIOVASCULAR MEDICINE

Lancée CT, ed: Echocardiology, 1979. ISBN 90-247-2209-8.

Baan J, Arntzenius AC, Yellin EL, eds: Cardiac dynamics. 1980. ISBN 90-247-2212-8.

Thalen HJT, Meere CC, eds: Fundamentals of cardiac pacing. 1970. ISBN 90-247-2245-4.

Kulbertus HE, Wellens HJJ, eds: Sudden death. 1980. ISBN 90-247-2290-X.

Dreifus LS, Brest AN, eds: Clinical applications of cardiovascular drugs. 1980. ISBN 90-247-2295-0.

Spencer MP, Reid JM, eds: Cerebrovascular evaluation with Doppler ultrasound. 1981. ISBN 90-247-2348-1.

Zipes DP, Bailey JC, Elharrar V, eds: The slow inward current and cardiac arrhythmias. 1980. ISBN 90-247-2380-9.

Kesteloot H, Joossens JV, eds: Epidemiology of arterial blood pressure. 1980. ISBN 90-247-2386-8.

Wackers FJT, ed: Thallium-201 and technetium-99m-pyrophosphate myocardial imaging in the coronary care unit. 1980. ISBN 90-247-2396-5.

Maseri A, Marchesi C, Chierchia S, Trivella MG, eds: Coronary care units. 1981. ISBN 90-247-2456-2.

Morganroth J, Moore EN, Dreifus LS, Michelson EL, eds: The evaluation of new antiarrhythmic drugs. 1981. ISBN 90-247-2474-0.

Alboni P: Intraventricular conduction disturbances. 1981. ISBN 90-247-2484-X.

Rijsterborgh H, ed: Echocardiology. 1981. ISBN 90-247-2491-0.

Wagner GS, ed: Myocardial infarction: Measurement and intervention. 1982. ISBN 90-247-2513-5.

Meltzer RS, Roelandt J, eds: Contrast echocardiography. 1982. ISBN 90-247-2531-3.

Amery A, Fagard R, Lijnen R, Staessen J, eds: Hypertensive cardiovascular disease; pathophysiology and treatment. 1982. ISBN 90-247-2534-8.

Bouman LN, Jongsma HJ, eds: Cardiac rate and rhythm. 1982. ISBN 90-247-2626-3.

Morganroth J, Moore EN, eds: The evaluation of beta blocker and calcium antagonist drugs. 1982. ISBN 90-247-2642-5.

Rosenbaum MB, ed: Frontiers of cardiac electrophysiology. 1982. ISBN 90-247-2663-8.

Roelandt J, Hugenholtz PG, eds: Long-term ambulatory electrocardiography. 1982. ISBN 90-247-2664-8.

Adgey AAJ, ed: Acute phase of ischemic heart disease and myocardial infarction. 1982. ISBN 90-247-2675-1.

Hanrath P, Bleifeld W, Souquet, J. eds: Cardiovascular diagnosis by ultrasound. Transesophageal, computerized, contrast, Doppler echocardiography. 1982. ISBN 90-247-2692-1.

Roelandt J, ed: The practice of M-mode and two-dimensional echocardiography. 1983. ISBN 90-247-2745-6.

Meyer J, Schweizer P, Erbel R, eds: Advances in noninvasive cardiology. 1983. ISBN 0-89838-576-8.

Morganroth J, Moore EN, eds: Sudden cardiac death and congestive heart failure: Diagnosis and treatment. 1983. ISBN 0-89838-580-6.

Perry HM, ed: Lifelong management of hypertension. 1983. ISBN 0-89838-582-2.

Jaffe EA, ed: Biology of endothelial cells. 1984. ISBN 0-89838-587-3.

Surawicz B, Reddy CP, Prystowsky EN, eds: Tachycardias. ISBN 0-89838-588-1.

Spencer MP, ed: Cardiac Doppler diagnosis. 1983. ISBN 0-89838-591-1.

Villarreal H, Sambhi MP, eds: Topics in pathophysiology of hypertension. 1984. ISBN 0-89838-595-4.

Messerli FH, ed: Cardiovascular disease in the elderly. 1984. ISBN 0-89838-596-2.

Simoons ML, Reiber JHC, eds: Nuclear imaging in clinical cardiology. 1984. ISBN 0-89838-599-7.

Ter Keurs HEDJ, Schipperheyn JJ, eds: Cardiac left ventricular hypertrophy. 1983. ISBN 0-89838-612-8.

Sperelakis N, ed: Physiology and pathophysiology of the heart. ISBN 0-89838-612-2.

Messerli FH, ed: Kidney in essential hypertension. ISBN 0-89838-616-0.

Sambhi MP, ed: Fundamental fault in hypertension. ISBN 0-89838-638-1.

Marchesi C, ed: Ambulatory monitoring: Cardiovascular system and allied applications. ISBN 0-89838-642-X.

Kupper W, MacAlpin RN, Bleifeld W, eds: Coronary tone in ischemic heart disease. ISBN 0-89838-646-2.

Sperelakis N, Caulfield JB, eds: Calcium antagonists: Mechanisms of action on cardiac muscle and vascular smooth muscle. ISBN 0-89838-655-1.

Godfraind T, Herman AG Wellens D, eds: Calcium entry blockers in cardiovascular and cerebral dysfunctions. ISBN 0-89838-658-1.

Morganroth J, Moore EN, eds: Interventions in the acute phase of myocardial infarction. ISBN 0-89838-659-4.

CALCIUM ENTRY BLOCKERS IN CARDIOVASCULAR AND CEREBRAL DYSFUNCTIONS

edited by

THÉOPHILE GODFRAIND, M.D.
Laboratoire de Pharmacodynamie Générale et de Pharmacologie
Université Catholique de Louvain,
Brussels, Belgium

ARNOLD G. HERMAN, M.D.
Department of Medicine, University of Antwerp, Wilrijk, Belgium

DONALD WELLENS, Dr. Sc.
Janssen Pharmaceutica, Beerse, Belgium

1984 **MARTINUS NIJHOFF PUBLISHERS**
a member of the KLUWER ACADEMIC PUBLISHERS GROUP
BOSTON / THE HAGUE / DORDRECHT / LANCASTER

Distributors

for the United States and Canada: Kluwer Boston, Inc., 190 Old Derby Street, Hingham, MA 02043, USA
for all other countries: Kluwer Academic Publishers Group, Distribution Center, P.O.Box 322, 3300 AH Dordrecht, The Netherlands

Library of Congress Cataloging in Publication Data

Main entry under title:

Calcium entry blockers in cardiovascular and cerebral
    dysfunction.

    (Developments in cardiovascular medicine)
    Text in Engl., with resumés in French, German, and
Spanish.
    Includes bibliographical references.
    1. Calcium--Antagonists--Therapeutic use. 2. Cardio-
vascular system--Diseases--Chemotherapy. 3. Cerebrovascu-
lar disease--Chemotherapy. I. Godfraind, T. (Théophile)
II. Herman, A. G. III. Wellens, Donald. IV. Series.
[DNLM: 1. Calcium Channel Blockers--pharmacodynamics.
2. Calcium Channel Blockers--therapeutic use. 3. Cardio-
vascular Diseases--drug therapy. 4. Cerebrovascular
Disorders--drug therapy. Wl DE997VME / QV 276 Cl429]
RC684.C34C36 1984   616.1'061   84-7968
ISBN 0-89838-658-6

ISBN-13: 978-94-009-6035-0   e-ISBN-13: 978-94-009-6033-6
DOI: 10.1007/978-94-009-6033-6

Copyright

Contents

Chapter I:

Introductory considerations

The major steps in the discovery of calcium entry blockers

A. G. Herman

Summary

The discovery of calcium entry blockers stresses the importance of the ubiquitous calcium gradient in all living cells.

The chemical structure as well as the functional selectivity of different calcium entry blockers may differ markedly. Some are primarily active on the myocardium, others on erythrocytes or on mast cells.

The potent antivasoconstrictor effect of some diphenylmethylderivatives was ascribed to Ca^{2+} entry blockade as early as 1968. The myocardial effects of verapamil and methoxyverapamil were also attributed to calcium entry blockade. The various mechanisms by which drugs can interfere with Ca^{2+} fluxes through the cell membrane are currently becoming more and more apparent.

There is no doubt that pharmacologists are getting a better insight into the basic mechanisms of cellular calcium homeostasis and that clinicians are obtaining new valuable medicines.

Résumé

La découverte de substances qui inhibent l'entrée intracellulaire des ions calciques confirme l'importance du gradient calcique transmembranaire qui caractérise toute cellule vivante.

Ce groupe de substances est très hétérogène aussi bien quant à leur structure chimique que quant à leur action fonctionnelle sélective. Certaines substances excellent par leur action sur le coeur, d'autres par leur action au niveau des érythrocytes ou des mastocytes. L'effet antivasoconstricteur très puissant de certains dérivés diphénylméthylés a déjà été attribué à un antagonisme calcique en 1968. Bientôt, les effets cardiaques du vérapamil et du méthoxyvérapamil furent aussi décrits comme étant le résultat d'un antagonisme calcique. Il devient de plus en plus clair que les inhibiteurs calciques peuvent interférer de plusieurs façons avec les voies de passage de Ca^{2+} à travers la membrane cellulaire. Indubitablement, les pharmacologues arrivent à mieux décrire les mécanismes fondamentaux de l'homéostasie calcique cellulaire tout en offrant de nouvelles thérapeutiques cliniques valables.

Resumen

El descubrimiento de inhibidores de la penetración intracelular de iones cálcicos acentúa la importancia del gradiente de calcio en toda célula viva.

Las estructuras químicas de las moléculas activas pueden ser muy diferentes y también sus efectos sobre varias funciones celulares. Unos fármacos son muy efectivos en el miocardio, otros en eritocitos o en mastocitos. La fuerte acción inhibidora de vasoespasmos causada por derivados de difenilmetil ya se la atribuyó a un antagonismo de calcio en 1968. Los efectos miocardíacos de verapamil y metoxiverapamil tampoco tardaron en atribuirse a un antagonismo de calcio. Se va observando cada día más que los fármacos pueden influir de varias maneras sobre el tránsito de Ca^{2+} a través de la membrana celular. Está claro que los farmacólogos van haciéndose una mejor idea de los mecanismos fundamentales de la homeostasis intracelular de calcio y que los investigadores clínicos van descubriendo mejores agentes terapéuticos.

Zusammenfassung

Die Entdeckung von Kalzium-Antagonisten hat die grosse Bedeutung des Kalzium-Membrangradienten in allen lebenden Zellen bestätigt.

Kalzium-Antagonisten können sowohl in der chemischen Struktur als auch in ihrer Interferenz mit bestimmten zellulären Prozessen verschiedenartig sein. Einige wirken stark am Myokard, andere an den Erythrozyten oder den Mastozyten. 1968 wurde zum ersten Male die kräftige antivasokonstriktorische Wirkung von Diphenylmethyl-Derivaten einer kalziumantagonistischen Wirkung zugeschrieben. Ebenso ist die Myokardbeeinflussung durch Verapamil und Methoxyverapamil auf eine kalziumantagonistische Wirkung zurückzuführen. Gegenwärtig wird zunehmend deutlich, dass die Arzneimittel an verschiedenen Punkten des Kalziumtransportes angreifen können. Die Substanzen dienen den Pharmakologen beim Verständnis der grundlegenden Mechanismen der zellulären Kalzium-Homöostase, während sie für den Therapeuten zweifellos neue, wertvolle Medikamente liefern können.

4

The discovery of calcium entry blockers has been an ongoing process for as long as 25 years now. As early as 1958 several drugs were already available either as pharmacological tools or as medicines.

The pharmacological insight that the major mechanism of action of these drugs was related to an inhibition of entry of calcium ions into the cells came only some 10 years later, ± 1968.

This situation contrasts sharply with the history of the detection of beta-blockers since the concept of the beta-receptor was already born in 1948 (Ahlquist, 1948), thus preceding the synthesis of the first beta receptor-blocking drug, dichloroisoproterenol, by about 10 years.

Diphenylmethyl-derivatives

The first calcium entry blockers were synthetized at the end of the fifties by pharmaceutical companies which were completely unaware of the mechanism of action of their own compounds.
Cinnarizine was initially described as an anti-histaminic agent (van Proosdij-Hartzema and de Jongh, 1959) and as an anti-motion-sickness drug (Philipszoon, 1959). In the following years, pharmacologists were impressed by the potent general antivasoconstrictor activity of cinnarizine. Some of them stressed e.g. the anti-angiotensine effects of the drug (Schaper et al., 1963; Van Nueten et al., 1964; Cession, et al. 1964).

In 1968 the antivasoconstrictor effect of cinnarizine was tentatively ascribed for the first time to an inhibition of calcium ion influx (Godfraind et al., 1968). The calcium entry blocking effect of cinnarizine was confirmed later on in a great variety of tissue cells by various authors. The same goes for other diphenylmethyl-derivatives, such as prenylamine, flunarizine, lidoflazine and many others, as can be seen in the listing further on in this book (Wellens, 1984).

It should be stressed however, that several compounds are devoid of any significant effect on the myocardial cells at the level of the so-called "slow channels". There is clear-cut experimental proof now that there are several quite different ways for calcium ions to enter various tissue cells (Peters, 1983). Consequently, calcium entry blockers often differ in their tissue-selective actions.

Verapamil-congeners

Methoxyverapamil (D 600) and verapamil have also been known for a long time. The basic pharmacology of the latter drug was published more than twenty years ago (Haas and Härtfelder, 1962). For several years verapamil was considered to be a peculiar beta-adrenergic blocker (Schamroth, 1981). Later on, in 1969, these drugs were described as competitive calcium antagonists and it was suggested that they interfered with the intracellular entry of calcium ions. Together with D 600 and verapamil, another drug belonging to the diphenylmethyl-derivatives, prenylamine, was also recognized as a calcium antagonist (Fleckenstein, et al., 1969).

Dihydropyridine derivatives

In the seventies another chemical group of calcium entry blockers was found. The most prominent members of this group are, simultaneously, potent general vasodilator drugs. Therefore, the final hemodynamic result of their action may be quite different from the cardiovascular effects which are normally expected, i.e. positive (instead of negative) inotropic and chronotropic reactions, flush reactions and eventually oedema instead of protection from oedema.

Influence of drugs on calcium fluxes through the cell membrane

Presently it is recognized that drugs may contribute to the maintenance of the Ca^{2+} gradient at the level of the cellular membrane by different mechanisms (Peters 1983):

1. by membrane stabilization, i.e. increasing or restoring the high degree of impermeability of the lipid bilayer to Ca^{2+}
2. by blockade of specific Ca^{2+}-channels (either voltage dependent or receptor operated channels) which serve physiologic functions in certain cells
3. by restoration or improvement of the Ca^{2+} extrusion pump which is ATP-dependent. This action, which also protects the cells from Ca^{2+} overload, does not involve calcium entry blockade.

A major step for the ongoing research will be to define more clearly to what extent these various membrane processes are modified by the existing calcium entry blockers.

References

Ahlquist, R.P. A study of the adrenotropic receptor. *Amer. J. Physiol.*, **153**, 586-600 (1948).

Cession, G., Lecomte, J. and Van Cauwenberghe, H. Action antagoniste de la cinnarizine vis-à-vis de l'angiotensine in vivo. *Compt. Rend. Soc. Biol.*, **158**, 1754-1756 (1964).

Fleckenstein, A., Tritthart, H. and Fleckenstein, B. A new group of competitive Ca-antagonists (iproveratril, D 600, prenylamine) with highly potent inhibitory effects on excitation-contraction coupling in mammalian myocardium. *Pflügers Arch. ges. Physiol.*, **307**, R 25 (1969).

Godfraind, R., Kaba, A. and Polster, P. Differences in sensitivity of arterial smooth muscles to inhibition of their contractile response to depolarization by potassium. *Arch. Intern. Pharmacodyn. Ther.*, **172**, 235-239 (1968).

Haas, H. and Härtfelder, G. α-Isopropyl- α[(N-methyl-N-homoveratryl)- γ-aminopropyl]-3,4-dimethoxyphenyl-acetonitril, eine Substanz mit coronargefässerweiternden Eigenschaften. *Arzneimittel - Forsch.*, **12**, 549-553 (1962).

Peters, T. Calcium-Antagonismus: Ein einheitlicher Begriff für uneinheitliche Wirkmechanismen. *Med. Klin.*, **78(11)**, 368-375 (1983).

Philipszoon, A.J. The effect of some drugs upon the labyrinth. A nystagmographical study of the action of anti-motion sickness drugs.
Thesis, Amsterdam, (1959).

Schamroth, L. The philosophy of calcium-ion antagonists. In: Calcium antagonism in cardiovascular therapy: experience with verapamil. p. 5-9. Eds. A. Zanchetti and D.M. Krikler, Excerpta Medica (1981).

Schaper, W.K.A., Jageneau, A.H.M., Xhonneux, R., Van Nueten, J. and Janssen, P.A.J. Cinnarizine (R 516), a specific angiotensine-blocking coronary vasodilator. *Life Sci.*, **2**, 963-974 (1963).

van Proosdij-Hartzema, E.G. and de Jongh, D.K. A new piperazine compound with antihistaminic activity. *Acta Physiol. Pharmacol. Neerlandica*, **8**, 337-342 (1959).

Van Nueten, J.M., Dresse, A. and Dony, J. Action antagoniste de la cinnarizine vis-à-vis de l'angiotensine in vitro. Comptes rendus des séances de la Société de Biologie, **158**, 1750-1754 (1964).

Wellens, D. Twenty-seven calcium entry blockers in development: a new chapter in pharmacology. In: "Calcium entry blockers in cardiovascular and cerebral dysfunctions", p. 25-42. Eds. T. Godfraind, A. Herman, D. Wellens. Martinus Nijhoff Publishers (1984).

Basic mechanisms and classification of calcium entry blockers

T. Godfraind

Summary

Calcium antagonists may exert the following actions at the level of the cell membrane:
1. they may interfere with specific Ca^{2+} channels e.g. the slow Ca^{2+} channels of the heart, voltage-operated or receptor-operated channels in smooth muscles;
2. they may diminish intracellular Ca^{2+} entry by blocking the continuous leakage of the cell membrane;
3. they might restore or improve Ca^{2+} extrusion via the Na-Ca exchange pump or the Ca-ATP pump.
Calcium antagonists may exert additional actions, related or not to calcium metabolism or to calcium function. Calcium entry blockers do specifically act on membrane Ca channels operated by depolarization or by receptors.

Résumé

Les antagonistes du calcium peuvent exercer les actions suivantes au niveau de la membrane cellulaire :
1. Ils peuvent interférer avec les canaux spécifiques de Ca^{2+}, par exemple les lents canaux de Ca^{2+} du coeur, les canaux activés par voltage ou par récepteur dans les muscles lisses.
2. Ils peuvent diminuer l'entrée de Ca^{2+} dans la cellule en bloquant l'infiltration s'effectuant par la membrane cellulaire.
3. Ils pourraient restaurer ou améliorer l'expulsion du Ca^{2+} via la pompe à échange Na-Ca ou la pompe Ca-ATP.
Les antagonistes du calcium peuvent exercer d'autres actions, reliées ou non au métabolisme du calcium ou à la fonction du calcium. Les agents bloqueurs de l'entrée de calcium agissent spécifiquement sur les canaux de calcium de la membrane activés par dépolarisation ou par des récepteurs.

Resumen

Los antagonistas de calcio pueden ejercer las acciones siguientes a nivel de la membrana celular :
1. pueden interferir con canales Ca^{2+} específicos p.ej. los canales Ca^{2+} "lentos" del corazón, los canales accionados por voltaje o por receptores en músculos lisos;
2. pueden disminuir la entrada intracelular de Ca^{2+} bloqueando la gota continua de la membrana celular;
3. podrían restablecer o mejorar la extrusión de Ca^{2+} via la bomba de cambio Na-Ca o la bomba Ca-ATP.
Los antagonistas de calcio pueden ejercer acciones adicionales, relacionadas o no con el metabolismo cálcico o con la función cálcica. Los inhibidores de la entrada de Ca^{2+} actúan específicamente en canales membranosos de Ca^{2+}, accionados por depolarización o por receptores.

Zusammenfassung

Kalzium-Einstromhemmer können an der Zellmembran die folgenden Wirkungen ausüben :
1. Beeinflussung spezifischer Ca^{2+}-Kanäle, z.B. der langsamen Ca^{2+}-Kanäle des Herzens, oder der potential- bzw. rezeptorabhängigen Kanäle glatter Muskeln ;
2. Herabsetzung des intrazellulären Ca^{2+}-Einstroms durch Hemmung des kontinuierlichen Durchlasses durch die Zellmembran ;
3. Wiederherstellung bzw. Verbesserung der Ca^{2+}-Ausfuhr über die Na-Ca-Austauschpumpe oder über die Ca-ATP-Pumpe.
Kalzium-Einstromhemmer können auch zusätzliche Wirkungen ausüben, die nicht unbedingt mit Calciummetabolismus oder Calciumfunktion zusammen-
hängen müssen. Sie wirken spezifisch auf Membran-Ca-Kanäle ein, die durch Depolarisierung oder Rezeptoren reguliert werden.

10

Basic mechanisms and terminology

No group of drugs has received so many names as the group which was originally called calcium antagonists and which is also referred to as calcium channel blockers, calcium entry blockers, calcium modulators or calcium overload inhibitors.

The concept of calcium antagonism in vascular smooth muscle cells emerged from earlier studies with lidoflazine and with cinnarizine (Godfraind et al., 1968; Godfraind and Polster, 1968), whereas the concept of calcium antagonism in heart muscle emerged from studies with verapamil (Fleckenstein, et al., 1969).

Presently, several basic mechanisms contributing to the calcium homeostasis in living cells, are identified. The information provided by physiological, pharmacologial and biochemical studies is summarized by the model illustrated in figure 1.

In a resting cell the concentration of calcium dissolved in the cytoplasmic sap only reaches 10^{-4} of the extracellular concentration. Since the intracellular potential is negative the electrochemical gradient pushes calcium ions inside the cell. The low internal/external calcium ratio is due to several cellular properties. The plasma membrane of the resting cell allows only a slow calcium influx. All the models representing the cell plasma membrane consider the existence of a lipid bilayer that is almost impermeable to polar molecules. The transfer across this barrier occurs generally 1) through channels or 2) when the ion or the molecule forms a complex with a carrier or 3) by endocytosis. Passage through channels is determined by the diameter of their opening and by the electrochemical gradient.

The best known channels are the sodium channels that are blocked by tetrodotoxin and other related drugs. Studies with these toxins have allowed to measure the density of the channels at the surface of the cell and to characterize some of their chemical properties. A large proportion of the sodium channels are open in the resting cell. Those channels allow the passage of ions ressembling sodium such as lithium, but not of ions that have other characteristics such as calcium (Caterall, 1980).

As far as calcium is concerned, few channels appear to be accessible when the membrane is polarized. Using ^{45}Ca, it is possible to observe that the radioactive ion will progressively replace the intracellular calcium. Because of the low permeability of the membrane, this process requires a prolonged incubation (Godfraind, 1976). However, it shows that the inward oriented calcium electrochemical gradient could, on the long run, allow a progressive increase of the intracellular calcium content, leading to a cellular calcium overload. The maintenance of the calcium steady-state requires calcium extrusion mechanisms located in the plasma membrane.

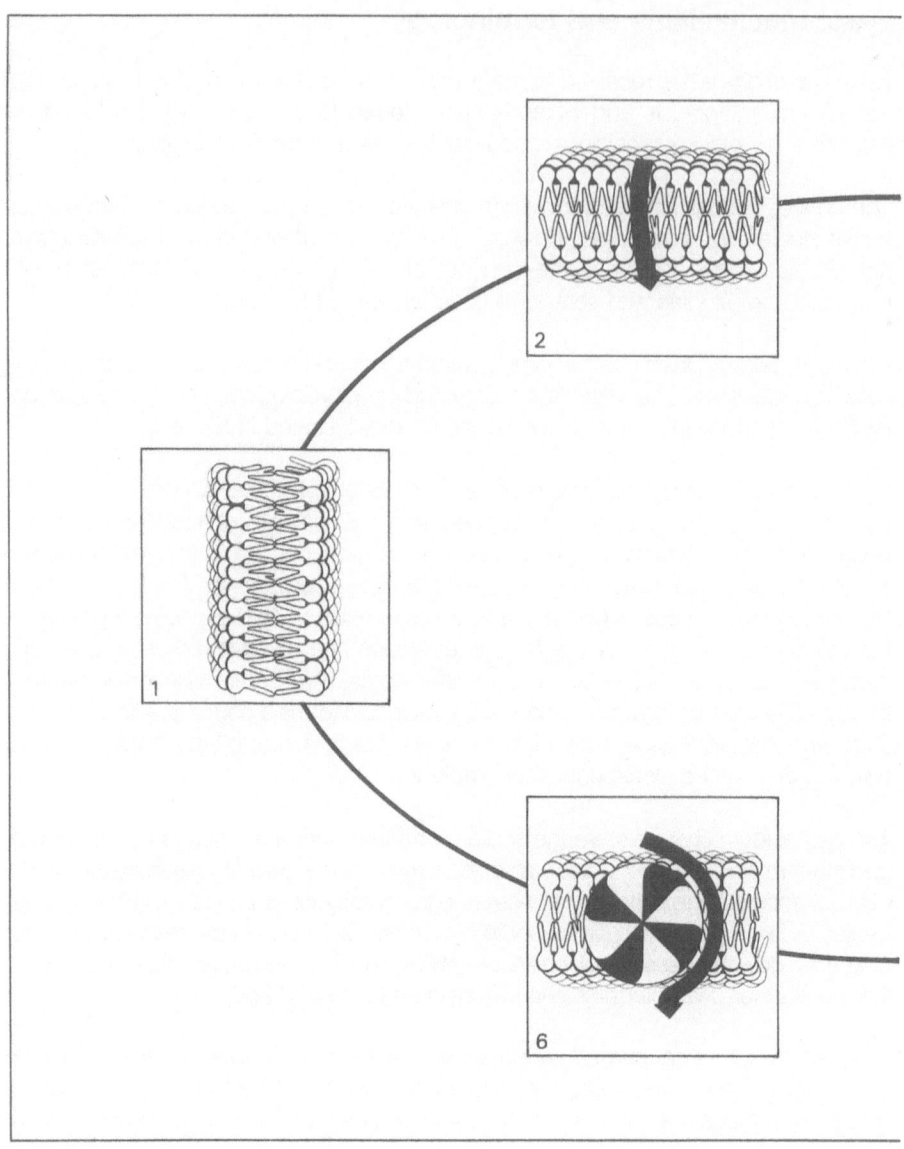

Figure 1. Schematic representation of calcium transport systems through the cell membrane.

From the left to the right:
1. Lipid double layer: basic structure of the cell membrane.
2. "Leak-flow" through the lipid double layer allowing a slow entry of extracellular Ca^{2+}.
3. "Voltage operated channel" in smooth muscle cells, highly sensitive to calcium entry blockers.

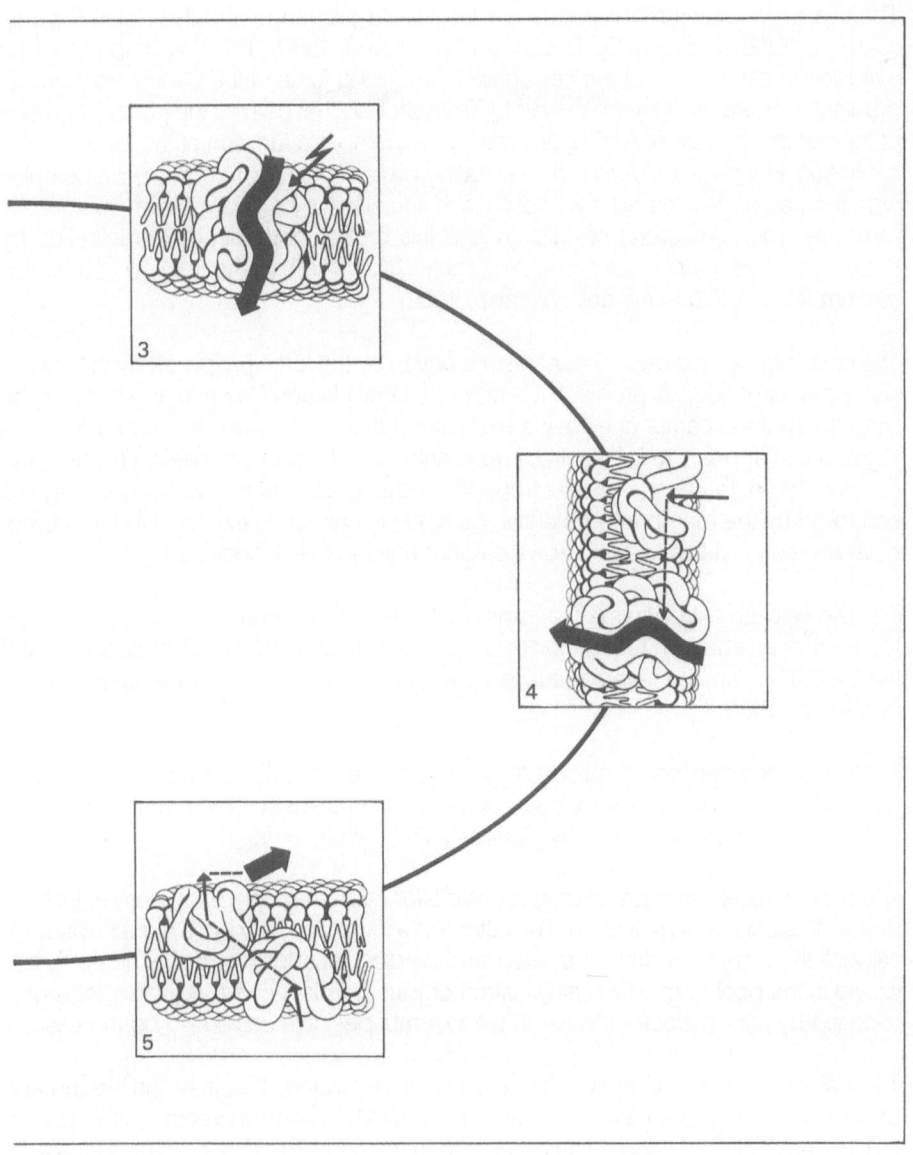

4. "Receptor operated channel", with receptor protein near the "channel".
5. System of release of Ca^{2+} from intracellular calcium stores through activation of a receptor protein at the outside of the cell membrane.
6. Calcium extrusion processes using energy which is derived a) either from the inward Na^+ electrochemical gradient b) or from the hydrolysis of ATP catalysed by a calmodulin-Ca-activated ATPase.

The two main known mechanisms are the Na-Ca exchange and the Ca-ATP pump (Carafoli, 1982; Godfraind-De Becker and Godfraind, 1980). The Ca-pump allows the extrusion of calcium out of the cell against the driving force of the Ca electrochemical gradient. It operates at the expense of ATP-hydrolysis that permits the phosphorylation of the pump. The rate of ATP hydrolysis by the pump is a function of the calcium concentration. However, calcium is not operating by itself but after formation of a complex with a small protein called calmodulin and identified by Cheung as an ubiquitous molecule. The interactions of calcium and this protein have been characterized by Kretsinger. This calcium-calmodulin complex (Ca-CAM) is the form under which calcium is operating in the cell (Vincenzi, 1982).

The other calcium extrusion mechanism is driven by the force produced by the inward sodium electrochemical gradient. It is proposed that Na and Ca have an affinity for the same membrane carrier (the Na-Ca exchanger) that binds one Ca^{2+} and 3 Na^+. Its function that appears to be electrogenic is enhanced by phosphorylation (Caroni and Carafoli, 1983). Because of its electrogenecity, the function of the Na-Ca exchanger is controlled by the membrane potential. As a result, calcium is extruded in the resting, polarized cell, but this system allows calcium entry in the depolarized cell.

The two calcium extrusion mechanisms are not equally distributed among the various tissues. For example, in heart, the Na-Ca exchange has a much higher capacity than the Ca-ATP pump, the reverse situation being found in the smooth muscle (Godfraind and Morel, 1983).

There is a compartmentalisation for calcium in the cell, this ion not being equally distributed within the cytosol but bound to buffering proteins such as parvalbumins and sequestered inside intracellular organelles (Gillis, 1982).

The main intracellular organelles responsible for calcium sequestration are mitochondria and sarcoplasmic reticulum. The latter has a lower capacity but a higher affinity for calcium than mitochondria. In striated and cardiac muscles, sarcoplasmic reticulum provides the pool from which all (striated) or part (cardiac) of the activator calcium is released by the contractile stimuli. In smooth muscles, this could also be the case.

The calcium scene changes when the cell is stimulated, because the membrane becomes abruptly permeable to calcium as shown by an increase in the rate of calcium entry after depolarization or receptor activation (Godfraind, 1976). It is assumed that the membrane of excitable cells contains Ca channels operated by membrane potential and by receptors and that they are open during depolarization or when an agonist interacts with its specific receptors (Bolton, 1979; Weiss, 1981). In the sixties, we have shown in smooth muscle that this increase in membrane permeability for calcium was prevented by cinnarizine and lidoflazine, polyvalent antagonists of vasoactive agents (Godfraind and Polster, 1968). Those drugs were at that time considered "calcium antagonists". We now have more information on their action, since it has been established that they act specifically on the potential and the receptor operated channels, the former being more sensitive than the latter to the blockade action of the drugs listed as calcium entry blockers (Table 1). Some of the drugs that block calcium channels in smooth muscles are also active on the heart where they block the slow Na-Ca channel responsible for the plateau phase of the action potential. The prototype of these drugs is verapamil (Fleckenstein, 1977). As shown in experimental studies, the three drugs active in hypertension (diltiazem, verapamil, nifedipine) have different actions on A-V mode conduction and on the general hemodynamic parameters (Taira et al., 1975).

Terminology and classification

As pointed out in the preceding section, some drugs act specifically on receptors and potential operated calcium channels, but some other drugs have additional actions related or not to calcium metabolism or to calcium function. The difficulty of the classification results from insufficient information on the pharmacological profile of most of the drugs listed in Table 1. The only common property shared by these drugs is their ability to inhibit the contraction evoked by K-depolarization of smooth muscle. Some of them have also an effect on the slow Na-Ca channel in the heart.

Table 1. Ca entry blockers with potential interest in therapy
(For Ref. see Godfraind 1982)

A. Specific Ca entry blockers
Angina
    Lidoflazine, verapamil, diltiazem, nifedipine
Hypertension
    Verapamil, nifedipine, diltiazem
Arrhythmia
    Verapamil
Cerebral and peripheral vascular disorders
    Cinnarizine, flunarizine, nimodipine
Under experimental study
    Nisoldipine, niludipine, nicardipine, tiapamil

B. Ca entry blockers with an additional action
1. On catecholamine receptors
    Chlorpromazine
    Rauwolscine and corynanthine
    Pimozide
2. On fast Ca channel
    Angina: Bepridil, perhexiline, prenylamine, fendiline, bencyclane
3. On Ca calmodulin
    Felodipine
4. On phosphodiesterase
    Papaverine
    Amrinone

If we consider intracellular actions, some drugs such as diltiazem interfere with the Ca-CAM complex, inhibit the release of calcium from sarcoplasmic reticulum and interfere with Na-Ca exchange in mitochondria (Cauvin et al., 1983). In a situation such as cardiac ischemia resulting in toxic calcium overload, the protective effect of diltiazem may be due to its action on calcium channels or on intracellular calcium metabolism (Millard *et al.*, 1983). However, if we consider spasm of coronary arteries, it seems fair to recognize that the action of nifedipine results from blockade of calcium channels (Godfraind and Miller, 1983). It is also likely that the action of flunarizine and cinnarizine in tissue hypoxia results from their blockade in vessels (Van Nueten, 1982; Vanhoutte, 1982). As far as these drugs are concerned, it must in addition be pointed out that they show a specificity of action for some vascular beds, which is the basis for the concept of tissue specificity. On the other hand, lidoflazine, flunarizine and cinnarizine, which are weak blockers of the slow Na-Ca channels in the heart, share with the potent blockers, verapamil and diltiazem, the property to protect myocytes against the necrotic action of factors such as hypoxia, ischemia, calcium paradox or catecholamines. In these conditions, cell death appears to be due to calcium overload. The cardioprotective mechanism still needs to be identified (Nayler *et al.*, 1980).

Recent studies using radioactive dihydropyridines have shown the existence of specific binding sites which are believed to be associated with calcium channels. The binding shows high affinity, saturability and is competed by calcium entry blockers of the same or of other chemical structure such as diltiazem or flunarizine (Glossmann *et al.*, 1982; Bolger *et al.*, 1983).

More recently, it has been shown that some dihydropyridines do not block but open the calcium channels producing smooth muscle contraction and cardiac positive inotropic effect. These agents interact with nifedipine binding sites. The field of drugs interfering with the function of calcium is now extending, raising new questions in Pharmacology and opening new possibilities in Therapy.

References

Bolger, G.T., Gengo, P., Klockowski, R., Luchowski, E., Siegel, H., Janis, R.A., Triggle, S.M. and Triggle, D.J. Characterization of binding of the Ca^{2+} channel antagonist, (^{3}H)-nitrendipine, to guinea-pig ileal smooth muscle. *J. Pharmacol. Exp. Ther.*, **225**, 291-309. (1983)

Bolton, R.B. Mechanisms of action of transmitters and other substances on smooth muscle. *Physiol. Rev.*, **59**, 606-718. (1979)

Caroni, P. and Carafoli, L. The regulation of the Na^+-Ca^{2+} exchange of heart sarcolemma. *Eur. J. Biochem.* **132**, 451-460. (1983)

Catteral, W.A. Neurotoxins that act on voltage-sensitive sodium channels in excitable membranes. *Ann. Rev. Pharmacol. Toxicol.*, **20**, 15-43. (1980)

Cauvin, C., Loutzenhiser, R. and van Breemen, C. Mechanisms of calcium antagonist-induced vasodilatation. *Ann. Rev. Pharmacol. Toxicol.*, **23**, 373-396. (1983)

Fleckenstein, A. Specific pharmacology of calcium in myocardium, cardiac pacemakers and vascular smooth muscle. *Ann. Rev. Pharmacol. Toxicol.*, **17**, 149-166. (1977)

Fleckenstein, A. Basic membrane actions of calcium antagonists with special reference to verapamil. In: Calcium Modulators. T. Godfraind, A. Albertini and R. Paoletti (Eds.)., pp. 297-310, Elsevier Biomedical Press, Amsterdam-New York-Oxford. (1982)

Fleckenstein, A. and Grun, G. Reversible Blockierung der elektromechanischen Koppelungsprozesse in der glatten Muskulatur des Rattenuterus mittels organischer Ca^{2+}-antagonisten (Iproveratril, D600, Prenylamin). *Pfluegers Arch.*, **307**, R26. (1969)

Fleckenstein, A., Tritthart, A., Fleckenstein, B., Herbst, A. and Grun, G. Elne neue Gruppe kompetitiver Ca^{2+}-antagonisten (Iproveratril, D600, Prenylamin), mit starken Hemmeffekten auf die electromekanische Koppelung in Warmblüter-myokard. *Pfluegers Arch.*, **307**, R25. (1969)

Gillis, J.M. Similarities and differences in excitation-contraction coupling in the various types of muscle cells. In: Calcium Modulators. T. Godfraind, A. Albertini and R. Paoletti (Eds.)., pp. 29-38, Elsevier Biomedical Press, Amsterdam-New York-Oxford. (1982)

Glossmann, H., Ferry, D.R., Lübbecke, F., Meeves, R., and Hofmann, F. Calcium channels: direct identification with radioligand binding studies. *TIPS*, 431-437. (1982)

Godfraind-De Becker, A. and Godfraind, T. Calcium transport system: a comparative study in different cells. *Int. Rev. Cytol.*, **67**, 141-170. (1980)

Godfraind, T. Calcium exchange in vascular smooth muscle, action of noradrenaline and lanthanum. *J. Physiol.* (London), **260**, 21-35. (1976)

Godfraind, T. Mechanisms of action of calcium entry blockers. *Fed. Proc.*, **40**, 2866-2871. (1982)

Godfraind, T. Pharmacology of calcium entry blockers. In: Calcium Modulators. T. Godfraind, A. Albertini and R. Paoletti (Eds.)., pp. 51-65, Elsevier Biomedical Press, Amsterdam-New York-Oxford. (1982)

Godfraind, T. Actions of nifedipine on calcium fluxes and contraction in isolated rat arteries. *J. Pharmacol. Exp. Ther.*, **224**, 443-450. (1983)

Godfraind, T. and Dieu, D. The inhibition by flunarizine of the norepinephrine-evoked contraction and calcium influx in rat aorta and mesenteric arteries. *J. Pharmacol. Exp. Ther.*, **217**, 510-515. (1981)

Godfraind, T. and Kaba, A. Blockade or reversal of the contraction induced by calcium and adrenaline in depolarized arterial smooth muscle. *Br. J. Pharmacol.*, **35**, 548-560. (1969)

Godfraind, T. and Miller, R.C. Specificity of action of Ca^{2+} entry blockers. Comparison of their actions in rat arteries and in human coronary arteries. *Circ. Res.*, **52**. (Suppl. 1), 181-192. (1983)

Godfraind, T. and Morel, N. Na-Ca exchange in guinea-pig and rat smooth muscle. *J. Physiol.* (London), **340**, 23P. (1983)

Godfraind, T. and Polster, P. Etude comparative de médicaments inhibant la réponse contractile de vaisseaux isolés d'origine humaine ou animale. *Thérapie*, **23**, 1209-1220. (1968)

Godfraind, T., Albertini, A. and Paoletti, R. (editors). Calcium Modulators. Elsevier Biomedical Press, Amsterdam-New York-Oxford. (1982)

Godfraind, T., Kaba, A. and Polster, P. Differences in sensitivity of arterial smooth muscles to inhibition of their contractile response to depolarization by potassium. *Arch. Int. Pharmacodyn. Ther.*, **172**, 235-239. (1968)

Lees, K.S. and Tsien, R.W. Mechanism of calcium channel blockade by verapamil, D600, diltiazem and nitrendipine in single dialyzed heart cells. *Nature*, **302**, 790-794. (1983)

Millard, R.W., Grupp, G., Grupp, I.L., Di Salvo, J., De Pover, A. and Schwartz, A. Chronotropic, inotropic and vasodilator actions of diltiazem, nifedipine and verapamil: a comparative study of physiological responses and membrane receptor activity. *Circ. Res.*, **52** (Suppl. I), 29-39. (1983)

Nayler, W.G., Ferrari, R. and Williams, A. Protective effect of pretreatment with verapamil, nifedipine and propranolol on mitochondrial function in the ischemic and reperfused myocardium. *Am. J. Cardiol.*, **46**, 242-248. (1980)

Rahwan, R.G., Piascik, M.F. and Witiak, D.T. The role of calcium antagonism in the therapeutic action of drugs. *Can. J. Physiol. Pharmacol.*, **57**, 443-460. (1979)

Saida, K. and van Breemen, C. Mechanism of Ca^{2+} antagonist-induced vasodilatation. Intracellular actions. *Circ. Res.*, **52**, 137-142. (1983)

Schramm, M., Thomas, G., Towart, R. and Franckowiak, G. Novel dihydropyridines with positive inotropic action through activation of Ca^{2+} channels. *Nature*, **303**, 535-537. (1983)

Singer, S.J. and Conrad, M.J. The structure of cell membranes. In: Cell membrane in function and dysfunction of vascular tissue. T. Godfraind and P. Meyer (Eds.), pp. 1-14, Elsevier Biomedical Press, Amsterdam-New York-Oxford. (1981)

Taira, N., Motomura, S., Narimatsu, A. and Fjima, T. Experimental pharmacological investigations of effects of nifedipine on atrioventricular conduction in comparison with those of other coronary vasodilators. In: The Second International Adalat Symposium. Lodner, W., Braasch, W. and Kroneberg, G. (Eds.), pp. 40-48, Springer Verlag. (1975)

Triggle, D.J. and Swamy, V.C. Pharmacology of agents that affect calcium: agonists and antagonists. *Chest*, **78** (Suppl.), 174-180. (1980)

Vanhoutte, P.M. Cinnarizine, flunarizine, lidoflazine. In: Calcium Modulators. T. Godfraind, A. Albertini and R. Paoletti (Eds।)., pp. 351-362, Elsevier Biomedical Press, Amsterdam-New York-Oxford. (1982)

Van Nueten, J.M. Selectivity of calcium entry blockers. In: Calcium Modulators. T. Godfraind, A. Albertini and R. Paoletti (Eds.)., pp. 199-208, Elsevier Biomedical Press, Amsterdam-New York-Oxford. (1982)

Vincenzi, F.F. Pharmacology of calmodulin antagonism. In: Calcium Modulators. T. Godfraind, A. Albertini and R. Paoletti (Eds.)., pp. 67-80, Elsevier Biomedical Press, Amsterdam-New York-Oxford. (1982)

Weiss, G. Sites of action of calcium antagonists in vascular smooth muscle. In: New perspectives on calcium antagonists. G. Weiss (Ed.), pp. 83-94, American Physiological Society, Bethesda, MD. (1981)

Weiss, B., Prozialeck, W.C. and Wallace, T.L. Interactions of drugs with calmodulin. Biochemical, pharmacological and clinical implications. *Biochem. Pharmacol.*, **31**, 2217-2226. (1982)

Zsoter, T.T. and Church, J.G. Calcium antagonists: pharmacodynamic effects and mechanism of action. *Drugs*, **25**, 93-112. (1983)

Calcium entry blockers: Perspectives

A. Schwartz

Summary

Some examples are mentioned to illustrate that the development of calcium antagonists increases our basic knowledge of cellular functions. Important clinical benefits may be obtained by developing calcium entry blockers with a highly selective action.

19

Résumé

Quelques exemples sont mentionnés pour illustrer le fait que le développement des bloqueurs de l'entrée de calcium amplifie nos connaissances de base sur les fonctions cellulaires. Des avantages cliniques importants peuvent être obtenus en développant des bloqueurs de l'entrée de calcium possédant une action hautement sélective.

Resumen

Algunos ejemplos se mencionan para ilustrar que el desarrollo de los antagonistas del calcio aumenta nuestros conocimientos básicos sobre las funciones celulares. Se pueden obtener importantes beneficios clínicos por el desarrollo de bloqueadores de la penetración intracelular del calcio con una actividad muy selectiva.

Zusammenfassung

Es wird an Beispielen gezeigt, dass die Entwicklung von Kalziumantagonisten zu einem verbesserten grundsätzlichen Verständnis der Zellfunktionen geführt hat. Bedeutende klinische Vorteile sind möglicherweise von der Entwicklung von Kalziumeintritthemmern mit stark selektiver Wirkung zu erwarten.

During the past 10 years, knowledge in the area of excitation-contraction-relaxation coupling in heart muscle has increased almost exponentially, so that we now have a basic understanding of how Ca^{2+} links these processes and how the cardiac cell may be regulated on a beat-to-beat level. While progress has been slower in vascular smooth muscle, recent developments have provided considerable information on a fundamental level. Thus, it is to be expected that pharmacological agents should emerge which have relatively selective effects on the movement of Ca^{2+}.

It is obvious that the cardiovascular drugs of the 1980's will be in the classification of "calcium antagonists" or "calcium entry blockers". As is the case with the development of all new classes of drugs, the situation has become much more complex than originally thought. There is no question that we are dealing with chemical structures that are not only different on paper, but even in a space-filling mode (Fig. 1). Accordingly, the fact that these agents share certain effects is interesting, but the fact that they do have qualitative and quantitative differences is to be expected (DePover, 1982; Schwartz, 1982).

In the United States, there are three Ca^{2+} channel blocking drugs on the market, verapamil, nifedipine, and diltiazem. These drugs have been approved for the treatment of variant (spasm) angina, as well as for stable angina pectoris. In addition, intravenous verapamil has been approved for the treatment of certain supraventricular cardiac arrhythmias. Those of us who deal with experimental animals, however, also recognize the potential for these drugs in a variety of clinical situatons is extremely high. Again, the reason is quite clear, namely that Ca^{2+} is the most important ionic link between processes involving excitation and biological processes. The drugs certainly interact with vascular smooth muscle and produce relaxation, hence the potential for treating certain types of hypertension is high. If, in some way, a "spasm" or change in contractile tone is involved in certain types of refractory migraine headaches, one could imagine that these drugs could be useful in that condition. For some years, alteration of Ca^{2+} metabolism in skeletal muscle associated with some types of muscular dystrophy has been an attractive hypothesis, and if so, again, one could imagine that these drugs might be useful in that debilitating illness. Preliminary evidence in this regard is encouraging. It is possible that some of the Ca^{2+} antagonists might inhibit the process of atherogenesis without altering serum cholesterol, but by somehow inhibiting the formation of free cholesterol and cholesterol esters inside the vascular smooth muscle cell and/or by inhibiting platelet aggregation.

As we continue to increase our knowledge base in this extremely important pharmacological area, I predict the synthesis of many drugs that will be selective for specific sites, such as cerebral blood vessels, peripheral blood vessels, secretory tissues, bronchiolar muscle, gastrointestinal muscle, uterine muscle, etc., so that these substances will surely find use in diseases which have been difficult to treat. Among these are certain allergies, stroke, dysmenorrhea, perhaps peptic ulcer, and certain endocrine disorders. Moreover, extending our receptor horizons from the cell membrane, where most of the available Ca^{2+} antagonists appear to act at the present, to the interior of the cell, we can predict the development of drugs that inhibit Ca^{2+} delivery to the contractile proteins and/or extrusion of Ca^{2+}; and these agents too, would have profound effects on a variety of processes.

We must keep in mind that the drugs we are dealing with are extraordinarily complex, that we are not dealing with a single class of drugs, and that when we do alter Ca^{2+}, we are manipulating perhaps the most fundamental component of life's processes. Even with the limited number of Ca^{2+} antagonists available at the present time, the complexities of their effects and the difficulties of interpretation are clearly demonstrated by examining the very recent [3H]-nitrendipine and nimodipine-binding data. The nifedipine-like drugs clearly inhibit the binding in a single site process, the verapamil-like drugs only inhibit the binding to about 50%, and diltiazem either has no effect or actually stimulates the binding (DePover, 1982; Schwartz, 1983). We have been able to show a "pharmacological synergism" between diltiazem and a dihydropyridine (DePover, 1983).

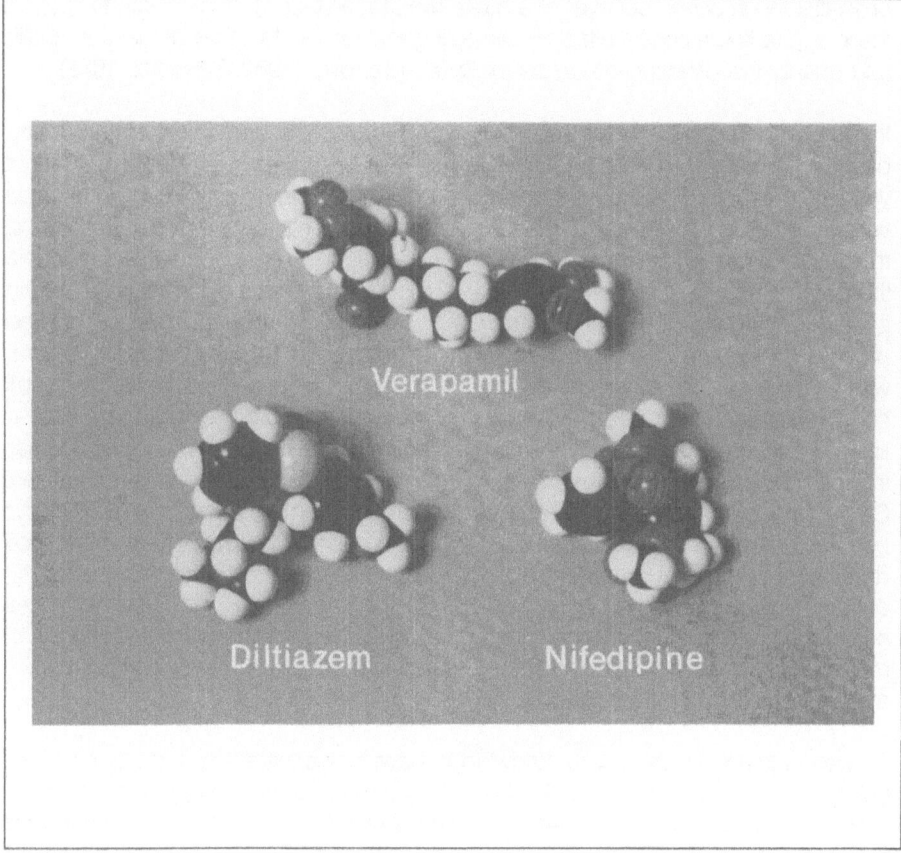

Figure 1.

My prediction is that the age of "calcium antagonists" will dominate cardiovascular pharmacology and perhaps other areas of pharmacology for years to come, and from the continued and hopefully increased basic and clinical activities, we will see emerge from these studies drugs that have highly selective actions and extraordinary important clinical benefits.

References

DePover, A., Matlib, M.A., Lee, S.W., Dube, G.P., Grupp, I.L., Grupp, G. and Schwartz, A. *Biochem. Biophys. Res. Commun.*, **108**, 110-117. (1982)

DePover, A., Grupp, I.L., Grupp, G. and Schwartz, A. *Biochem. Biophys. Res. Commun.*, **114**, 922-929. (1983)

Schwartz, A. *Am. J. Cardiol.*, **49**, 497-498. (1982)

Schwartz, A. and Taira, N. *Circ. Res.*, **52**, (Supp. 1), 11-12. (1983)

Twenty-seven calcium entry blockers in development: a new chapter in pharmacology

D. Wellens

Summary

Intracellular calcium overload can be prevented or antagonized by drugs which restore the impermeability of the lipid bilayer of the cell membrane, which block specific Ca^{2+}-channels or which enhance the Ca^{2+} extrusion pump. The chemically heterogeneous calcium entry blockers are tools which further our insight into the mechanisms of passage of calcium ions through cell membranes. The continuous interest in calcium entry blockers is due in the first place to their potentials as cardiovascular drugs. Their pharmacological characterization and their clinical applications in this respect are briefly reviewed in two listings. It is clear, however, that many other cell functions, outside the cardiovascular area, can be influenced by selective calcium entry blockers as well.

Résumé

L'excès d'ions calciques intracellulaires peut être prévenu ou remédié par des drogues qui restorent l'imperméabilité relative de la structure lipidique de la membrane cellulaire aux ions calciques, qui interfèrent avec des canaux calciques spécifiques existants dans certaines cellules ou qui activent la pompe d'extrusion cellulaire de Ca^{2+}. Le groupe des inhibiteurs de l'influx calcique, qui est chimiquement très hétérogène, mène à une meilleure évaluation des divers mécanismes de base réglant le passage de Ca^{2+} à travers les membranes cellulaires.

Les inhibiteurs de l'entrée calcique intracellulaire ont soulevé un intérêt majeur, en premier lieu dans le domaine de la pharmacothérapie cardiovasculaire. La caractérisation pharmacologique et les applications cliniques dans ce domaine sont décrits dans deux tableaux synoptiques. Il est clair, cependant, qu'il y a des fonctions cellulaires importantes, en dehors du domaine cardiovasculaire, susceptibles d'être influencées par des inhibiteurs sélectifs de l'entrée calcique.

Resumen

El exceso de los iones cálcicos intracelulares puede ser prevenido o remediado por drogas que restauran la impermeabilidad relativa de la estructura lípida de la membrana celular, que interfieren con canales cálcicos específicos presentes en ciertas células o que activan la bomba de extrusión de Ca^{2+}. Los inhibidores de la penetración intracelular de Ca^{2+}, muy heterogéneos desde el punto de vista químico, son medios que mejoran la evaluación de los diversos mecanismos de pasaje de los iones cálcicos a través de las membranas celulares. El continuo interés en los inhibidores de la penetración intracelular de Ca^{2+} es debido, en primer lugar, a sus aplicaciones como drogas cardiovasculares. Se examina su caracterización farmacológica y sus aplicaciones clínicas cardiovasculares en dos tablas sinópticas. Está claro, no obstante, que muchas otras funciones celulares, fuera del área cardiovascular, pueden ser influidas por inhibidores selectivos de la penetración intracelular de Ca^{2+} también.

Zusammenfassung

Ein Überschuss an intrazellulären Kalziumionen kann durch Arzneimittel entweder gehemmt oder antagonisiert werden. Dazu wird die relative Undurchdringlichkeit der Lipiddoppelschicht der Zellmembran wiederhergestellt, werden die spezifischen Ca^{2+}-Kanäle in bestimmten Zellen blockiert, oder wird die Aktivität der Kalziumpumpe gegen den Gradienten gesteigert. Die chemisch sehr heterogene Gruppe der Kalziumeinstromhemmer führt zu einer besseren Beurteilung der verschiedenen Basismechanismen, die den Durchgang von Kalzium durch Zellmembranen regeln. Besonders auf dem Gebiet der kardiovaskulären Pharmakotherapie liegt ein grosses Interesse an den Kalziumeinstromhemmern vor. Die pharmakologische Charakterisierung und die klinischen Anwendungen werden zu diesem Zweck in 2 Übersichtstabellen kurz beschrieben. Es ist jedoch klar, dass viele andere wichtige Zellfunktionen ausserhalb des kardiovaskulären Gebietes von selektiven Inhibitoren des Kalziumeintritts beeinflusst werden können.

There are two sound reasons for the overwhelming amount of continuing research work and for the avalanche of scientific publications on calcium entry blockers.

The first reason is that the enormous gradient of intracellular to extracellular calcium ion concentration is indeed a basic fact of life. This gradient is of crucial importance for the majority of biological processes.

The second reason is that the deciphering of this central point of the living machinery is being tackled intensively with a reasonable amount of success. A significant contribution to this success stems from the growing list of calcium entry blockers, providing valuable tools for this area of research.

1. The calcium ion gradient: the cornerstone of cellular life

The concentration of free calcium ions in the cytoplasm of living cells is approximately 10^{-7} M, whereas it is some 10,000 times higher in the surrounding extracellular fluid. This situation is visualised in figure 1. In some living cells important oscillations occur along with biological processes. For instance, in the myocardial cells the cytoplasmic Ca^{2+} concentration rises to some 10^{-5} M at each heart beat. Also in vascular smooth muscle cells vasoconstriction is accompanied by an elevation of cytoplasmic Ca^{2+}. This can be visualised by cytochemistry and measured e.g. with laser microprobe mass analysis (LAMMA). The LAMMA-method has shown that calcium entry blockers, which inhibit vasospasms provoked by high extracellular K^+ and Ca^{2+} concentrations, indeed also prevent the elevation of cytoplasmic Ca^{2+} (see De Nollin e.a. further in this book).

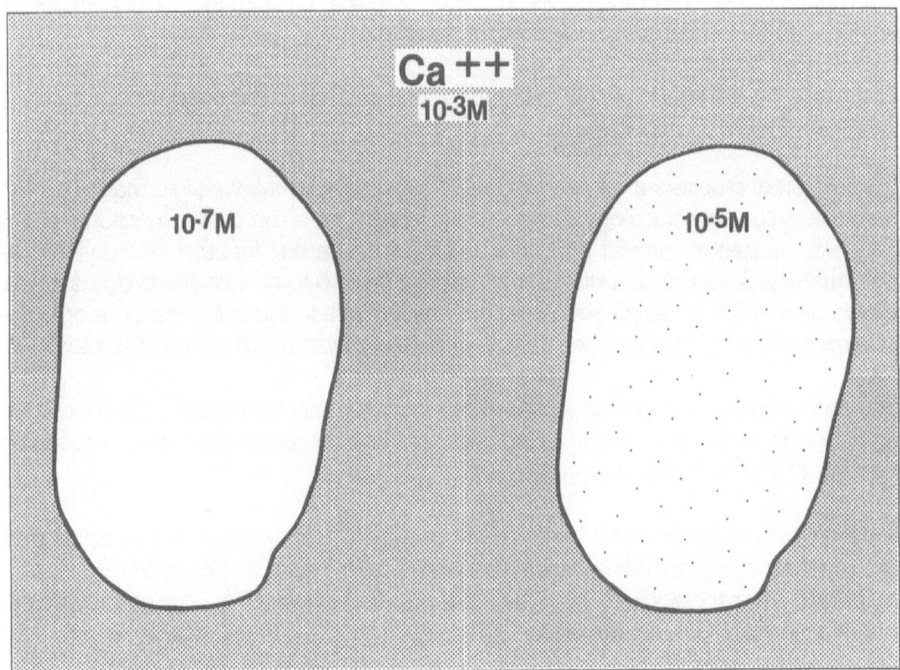

Figure 1: Relative concentrations of calcium ions in the extracellular fluid and in myocardial cells during diastole (relaxation: left side) or systole (contraction: right side).

The calcium ion gradient is maintained by the special lipid structure of the cell membrane, which is positively charged at the outside and negatively charged at the inside of the cell. The extremely small amount of leakage through the cell membrane is balanced by an ATP-dependent system pumping Ca^{2+} to the outside via a protein incorporated in the cell wall. The intracellular entry of Ca^{2+} will be excessive when the cell membrane loses its relative impermeability (e.g. depolarization due to elevation of extracellular $K+$; calcium-ionophores) or when the extrusion pump fails (e.g. shortage of ATP). Drugs can restore the basic impermeability of the cell membrane (calcium entry blockers) or the function of the extrusion pump (calcium overload blockers). The above applies to all cells, including red blood cells. In addition, specific calcium entry channels have been described in particular cells (e.g. slow channels in the myocardial cells). These channels (receptor operated or voltage operated) serve specific biological functions (e.g. myocardial contraction) and they can also be blocked by drugs (calcium channel blockers). This means that there are at least three mechanisms by which drugs provide protection against intracellular calcium overload.

2. The growing list of calcium entry blockers, calcium overload blockers and/or calcium channel blockers

Although the use of calcium entry blockers is mainly pointed at cardiovascular therapy, it is obvious that these agents contribute to a better understanding of physiological and pathological mechanisms in many other domains as well. A few topics are the Ca^{2+}-regulated processes in peripheral and central neurones, in mastocytes and in the various phases of cellular division. Some selective calcium entry blockers, for instance, can have interesting anti-allergic properties.

The major breakthrough of this category of drugs in the cardiovascular domain is illustrated in tables 1 and 2.

Calcium entry blockers are listed in Table 1 together with relevant information on the cardiovascular pharmacology of these compounds, focusing on the functional selectivity with respect to arterial and venous tone, myocardial function and erythrocyte deformability. A rough indication of the potency (from 0 to + +) of the drugs is given. Open cases in the table mean that no information was found in the literature or at the pharmaceutical companies that were very helpful in the compilation of the data.

The compounds are classified alphabetically according to their generic names. Some compounds at the end of the listing are only known, at present, by the research number of the company of origin.

Most calcium entry blockers have clearly divergent chemical structures, the largest group being dihydropyridine-derivatives. Some cardiovascular properties are shared by all calcium entry blockers, but others are not. The following relevant cardiovascular pharmacological features are listed:

1. "In vitro" antagonism of either KCl- or noradrenaline-induced arterial vasoconstriction. Calcium entry blockers are potent antagonists in both tests. However, the initial constrictor phase elicited by noradrenaline, is ascribed to a receptor-mediated release of intracellular calcium. This phase is not antagonized by calcium entry blockers, unless they also interfere with intracellular Ca^{2+}-mobilization. It should be stressed that tonic noradrenergic vasoconstrictions "in vivo" are readily inhibited by calcium entry blockers.

2. The myogenic contractions of venous preparations (especially the portal vein of the rat), which ultimately also depend on calcium ions, are not inhibited to the same extent by the calcium entry blockers. The compounds which inhibit the myogenic venous tone may reduce the preload of the heart. This would be helpful in anginal patients, whereas it could be harmful in patients with peripheral vascular disorders when venous return is hampered.

3. In various experimental and clinical conditions excessive Ca^{2+} entry in erythrocytes impedes the deformability of their cell membranes. Some calcium entry blockers are shown to antagonise these effects.

4. The entry of calcium ions in the myocardial cells during the depolarisation phase is known as the "slow channel entry". Many calcium entry blockers are potent slow channel blockers and they exert significant negative inotropic and chronotropic effects. By this mechanism the oxygen requirement of the heart is lowered along with the cardiac output and the total peripheral circulation. Slow channel blockers are mainly used for their anti-anginal and/or antiarrhythmic effects. Calcium entry blockers which are devoid of significant negative inotropic and chronotropic effects are found to have clinical applications as anti-hypoxic agents in peripheral and/or cerebral vascular disturbances.

5. Several calcium entry blockers were shown to provide special myocardial protection in pharmacological tests as well as in clinical conditions, e.g. during open heart surgery. Similarly, some calcium entry blockers were shown to protect cerebral function against hypoxia.

6. Some additional characteristics are mentioned in as far as they may have a major cardiovascular impact.

It goes without saying that new data are continuously added due to continued research in this area. Therefore Table 2 comprises the addresses of the research laboratories where the drugs are (being) developed and where updating of information can be obtained. It also gives the major trade names as well as the fields of clinical applications of the drugs. The originating companies or the official drug leaflets should be consulted for further specification of the clinical use (e.g. what type of arrhythmias can be treated).

When the registration of the drug has been approved in one or more countries, the generic name is indicated in the appropriate column(s) of the fields of clinical applications of Table 2.
When the drug is currently in development, this is indicated by "i.d.".

Table 1: Cardiovascular pharmacology of calcium entry blockers.

Generic name and formula	Inhibition of arterial vasoconstriction		Inhibition of myogenic venous tone	Inhibition of red blood cell crenation	Blockade of slow channels (depression of myocardial contractility)	Protection of myocardial function	Protection of cerebral function	Special characteristics
	KCl depol.	Noradr. constr.						
bencyclan	+ +	(+)	+ +		+ +			
bepridil	+ +	+			+	+ +	+	
cetiedil citrate	+ +	(+)		+	(+)		+	
cinnarizine	+ +	+	(+)	+	(+)	+	+	

	peripheral vasodilatation						
diltiazem	(+)	++	++	(+)	++	(+)	++
felodipine			(+)		+	+	++
fendiline		+	++				++
flunarizine	+	+	(+)	++	0	+	++
gallopamil (D 600, methoxyverapamil)	+	++	++	+	++	+	++

Table 1 : continued

Generic name and formula	Inhibition of arterial vasoconstriction		Inhibition of myogenic venous tone	Inhibition of red blood cell crenation	Blockade of slow channels (depression of myocardial contractility)	Protection of myocardial function	Protection of cerebral function	Special characteristics
	KCl depol.	Noradr. constr.						
lidoflazine	++	++	+	+	(+)	++	(+)	adenosine potentiation
mesudipine SKF-101,113	++	+			++			
nicardipine	++	(+)			(+)	++	++	
nifedipine	++	(+)	++	0	++	++	+	- potent vasodilatation - reflexogenic tachycardia

niludipine				++	0			++
nimodipine		+		++			(+)	++
nisoldipine				+				++
nitrendipine				+				++
perhexiline				++				++

Generic name and formula	Inhibition of arterial vasoconstriction		Inhibition of myogenic venous tone	Inhibition of red blood cell crenation	Blockade of slow channels (depression of myocardial contractility)	Protection of myocardial function	Protection of cerebral function	Special characteristics
	KCl depol.	Noradr. constr.						
prenylamine	+			0	+ +	+ +		catecholamine depletion and inhibition of reuptake
terodiline		+				+		
tiapamil	+ +	+	+ +	+	+ +	+ +		- peripheral vasodilatation - antagonism of ventricular and supraventricular types of arrhythmias
verapamil	+ +	+		(+)	+ +	+ +	+	inhibits reflex tachycardia

Compound								Remarks
KB-944 (fostedil) A-53986	++	(+)			+			
FR 34235	++	+			(+)			
PY-108-068	++	(+)			(+)		++	potent vasodilatation; inhibits reflex tachycardia
PN-200-110	++	(+)			(+)			potent vasodilatation
BRL-40015	++	(+)	+	0	+	+		no peripheral vasodilatation

Table 2: Clinical applications of calcium entry blockers.

Generic name and Major trade names	Originating company	Fields of clinical applications					
		Arrhythmias	Coronary heart disease	Peripheral and/or cerebral vascular disorders	Vertigo	Migraine	Hypertension
bencyclan - FLUDILAT, HALIDOR	Dr. Thiemann GmbH, Postfach 2080, 4670 Lünen, Westfalen, W. Germany			bencyclan			
bepridil - CORDIUM	Organon International BV, Oss, The Netherlands	i.d.	bepridil				i.d.
cetiedil citrate - STRATENE - VASOCET	Innothera S.A., 10 Av. Paul Vaillant Couturier 94117 Arcueil, France	i.d.	i.d.	cetiedil			
cinnarizine - STUGERON	Janssen Pharmaceutica N.V. Turnhoutseweg 30, B-2340 Beerse, Belgium			cinnarizine	cinnarizine		

- "i.d." = in development.

diltiazem - TILDIEM, - HERBESSER, - CARDIZEM	Tanabe Seiyaku Co. Ltd., 21 Dosho-machi 3-chome, Higashi-ku, Osaka 541, Japan		diltiazem				diltiazem
felodipine	A.B. Hässle, S-431 83 Mölndal, Sweden		i.d.				i.d.
fendiline - SENSIT	Dr. Thiemann GmbH, Postfach 2080, 4670 Lünen, Westfalen W. Germany	Fendiline	Fendiline				
flunarizine - SIBELIUM	Janssen Pharmaceutica N.V. Turnhoutseweg 30, B-2340 Beerse, Belgium			flunarizine	flunarizine	flunarizine	
gallopamil (D 600, methoxyverapamil) - PROCORUM	Knoll AG, Knollstrasse 50, Postfach 210805, 6700 Ludwigshafen, W. Germany		i.d.				i.d.

Table 2 :continued

Generic name and Major trade names	Originating company	Fields of clinical applications					
		Arrhythmias	Coronary heart disease	Peripheral and/ or cerebral vascular disorders	Vertigo	Migraine	Hypertension
lidoflazine - CLINIUM	Janssen Pharmaceutica N.V. Turnhoutseweg 30, B-2340 Beerse, Belgium		lidoflazine				
mesudipine SKF-101,113	UPSA-laboratories, 128 Rue Danton, 92506 Reuil-Malmaison, France						i.d.
nicardipine - PERDIPINE	Yamanouchi Pharmaceutical Co Ltd., No. 5, 2-chome, Nihonbashi-Honcho, Chuo-ku, Tokyo, Japan		i.d.	nicardipine			nicardipine
nifedipine - ADALAT, CORINFAR PROCARDIA	Bayer AG, Wuppertal, W. Germany		nifedipine	i.d.			i.d.

niludipine	Bayer AG, Wuppertal, W. Germany	i.d.	i.d.		i.d.	
nimodipine	Bayer AG, Wuppertal W. Germany			i.d.		i.d.
nisoldipine	Bayer AG, Wuppertal W. Germany	i.d.	i.d.			
nitrendipine	Bayer AG, Wuppertal, W. Germany					i.d.
perhexiline - PEXID	Merrell Dow Pharmaceutical Inc. 2110 East Galbraith Road, Cincinnati, Ohio 45215, U.S.A.	perhexiline				

Table 2 : continued

Generic name and Major trade names	Originating company	Fields of clinical applications					
		Arrhythmias	Coronary heart disease	Peripheral and/or cerebral vascular disorders	Vertigo	Migraine	Hypertension
prenylamine - SEGONTIN, BIOCOR, AMINOCOR, CORPAX	Albert-Roussel Pharma GmbH Abraham Lincoln strasse 38-42, 6200-Wiesbaden, W.Germany	prenylamine	prenylamine				
terodiline - BICOR	Merrell Dow Pharmaceutical Inc. 2110 East Galbraith Road, Cincinnati, Ohio 45215, U.S.A.		i.d.				
tiapamil - LAROCORD, Ro-11-1781	F. Hoffmann- La Roche & Co AG, Grenzacherstrasse 124, 4058 Basle, Switzerland	i.d.	i.d.				
verapamil - ISOPTIN, DILACORAN CALAN, CORDILOX, VASOLAN, MANIDON, IKACOR	Knoll AG, Knollstrasse 50, Postfach 210805, 6700 Ludwigshafen, W.Germany	verapamil	verapamil	i.d.	i.d.	i.d.	verapamil

Compound	Company				
KB-944 (fostedil) A-53986	Kanebo, Ltd., 3-80 Tomobuchi-cho 1-chome Miyakojima-ku Osaka 534, Japan		i.d.		i.d.
FR 34235	Fujisawa Pharmaceutical Co Ltd., 3 doshomachi 4-chome, Higashi-ku, Osaka 541, Japan		i.d.	i.d.	i.d.
PY-108-068	Sandoz AG, CH-4002 Basel, Switzerland		i.d.	i.d.	
PN 200-110	Sandoz AG, CH-4002 Basel, Switzerland		i.d.		i.d.
BRL-40015	Centre de Recherches et d'Etudes, Sobio, 4 Rue du Chesnay Beauregard B.P. 45, 35760 St.Grégoire, France (French branch of Beecham Laboratories)		i.d.		

Conclusion

After 25 years of abundant research, calcium entry blockers became an important new chapter of cardiovascular pharmacology and therapy.

This class of drugs has been developped much earlier in Europe (Gunawan *et al.*, 1981) but in the end has also gained full recognition in North America (e.g. Hoffman, 1982, Rahwan, 1983).

Calcium entry blockers, most certainly, show important differences with regard to the pharmacological profile of their effects as well as to their clinical applications. This is often attributed to a difference of tissue selectivity (Janis and Riggle, 1983). It is of fundamental interest that the drugs which protect the cells against calcium overload often also protect physiological functions and tissues against hypoxia (Rose and Amery, 1982; Wauquier *et al.*, 1982). The clinical usefulness of these findings is not at all limited to the cardiovascular system.

Acknowledgement

The information provided by various pharmaceutical companies for the compilation of Tables 1 and 2 is gratefully acknowledged.

References

Gunawan, A., Masumi, A. and Hall, R.J. Calcium antagonists: a new class of therapeutic agents. *Cardiovasc. Dis. Bull. Texas Heart Inst.*, **8**, 413-420. (1981)

Hoffman, B.F. (editor). Calcium antagonists: the state of the art and role in cardiovascular disease. Symposia on Frontiers of Pharmacology, Vol. II, American College of Clinical Pharmacology. (1983)

Janis, R.A. and Triggle, D.J. New developments in Ca^{2+} channel antagonists. *J. Med. Chem.*, **26**, 775-785. (1983)

Rahwan, R.G. Mechanisms of action of membrane calcium channel blockers and intracellular calcium antagonists. *Med. Res. Rev.*, **3**, 21-42. (1983)

Rose, F.C. and Amery, W.K. (editors). Cerebral hypoxia in the pathogenesis of migraine. Progress in Neurology Series, Pitman. (1982)

Wauquier, A., Borgers, M. and Amery, W.K. (editors). Protection of tissues against hypoxia. Elsevier Biomedial Press. (1982)

Chapter II:

Calcium entry blockers and peripheral circulatory function

Calcium-ions and excitation contraction coupling in vascular smooth muscle cells

R. Casteels

Summary

Calcium entry, release and extrusion are essential parameters in determining the activity of smooth muscle cells. Modification of any of these parameters by pharmacological means could have important therapeutic implications. However, we should also be aware of the fact that Ca^{2+} is not the only secondary messenger in smooth muscle, and that therefore pharmacological agents not necessarily always act by changing the Ca metabolism of smooth muscle cells.

Résumé

L'entrée des ions calciques, leur libération et leur extrusion sont des processus essentiels déterminant l'activité des muscles lisses. La modification d'un de ces processus par des agents pharmacologiques peut mener à des implications thérapeutiques importantes. Cependant, le Ca^{2+} n'est pas le seul messager secondaire dans le muscle lisse et, par conséquent, l'effet des agents pharmacologiques n'y est pas toujours nécessairement dû à un changement du métabolisme calcique.

Resumen

La penetración, liberación y expulsión de calcio son parámetros esenciales en la determinación de la actividad de las células musculares lisas. La modificación de cualquier de estos parámetros por medio de fármacos podría tener implicaciones terapéuticas importantes. No obstante, ha de tenerse en cuenta el hecho de que Ca^{2+} no es el único agente secundario en el músculo liso, y que por eso los agentes farmacológicos no siempre actúan necesariamente cambiando el metabolismo de calcio en las células musculares lisas.

Zusammenfassung

Kalziumeintritt, -freisetzung und -verdrängung sind essentielle Parameter, die die Aktivität der glatten Muskeln bestimmen. Die Veränderung eines dieser Parameter durch pharmakologischen Mittel kann wichtige therapeutische Folgen haben. Wir sollen jedoch berücksichtigen, dass Ca^{2+} nicht der einzige sekundäre Botenstoff in den glatten Muskeln ist und dass pharmakologische Stoffe daher nicht immer notwendigerweise dadurch wirken, dass sie den Ca-Stoffwechsel in der glatten Muskulatur ändern.

The regulation of the force development in smooth muscle cells depends largely on changes of the intracellular concentration of ionized Ca. However also other factors, such as cAMP, can play a role in modulating this fundamental mechanism (Adelstein & Eisenberg, 1980). Although the biochemical pathways which are activated by changes of $(Ca^{2+})_{cyt}$ in smooth muscle are different from those in striated muscle (Nonomura & Ebashi, 1980), changes of $(Ca^{2+})_{cyt}$ are in both tissues the primary trigger in the activation of the contractile proteins. It is therefore absolutely essential to have a clear insight in the mechanisms which are responsible for the increase and the decrease of the cytoplasmic Ca concentration. In describing our present views of these regulatory systems we consider the smooth muscle cell as a compartment surrounded by a plasma membrane, which limits the entry of external Ca to a minimum in resting conditions, and which is able to extrude Ca from the cytoplasm. Comparing the dependence of the activation of smooth muscle and skeletal muscle on external Ca we observe a fundamental difference. In the contraction-relaxation cycle of skeletal muscle, Ca is largely recycled between the sarcoplasmic reticulum and the cytoplasm and consequently the supply of Ca from the outer medium is of limited importance (Caputo, 1978). But in smooth muscle the role of the intracellular Ca stores is found to be less important. In these tissues the intracellular recycling of Ca does not seem to be very important, as can be deduced from experiments in Ca-free medium (van Breemen et al., 1972; Droogmans et al., 1977). Smooth muscle depends for the activation of its contractile proteins to a much larger extent on the supply of Ca from the outer medium than skeletal muscle. This supply has to occur across the smooth muscle membrane by an increase of its Ca-permeability induced by pharmacological and physiological substances and also cellular Ca can be mobilized for activation of the contractile proteins.

The cellular Ca compartments are mostly studied in a Ca-free medium containing EGTA because of the large value of the extracellular space and the binding sites for Ca in this space. Such exposure to Ca-free medium certainly affects the membrane potential and the ion permeabilities of the membrane and leads to a depletion of the intracellular Ca-stores at a variable rate. The major advantage of this approach is however that the function of the intracellular stores can be studied without direct interference of the external Ca.

It should be pointed out that the largest part of the Ca remaining in a smooth muscle tissue after prolonged exposure to a Ca-free medium, does not exchange with ^{45}Ca (van Breemen et al., 1975) but nothing is known about the localisation and the function of this Ca-fraction.

The cellular Ca which exchanges with ^{45}Ca is distributed over various compartments. A first one is the store from which Ca can be released by addition of an agonist to the bathing medium (Deth & van Breemen, 1974; Droogmans et al., 1977). This compartment probably corresponds to the sarcoplasmic reticulum (SR) of smooth muscle, but it can also be described as the agonist-sensitive Ca compartment (Casteels & Droogmans, 1981). The Ca present in the mitochondria corresponds to a second compartment. The studies of Somlyo et al. (1979) have revealed that the Ca content of the mitochondria is low in undamaged smooth muscle cells. This Ca can be released by uncouplers of the oxidative phosphorylation as DNP or FCCP (Deth & Casteels, 1977) and it has probably no function for regulation of the excitation-contraction coupling. Also the Ca bound to the contractile proteins and other Ca-binding proteins can be considered as another Ca-compartment. ^{45}Ca present in this compartment can exchange rapidly with ^{40}Ca which enters into the cells during K-depolarization (van Breemen et al., 1975).

It can be accepted that the agonist-sensitive Ca store is the only compartment which can contribute to an increase of $(Ca^{2+})_{cyt}$ during physiological activation. This Ca-store seems to exist in all smooth muscle tissues, but there is a large variability of the rate at which Ca is lost from this store during exposure of the tissue to Ca-free medium. In taenia coli at 35°C this store is depleted after 3 min exposure to Ca-free medium (Casteels & Raeymaekers, 1979), while in the ear artery and the main pulmonary artery of the rabbit sufficient Ca remains in this store after 60 min exposure to the Ca-free solution to induce contraction (Droogmans et al., 1977). The Ca which is released from this store also activates the Ca-extrusion pump rather than being reaccumulated into the sarcoplasmic reticulum. Hereby the fractional loss of ^{45}Ca from the tissue increases transiently. The addition of a supramaximal concentration of the agonist to Ca-free medium depletes this Ca-compartment. This sequence of events could be due to the higher affinity for Ca of the Ca extrusion mechanism as compared to that of the Ca-pump of the sarcoplasmic reticulum.
This hypothesis is also supported by the finding that after depletion of the SR in a Ca free medium, Ca is further lost from the cells, but no more accumulated in the SR. It could also explain the absence of recycling of Ca between the SR and the cytoplasm as occurs in skeletal muscle. These findings raise the question how the agonist-sensitive stores are refilled with Ca. It is likely that these mechanisms of filling vary according to the experimental conditions and the type of smooth muscle. A large supply of Ca to the cytoplasm as occurs during K-depolarization will induce in taenia coli and in the ear artery a more pronounced filling of the agonist-sensitive store, probably because the higher value of $(Ca^{2+})_{cyt}$ under these conditions stimulates the CaMg ATPase of the SR. Also β-agonists can stimulate the Ca uptake by the SR, but this effect is more obvious in taenia coli than in the ear artery (Casteels & Raeymaekers, 1979).

The filling of the agonist-sensitive Ca store of the ear artery in a Ca containing medium proceeds at a much faster rate than the depletion in Ca-free medium (Casteels & Droogmans, 1981). Moreover the final amount of Ca taken up by this store depends on the external Ca-concentration. These observations suggest the existence of a direct pathway between the extracellular space and the agonist-sensitive store. The permeability of this pathway could depend either on the direction of the electrochemical gradient or on the degree of filling of the store and thereby explain the discrepancy between the rate of filling and the rate of depletion. This assumption has lead to an alternative hypothesis on the receptor-operated channels, as discussed below.

Because external calcium is essential for the maintenance of force development by smooth muscle only a transient phasic contraction can be induced by addition of an agonist during the exposure of the tissue to Ca-free medium or to a medium containing

La^{3+} or Mn^{2+} (van Breemen et al., 1972). If however the membrane function is not modified by such substances a stimulus applied to the smooth muscle cells will induce a Ca-influx and a force development which last as long as the stimulus is applied.

This stimulus can be either a membrane depolarization or the activation of receptors by an agonist. The occurrence of this Ca-influx implies the opening of membrane pores which allow the entry of external Ca down its electrochemical gradient. These pores are classified in potential-dependent pores and receptor-operated channels (Bolton, 1979).

The potential-dependent pores, are opened by action potentials and are also activated by K-depolarization. One of the arguments to accept that both activation procedures depend on the same type of channel, is the effect of various Ca-antagonists on the contractions induced by action potentials and those induced by exposure to a Ca-containing, K-rich solution.

The action of an agonist on smooth muscle cells is at least twofold: it increases the Ca permeability of the membrane by opening the so-called receptor-operated channels and in addition these agonists release Ca from the agonist-sensitive compartment as described earlier. The opening of receptor-operated channels by an agonist can occur independently of changes of the resting potential (Droogmans et al., 1977; Kitamura & Kuriyama, 1979). An increased influx of Ca can occur concomitantly with either depolarization, or hyperpolarization or no change of the membrane potential. It is for this reason that the opening of ROC has been called pharmaco-mechanical coupling (Somlyo & Somlyo, 1968) in contrast with the electro-mechanical coupling which depends on the opening of the potential dependent pores. It is also generally accepted that the R.O.C. are not blocked as easily by the Ca-antagonists as the potential-dependent pores, while Mn^{2+} and La^{3+} block both types of channels. (Golenhofen & Hermstein, 1975; van Breemen et al., 1972).

It has been mentioned already that the agonist-sensitive Ca-compartment is filled at a fast rate after depletion by noradrenaline in a Ca-free medium and that the degree of filling depends on the external Ca-concentration. From these studies (Casteels & Droogmans, 1981) it can be deduced that the agonist-sensitive store can be replenished very rapidly from the outside, while the Ca-uptake from the cytoplasm seems to be only important if $(Ca^{2+})_{cyt}$ is increased by exposure to a Ca-containing depolarizing solution. These observations might be related to the morphological findings of Somlyo et al. (1971) on the close connections between part of the SR and the surface membrane. It is therefore proposed to integrate the receptor-operated channels and these plasma membrane-SR connections, and to speculate that agonists by releasing Ca from the agonist-sensitive compartment and depleting this store, would induce a faster influx of external Ca in this store. The initial phasic contraction induced by noradrenaline would depend on the release of Ca present in the store while the ensuing maintained tonic contraction would according to this hypothesis be due to a continuous influx of external Ca over the sarcoplasmic reticulum to the cytoplasmic compartment. This model which has to be considered as a working hypothesis should be further investigated because the junction between the plasma membrane and the SR could be an interesting site of action for pharmacological substances.

The important contribution of external calcium to the maintained force development of smooth muscle cells under all experimental conditions implies that those cells should also have a very efficient Ca-extrusion pump. This extrusion is essential for maintaining the homeostasis of the cells, but in view of the limited capacity of the sarcoplasmic reticulum and other intracellular Ca compartments, it can be proposed that relaxation itself could ultimately depend on the transmembrane Ca pump. Concerning the nature of the calcium extrusion system, two mechanisms have been proposed: a Na/Ca exchange and an ATP-dependent Ca pump (Reuter et al., 1973; Casteels et al., 1973). The Na/Ca exchange is attractive because it relates the Ca-homeostasis to the maintenance of a high value of the transmembrane electrochemical gradient for Na. This hypothesis not only seems to explain rather well the force development induced in some smooth muscles by Na-deficient, K-free or ouabain-containing solutions, but would also imply that $(Ca^{2+})_{cyt}$ and the ensuing tonic force development could be modified by slight changes of the electrochemical gradient for Na. Because of the important physiological and therapeutic implications, we have examined in detail this hypothesis in two smooth muscle tissues, i.e. in the taenia coli of the guinea-pig and in the ear artery of the rabbit. The results of these experiments cannot be reconciled with the Na/Ca exchange hypothesis (Raeymaekers et al., 1975; Droogmans & Casteels, 1979). Although it cannot be excluded that under some experimental conditions Na-Ca exchange could play a role, it seems rather unlikely that it could be the primary regulatory system for $(Ca^{2+})_{cyt}$. It has not been possible up till now to provide a direct proof of an ATP-dependent Ca pump in the plasma membrane. A complete metabolic inhibition of the cells by monoiodoacetic acid and DNP or FCCP not only results in a reduction of the ATP supply to the transport enzyme, but it also results in a release of Ca from cellular compartments, and could modify the membrane permeabilities. All these simulataneous changes make an interpretation of the ^{45}Ca efflux under these experiments impossible. Because no specific inhibitor for CaMg ATPase is available either, we have tried to isolate CaMg ATPase from smooth muscle tissues and to specify the properties of this enzyme (Wuytack & Casteels, 1980). Two CaMg AT-Pases, which are related to Ca transport systems have been extracted from smooth muscle microsomes. One of these ATPases is activated by calmodulin (Wuytack et al., 1980, 1981a, b) and the purified enzyme has a molecular weight of 130000.

These two properties make this ATPase resemble the CaMg ATPase of human erythrocytes. The other CaMg ATPase is not activated by calmodulin and has a molecular weight of 100.000. It resembles thereby the transport enzyme of the sarcoplasmic reticulum. This knowledge has now to be further expanded and integrated in the function of smooth muscle cells, because a more detailed knowledge of the enzymes and of the Ca extrusion pump will provide new approaches to study the role of the Ca pumps in the relaxation process. The only factor which was found to affect ^{45}Ca extrusion and the corresponding tension response was a change of temperature. It was observed that on releasing the same amount of Ca from the noradrenaline-sensitive store the force development is higher at 20°C than at 35°C because the Ca is extruded at a slower rate at 20°C and because consequently $(Ca^{2+})_{cyt}$ will rise to a higher value at 20°C than at 35°C. These results strongly suggest a direct regulatory role of the Ca pump in the relaxation process (Droogmans & Casteels, 1981).

Acknowledgement

This work has been supported by grant nr. 3.0087.74 of the FWGO (Belgium).

References

Adelstein, R.S., and E. Eisenberg. Regulation and kinetics of the actin-myosin-ATP interaction. *Ann. Rev. Biochem.*, **49**, 921-956. (1980)

Bolton, T.B. Mechanisms of action of transmitters and other substances on smooth muscle. *Physiol. Rev.*, **59**, 606-718. (1979)

Caputo, C. Excitation and contraction processes in muscle. *Ann. Rev. Biophys. Bioeng.*, **7**, 63-84. (1978)

Casteels, R., and G. Droogmans. Exchange characteristics of the noradrenaline-sensitive calcium store in vascular smooth muscle cells of rabbit ear artery. *J. Physiol.*, **317**, 263-279. (1981)

Casteels, R., J. Goffin, L. Raeymaekers and F. Wuytack. Calcium pumping in the smooth muscle cells of the taenia coli. *J. Physiol.*, **231**, 19-20P. (1973)

Casteels, R. and L. Raeymaekers. The action of acetylcholine and catecholamines on an intracellular calcium store in the smooth muscle cells of the guinea-pig taenia coli. *J. Physiol.*, **294**, 51-68. (1979)

Deth, R. and C. van Breemen. Relative contributions of Ca^{2+} release during drug induced activation of the rabbit aorta. *Pflugers Arch.*, **348**, 13-22. (1974)

Deth, R. and R. Casteels. A study of releasable Ca fractions in smooth muscle cells of the rabbit aorta. *J. Gen. Physiol.*, **69**, 401-416. (1977)

Droogmans, G. and R. Casteels. Temperature-dependence of ^{45}Ca fluxes and contraction in vascular smooth muscle cells of rabbit ear artery. *Pflugers Arch.*, **391**, 183-189. (1981)

Droogmans, G., L. Raeymaekers and R. Casteels. Electro- and pharmacomechanical coupling in the smooth muscle cells of the rabbit ear artery. *J. Gen. Physiol.*, **70**, 129-158. (1977)

Golenhofen, K. and N. Hermstein. Differentiation of calcium activation mechanisms in vascular smooth muscle by selective suppression with verapamil and D600. *Blood Vessels*, **12**, 21-37. (1975)

Kitamura, K. and H. Kuriyama. Effects of acetylcholine on the smooth muscle cell of isolated main coronary artery of the guinea-pig. *J. Physiol.*, **293**, 119-133. (1977)

Nonomura, Y. and S. Ebashi. Calcium regulatory mechanism in vertebrate smooth muscle. *Biomed. Res.*, **1**, 1-14. (1980)

Raeymaekers, L., F. Wuytack and R. Casteels. Na-Ca exchange in taenia coli of the guinea-pig. *Pflugers Arch.*, **347**, 329-340. (1975)

Reuter, H., M.P. Blaustein and G. Haeusler. Na-Ca exchange and tension development in arterial smooth muscle *Phil. Trans. R. Soc. B.*, **265**, 87-98. (1973)

Somlyo, A.P., C.E. Devine, A.V. Somlyo, S.R. North. Sarcoplasmic reticulum and the temperature-dependent contraction of smooth muscle in calcium-free solutions. *J. Cell. Biol.*, **51**, 722-741. (1971)

Somlyo, A.V. and A.P. Somlyo. Electromechanical and pharmacomechanical coupling in vascular smooth muscle. *J. Pharmac. exp. Ther.*, **159**, 129-145. (1968)

Somlyo, A.P., A.V. Somlyo and H. Shuman. Electron probe analysis of vascular smooth muscle. Composition of mitochondria, nuclei and cytoplasm. *J. Cell. Biol.*, **81**, 316-335. (1979)

van Breemen, C., B.R. Farinas, P. Gerba and E.D. McNaughton. Excitation-contraction coupling in rabbit aorta studied by the lanthanum method for measuring cellular calcium influx. *Circul. Res.*, **30**, 44-54. (1972)

van Breemen, C., F. Wuytack and R. Casteels. Stimulation of ^{45}Ca efflux from smooth muscle cells by metabolic inhibition and high K depolarization. *Pflugers Arch.*, **359**, 183-196. (1975)

Wuytack, F. and R. Casteels. Demonstration of A($Ca^{2+} + Mg^{2+}$)-ATPase activity probably related to Ca^{2+}-transport in the microsomal fraction of porcine coronary artery smooth muscle. *Biochim. Biophys. Acta*, **595**, 257-263. (1980)

Wuytack, F., G. De Schutter and R. Casteels. The effect of calmodulin on the active calcium-ion transport and ($Ca^{2+} + Mg^{2+}$)-dependent ATPase in microsomal fractions of smooth muscle compared with that in erythrocytes and cardiac muscle. *Biochem. J.*, **190**, 827-831. (1980)

Wuytack, F., G. De Schutter and R. Casteels. Partial purification of ($Ca^{2+} + Mg^{2+}$)-dependent ATPase from pig smooth muscle and reconstitution of an ATP-dependent Ca^{2+}-transport system. *Biochem. J.*, **198**, 265-271. (1981a)

Wuytack, F., G. De Schutter and R. Casteels. Purification of ($Ca^{2+} + Mg^{2+}$)-ATPase from smooth muscle by calmodulin affinity chromatography. *Febs Letters*, **129**, 297-300. (1981b)

Laser microprobe mass analysis (LAMMA) as a technique to quantitate Ca²⁺ ions

S. De Nollin, W. Jacob, and R. Hertsens

Summary

The LAMMA technique provides good evidence that the cytochemical oxalate-pyroantimonate method may be reliably used to visualise the presence of calcium ions in cells and tissues. This has been shown in vascular smooth muscles and in myocardial cells. It has also been confirmed that flunarizine inhibits the entry of Ca²⁺ in depolarized vascular smooth muscle preparations.

Résumé

La technique de l'analyse de masse d'échantillons ultramicroscopiques prélevées par laser confirme que la méthode cytochimique, utilisant l'oxalate-pyroantimonate, est fiable dans le but de visualiser la présence des ions calciques dans les cellules cardiaques et musculaires lisses vasculaires. Il a été confirmé également que la flunarizine inhibe l'entrée des ions calciques dans des préparations de muscle lisse vasculaire dépolarisé.

Resumen

La técnica LAMMA confirma que el método citoquímico oscalato-piroantimoniato es de gran fiabilidad para hacer visible la presencia de iones cálcicos en células y tejidos. Esto se ha demostrado en células musculares lisas vasculares y en células miocardíacas. También se ha confirmado que flunarizina inhibe la penetración de Ca^{2+} en preparados de músculos lisos vasculares despolarizados.

Zusammenfassung

Die LAMMA Technik bestätigt, dass die zytochemische Oxalat-Pyroantimonat-Methode zuverlässig gebraucht werden kann, um die Anwesenheit von Kalziumionen in den Zellen und Geweben sichtbar zu machen. Das wurde in glatter Gefässmuskulatur und in Herzmuskelzellen gezeigt. Es wird ebenfalls bestätigt, dass Flunarizin den Eintritt von Kalziumionen in depolarisierte glatte Gefässmuskelpräparate hemmt.

Ca^{2+} ions play an important role in many cellular processes. The subcellular stores of Ca^{2+} can be localized by cytochemical means and visualized as electron dense precipitate after assessment with a combined oxalate-pyroantimonate (OPA) method (Borgers et al., 1981; Jacob et al., submitted).

It can be demonstrated that black precipitate in the cells is almost totally due to the presence of Ca^{2+} and not to other cations such as Na^+ and Mg^{++}. The LAMMA technique provides indeed an adequate quantitative control for the cytochemical Ca^{2+} localization. It has a high speed of operation, a sensitivity of about $10^{-20}g$ and a spatial resolution of about 1 μm.

I. Technique

The LAMMA-500 instrument (Leybold-Hereaus, GmbH, Köln, FRG) has been fully described previously (De Noyer et al., 1982). A high energy laser pulse is focused on the specimen by means of UV transmitting optics. In this way a small amount of the specimen is vaporized and ionized. The created ions are accelerated in an electric field and analysed according to their velocity. Ion masses are displayed in either positive or negative spectra by switching the polarity of the electric field.

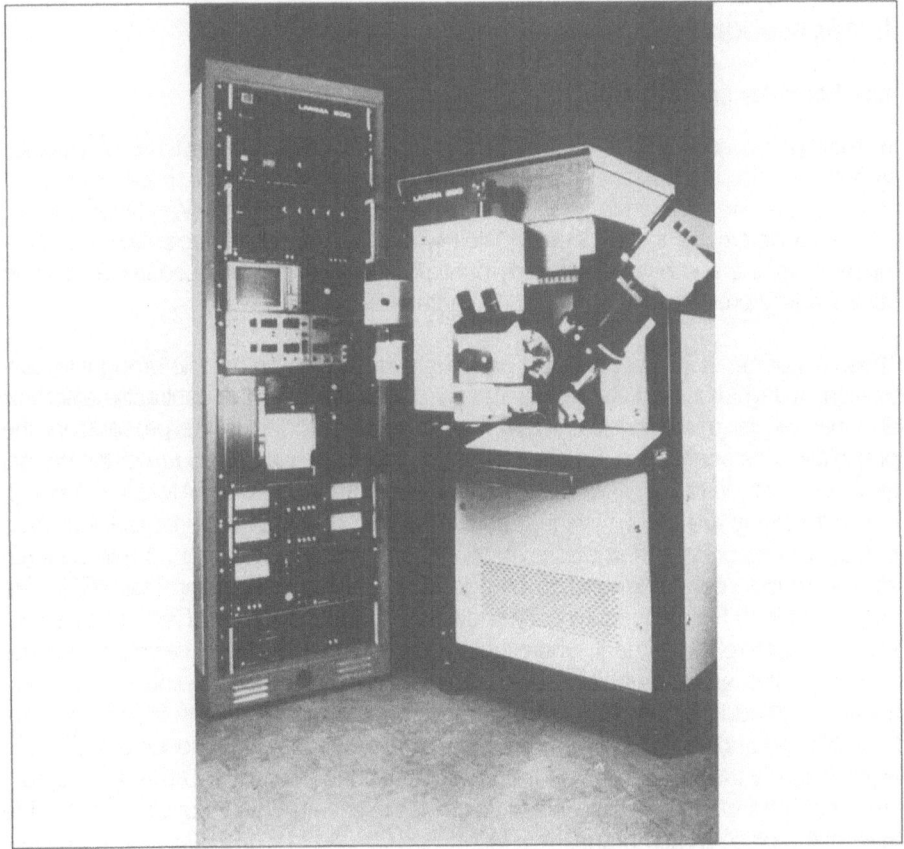

Figure 1.

In our study, sections of 0.25 μm are collected on copper finder-grids. The grid is mounted in the vacuum chamber of the instrument, which is equipped with 2 lasers (Fig. 1). One is a low powered He/Ne search laser, which can be focused on a spot for illuminating the analytical region (pilot laser). The other laser is a Neodymium-YAG laser, whose output is quadrupled in frequency to provide a high power density for vaporization and ionization (pulse laser).

The sample may be viewed with a binocular light microscope using top-or transillumination. Magnifications in the range between 100 and 1250 are available. For selection of comparable physiological situations and of cytochemical Ca^{2+} precipitate pattern, electron micrographs of these 0.25 μm sections were made at a final magnification of 3800. Once the region to be analysed is recognized, a laser pulse is given leaving a perforation of about 1 μm diameter. Immediately a mass spectrum is displayed on the oscilloscope which can be recorded on paper or transferred to a computer for storage or data-treatment. To study Ca^{2+} concentrations, positive spectra covering the mass range from 20-90 are recorded.

To allow a correct localization of the evaporated region after LAMMA analysis, the perforations are recorded electron micrographically.

II. Applications

II. a. Vascular smooth muscle

Increasing the extracellular Ca^{2+} concentration provokes contractions of vascular smooth muscle preparations in a dose-dependent way. Flunarizine, a selective Ca^{2+} entry blocker, was shown to suppress these muscle contractions (Van Nueten et al., 1978). To determine the subcellular sites where flunarizine interacts with the Ca^{2+} movements, the combined oxalate-pyroantimonate method was used in depolarized caudal artery preparations of the rat (Borgers et al., 1980).

These experiments showed that the precipitate in the smooth muscle brought to contraction by high K^+ and Ca^{2+}, was mainly distributed over the contractile elements and intracellular microvesicles. When flunarizine was added to the preparation, the precipitate was confined to the extracellular space. Sections of 0.25 μm of the caudal artery preparation of the rat were taken to be mass analysed with LAMMA. On Fig. 2, the perforations are shown in the 0.25 μm section of the smooth muscle. For morphological interpretations, a discrimination was made between light (L) and dark (D) smooth muscle cells, surrounding collagen (C) and the embedding resin (ER). The spectra seen in Fig. 3 unequivocally show that a high intracellular Ca^{2+} peak is present in the control experiment, where the muscle cells are strongly contracted and bear a considerable amount of black, cytochemical precipitate. On the other hand, when flunarizine is added to the Ca^{2+} rich incubation medium, the smooth muscle cells remain relaxed and show hardly any precipitate. The intracellular presence of Ca^{2+} ions is indeed very low as shown with the LAMMA (De Nollin et al., submitted). This confirms that flunarizine exerts its effect of blocking the excessive entry of Ca^{2+} ions at the level of the plasma membrane.

Figure 2

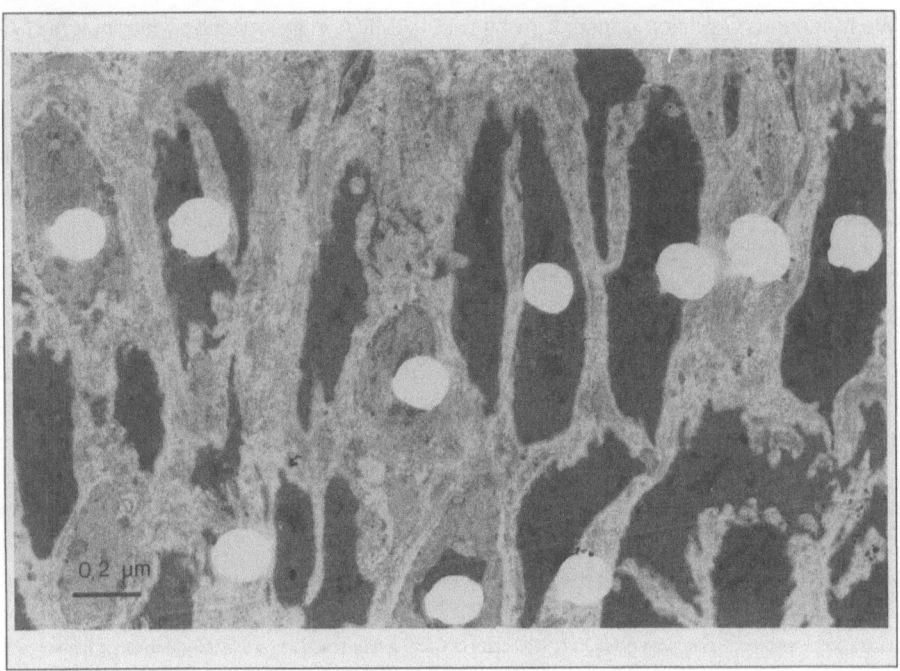

Figure 3

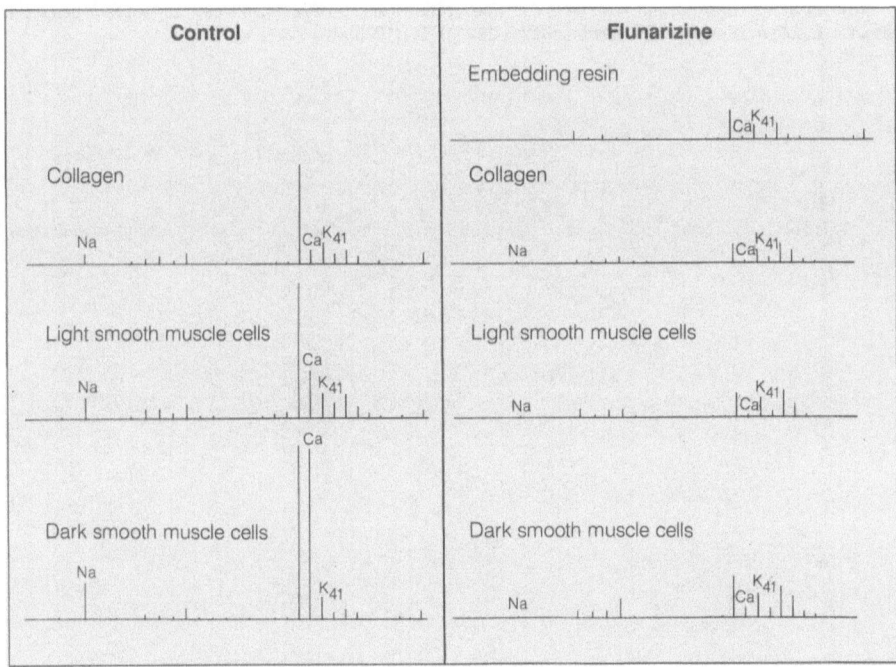

II. b. Heart muscle

We measured Ca^{2+} ion concentrations with LAMMA in the mitochondria, in I- and A-bands and in the sarcoplasm.

After noradrenaline stimulation of the heart, the individual myocardial cells exhibit different degrees of Ca^{2+} overload, which are shown by the oxalate-pyroantimonate precipitation method. The LAMMA measurements parallel completely the cytochemical observations (Jacob, Hertsens and van Bogaert, submitted).

References

Borgers, M., Thoné, F. and Van Nueten, J. The subcellular distribution of Ca^{2+} and the effects of Ca^{2+} antagonists as evaluated with a combined oxalate-pyroantimonate method. *Acta Histochemica*, **Suppl. 24**, 327-332. (1981)

Borgers, M., Ghoos, E., Thoné, F. and Van Nueten, J. Effects of flunarizine on the distribution of calcium in vascular smooth muscle. *Blood Vessels*, **17**, 123-130. (1980)

De Nollin, S., Borgers, M., Jacobs, W. and Wellens, D.. The prevention of Ca^{2+} overload in vascular smooth muscle by flunarizine, as detected by L'AMMA. *Angiology* (submitted).

De Noyer, E., Van Grieken, R., Adams, F. and Natusch. Laser Microprobe Mass Analysis. *Analytical Chemistry*, **54**, A26-A43. (1982)

Jacob, W., Hertsens, R. and Van Bogaert A. Detection of Ca^{2+} in heart muscle by LAMMA. *Angiology* (submitted).

Jacob, W., De Smedt, M., Borgers, M. and De Nollin, S. Ultrastructural localization of Ca^{2+} ions with a combined oxalate pyroantimonate method. Laser Microprobe Mass Analysis controlled specificity. (Submitted).

Van Nueten, J., Van Beek, J. and Janssen, P.A.J. Effect of flunarizine on calcium-induced responses of peripheral vascular smooth muscle. *Arch. int. Pharmacodyn.*, **232**, 42-52. (1978)

Vascular pharmacology of calcium entry blockers

J.M. Van Nueten

Summary

Vasoconstriction results from an exaggerated increase of intracellular calcium ions which initiate the contractile process within the vascular smooth muscle cells. One of the major sources of the activator calcium ions is the influx of extracellular Ca^{2+}, which, particularly in precapillary vessels, can be inhibited by calcium entry blockers. The dependency of the vascular smooth muscle cells on extracellular Ca^{2+} to trigger the contractile process when exposed to naturally occurring vasoconstrictors is variable in different vascular areas. This determines the different sensitivity to various calcium entry blockers. Tissue selectivity of calcium entry blockers is also observed when the excitation-contraction coupling is triggered during K^+-depolarization, either in vascular or non-vascular (e.g. myocardial) tissues. Such selectivity, observed with certain calcium entry blockers (e.g. cinnarizine, flunarizine and lidoflazine) can be understood if the access to the calcium-channels or/and the characteristics of these channels within the cell membrane vary among different vascular and non-vascular tissue cells. Finally, differences between calcium entry blockers in time of onset and duration of effects reflect different kinetic properties and probably a different access to the calcium channels within the cell membrane. All these findings may help explain pharmacokinetic and therapeutic differences between the available Ca^{2+} entry blockers.

Résumé

Une augmentation excessive de Ca^{2+} intracellulaire déclenche la contraction des muscles lisses vasculaires et donc la vasoconstriction. Une des sources majeures d'ions calciques activateurs est l'entrée de Ca^{2+} extracellulaire, qui peut être inhibée par des drogues, particulièrement au niveau des vaisseaux précapillaires. L'influence du Ca^{2+} extracellulaire sur le déclenchement de la contraction des muscles lisses vasculaires exposés à des agents vasoconstricteurs biogènes est variable d'un territoire vasculaire à l'autre. Ceci détermine la différence de sensibilité de ces territoires envers divers inhibiteurs d'entrée calcique.

On observe aussi une sélectivité tissulaire quant au déclenchement de la contraction pendant la dépolarisation potassique selon qu'il s'agit de tissu vasculaire et non-vasculaire (p.ex. myocardique). Une pareille sélectivité, observée en utilisant certains inhibiteurs d'entrée calcique (p.ex. cinnarizine, flunarizine et lidoflazine) se comprend si l'accessibilité des canaux calciques et/ou les caractéristiques de ces canaux dans la membrane cellulaire varient dans les différentes cellules tissulaires vasculaires et non-vasculaires. Finalement, il y a des différences entre les inhibiteurs d'entrée calcique en ce qui concerne la rapidité et la durée de leur action, reflétant des différences pharmacocinétiques et probablement d'accessibilité des canaux calciques dans la membrane cellulaire. Toutes ces observations contribuent à expliquer les différences pharmacocinétiques et thérapeutiques parmi les inhibiteurs d'entrée calcique disponibles en ce moment.

Resumen

La vasoconstricción resulta de un aumento excesivo de Ca^{2+} intracelular que inicia el proceso contráctil dentro de las células musculares lisas de la pared vascular. Una de las fuentes más importantes del activador Ca^{2+} es la penetración de Ca^{2+} extracelular que, particularmente en vasos precapilares, puede ser frenada por inhibidores específicos. La dependencia de las células vasculares musculares lisas de Ca^{2+} extracelular, en cuanto al desencadenamiento del proceso contráctil por vasoconstrictores endógenos, es variable en distintas áreas vasculares. Esto determina la distinta sensibilidad a los diversos inhibidores de la penetración del calcio. La selectividad de estos inhibidores en cuanto al tejido se observa también cuando se inicia el acoplamiento excitación - contracción durante la depolarización K^+, sea en tejidos vasculares o otros (p. ej. miocardíaco). Dicha selectividad, observada con ciertos inhibidores (p. ej. cinarizina, flunarizine y lidoflazina), puede entenderse si el acceso a los canales Ca^{2+} y / o las características de estos canales mismos varían entre células de tejidos vasculares y no vasculares. Finalmente, diferencias entre inhibidores de la penetración del calcio en cuanto a la rapidez del comienzo y la duración de los efectos reflejan propiedades cinéticas diferentes y, probablemente, un acceso diferente a los canales Ca^{2+} dentro de la membrana celular. Todos estos factores pueden ayudar a explicar las diferencias farmacocinéticas y terapéuticas entre los inhibidores de la penetración del calcio disponibles.

Zusammenfassung

Eine starke Zunahme der intrazellulären Kalziumionen verursacht Kontraktion der glatten Gefässmuskulatur und damit Vasokonstriktion. Eine der bedeutendsten Quellen von aktivierenden Kalziumionen ist der Einstrom von extrazellulärem Ca^{2+}, der besonders in den Präkapilaren durch Arzneimittel gehemmt werden kann. Der Einfluss des extrazellulären Ca^{2+} auf die Kontraktion der glatten Gefässmuskulatur in Anwesenheit natürlich vorkommender Vasokonstriktoren, ist von einem Gefässbereich zu dem anderen verschieden. Dies bestimmt die verschiedenartige Empfindlichkeit dieser Bereiche für verschiedene Kalziumeinstromhemmer. Eine Selektivität des Gewebes wird auch festgestellt, wenn der Erregungs-Kontraktionsmechanismus während K^+-Depolarisierung geschieht, sowohl in Gefässgewebe als auch in nicht-vaskulärem Gewebe (z.B. Herzmuskelgewebe). Eine solche Selektivität, die bei gewissen Kalziumeinstromhemmern vorkommt (z.B. Cinnarizin, Flunarizin und Lidoflazin), kann man verstehen, wenn der Zugang zu den Kalziumkanälen und/oder die Charakteristika dieser Kanäle innerhalb der Zellmembran in den verschiedenen vaskulären und nicht-vaskulären Zellen des Gewebes unterschiedlich sind. Schliesslich bestehen Unterschiede zwischen den Kalziumeinstromhemmern in Bezug auf die Eintrittsgeschwindigkeit und die Dauer ihrer Wirkung. Dies spiegelt pharmakokinetische Unterschiede und wahrscheinlich auch die verschiedenartige Zugänglichkeit der Kalziumkanäle in die Zellmembran wider. Alle diese Ergebnisse können helfen, die pharmakokinetischen und therapeutischen Unterschiede zwischen den zur Zeit verfügbaren Kalziumeinstromhemmern zu erläutern.

Sustained vasoconstriction may lead to underperfusion of the tissues. The appropriate supply of oxygen and substrates, and the continuous wash-out of metabolites can no longer be assured; tissue ischemia and dysfunction become unavoidable. In such case drugs which prevent or inhibit vasoconstrictor episodes, may be helpful to normalize tissue perfusion. This is the case for the calcium entry blockers, a chemically heterogeneous group of compounds which are able to inhibit Ca^{2+}-dependent processes in various tissues. Their inhibitory action depends on their potential, to decrease the level of free intracellular Ca^{2+} (Church and Zsotér, 1980; Rahwan et al., 1979; Vanhoutte, 1981, 1982a, 1982b; Van Nueten and Vanhoutte, 1980a; Weiss, 1981;). This chapter will review the action of the available calcium entry blockers in vascular smooth muscle tissue with special focus on heterogeneity of some of their effects.

1. Contractile activity of vascular smooth muscle

Contraction of vascular smooth muscle cells leads to vasoconstriction and, when exaggerated, to vasospasm. It is triggered by an increase in cytoplasmic concentration of calcium ions (Ca^{2+}). Although at rest the concentration of intracellular Ca^{2+} is less than 10^{-7} M, while the concentration of extracellular free Ca^{2+} is about 1.5×10^{-3} M, the low permeability of the cell membrane to Ca^{2+} prevents excessive influx of Ca^{2+}. At rest, equilibrium between inward and outward transport of Ca^{2+} is maintained by the existence of an active extrusion pump in the cell membrane, thus assuring the homeostasis of intracellular Ca^{2+}.

During activation of the vascular smooth muscle cell the intracellular concentration raises by a factor of 100, thus triggering the excitation-contraction coupling mechanism (Bohr, 1964, 1973; Bolton, 1979; Borgers et al., 1982; Casteels and Van Breemen, 1975; Johansson, 1978; Somlyo and Somlyo, 1968a, 1968b, 1970; Van Breemen, 1977; Van Breemen et al., 1980; Van Nueten and Vanhoutte, 1980a). The sources of Ca^{2+} used in excitation-contraction coupling include extracellular, membrane bound and intracellularly stored Ca^{2+}; different stimulants may employ different Ca^{2+}-sources (Fig. 1). The relative quantities of Ca^{2+} delivered from extra- and intracellular sources not only depend on the mode of activation, but may vary with the blood vessels studied (Bevan, 1979; Bolton, 1979; Johansson, 1978; Triggle and Swamy, 1980; Van Breemen et al., 1980; Vanhoutte, 1982a; Van Nueten and Vanhoutte, 1980, 1981a,b; Weiss, 1981).

In most cases, the activation of vascular smooth muscle cells is accompanied by opening of "Ca^{2+} channels" within the cell membrane and entry of extracellular Ca^{2+} into the cells. Such Ca^{2+} channels are classified into two major types: channels linked to specific receptors (receptor-operated channels) predominantly responsible for vascular smooth muscle contraction, and in some vascular tissue, channels coupled with membrane depolarization (potential operated channels). The latter type of channel is also present in heart muscle. The opening of receptor-operated channels can be triggered by various agents including norepinephrine, histamine, angiotensin II, prostaglandins, 5-hydroxytryptamine; it is not necessarily accompanied by changes of membrane potential. Receptor activation especially at high concentrations of agonist, also leads to release of Ca^{2+} from a limited intracellular pool which is superficially located and has to

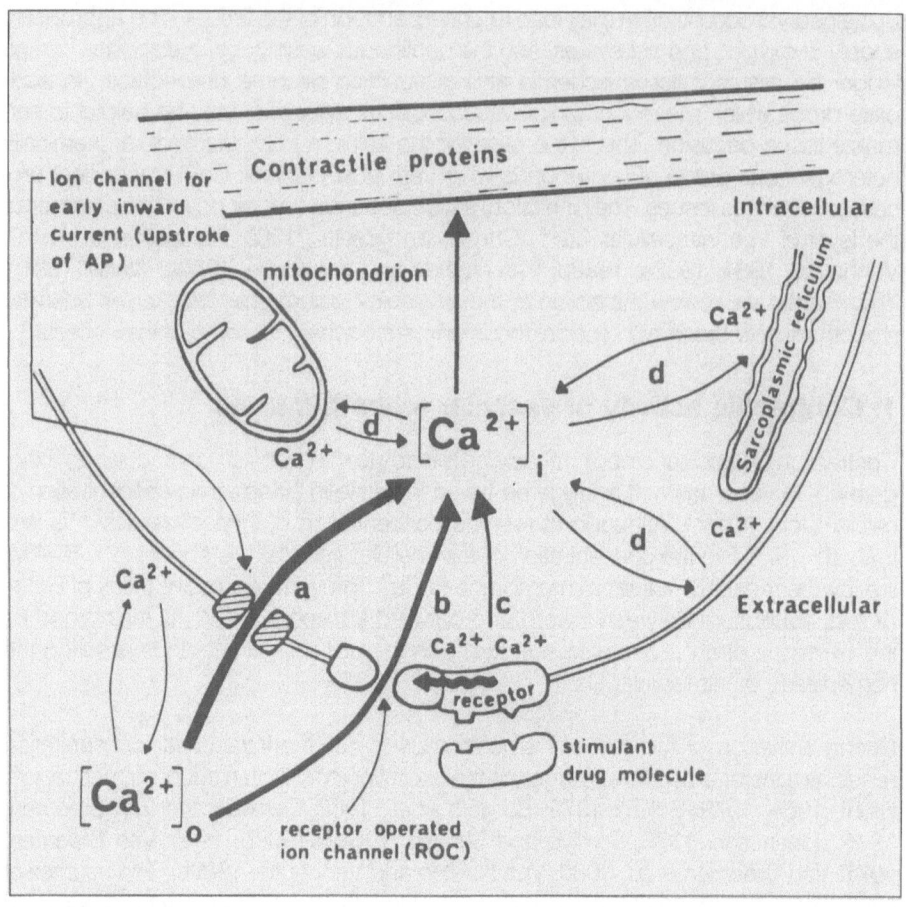

Figure 1: Schematic representation of postulated calcium sources involved in contraction of smooth muscle tissues (Bolton, 1979, with permission).

be refilled from the outside. Channels coupled with membrane depolarization (potential operated channels) can be activated by exposure to relatively high concentrations of potassium and are present in myogenically active blood vessels characterized by spontaneous development of action potentials.

However, in given vascular tissues K-depolarization will also induce the release of endogenous norepinephrine, thus indirectly activating receptor-operated channels. It is uncertain whether the channels coupled with depolarization of the membrane of the vascular smooth muscle cell are equivalent to the "slow" voltage dependent channels described in heart muscle. The relative importance of activation of the two calcium channels depends on the anatomical origin of the vascular tissue (Bolton, 1979; Casteels, 1980; Droogmans *et al.*, 1977; Kitamara and Kuriyama, 1979; Somlyo and Somlyo, 1968b; Uchida and Bohr, 1969; Van Breemen, 1977; Van Breemen *et al.*, 1980; Vanhoutte, 1978; Vanhoutte *et al.*, 1981; Van Nueten, 1978).

2. Effects of calcium entry blockers

Drugs such as bepridil, cinnarizine, diltiazem, D600, flunarizine, lidoflazine, nicardipine, nifedipine, niludipine, nimodipine and verapamil share the property to inhibit the entry of Ca^{2+} into vascular smooth muscle. Their chemical heterogeneity together with the varying importance of the different sources, of activator Ca^{2+}, depending on the anatomical origin of the vascular tissue, explain the variability in the ability of these drugs to inhibit vasoconstrictor responses. For example, flunarizine is particularly potent in inhibiting Ca^{2+}-induced contractions of brain arteries and gastrosplenic veins. Differences also exist among the individual compounds regarding the time-course of their effect. Thus the inhibitory action of nifedipine, D600, verapamil and diltiazem is characterized by a rapid onset and short duration; in contrast the calcium entry blocking effects of cinnarizine, flunarizine and lidoflazine are progressive and sustained for a long period of time.

These pharmacological differences explain in part the individual pharmacodynamic and pharmacokinetic profiles of calcium entry blockers (Table 1). They must reflect different kinetic properties of the interaction of the various substances with the calcium channels of the cell membrane (Church and Zsotér, 1980; Fleckenstein, 1977; Godfraind and Morel, 1978; Godfraind, 1981a,b; Grün and Fleckenstein, 1972; Kazda et al., 1979; Labrid et al., 1979; Rahwan et al., 1979; Triggle and Swamy, 1980; Vanhoutte, 1981, 1982b; Van Nueten, 1969; Van Nueten et al., 1978; Van Nueten and Vanhoutte, 1981a,b; Weiss, 1981).

2.1. Vasoconstrictor substances

Naturally occurring vasoconstrictor substances can be endogenously formed and released or they can be administered exogenously. A good example is norepinephrine, present as the normal transmitter in the blood vessel wall, which is released when the sympathetic nerves are excited. The sympathetic nervous system is one of the most important determinants of vascular function in the living organism (Bohr, 1973; Godfraind, 1981a; Johannson, 1978; Rahwan et al., 1979; Robinson and Collier, 1979; Van Breemen, 1977; Vanhoutte, 1978, 1982b; Van Nueten and Wellens, 1979; Van Nueten et al., 1980).

The contraction of vascular smooth muscle in response to sympathetic nerve stimulation is initiated by the binding of norepinephrine released from adrenergic nerves, to alpha-adrenergic receptors of the cell membrane. The inhibitory effect of different calcium entry blockers on norepinephrine-induced contractions may vary among different blood vessels. For example, lidoflazine inhibits norepinephrine-induced contractions, more in splanchnic veins and precapillary vessels than in cutaneous veins; this must be due to basic differences in the characteristics of the cell membranes involved including the pharmacological properties of the postjunctional alpha-adrenoceptor. In the rat caudal artery, the effect of increasing concentrations of various calcium entry blockers was investigated on the contractile response evoked either by norepinephrine or by Ca^{2+} containing depolarizing solution. While some antagonists were equiactive on norepinephrine- or Ca^{2+}-induced contractions (e.g. diltiazem, flunarizine, lidoflazine), other Ca^{2+}-entry blockers inhibited Ca^{2+}-induced contractions significantly more than the contractile response to norepinephrine (e.g. cinnarizine, verapamil). Some others (e.g. nifedipine) were particularly weak in antagonizing the response to norepinephrine (Fig. 2) (Vanhoutte et al., 1980; Van Nueten, 1978, 1982; Van Nueten and Vanhoutte, 1981b).

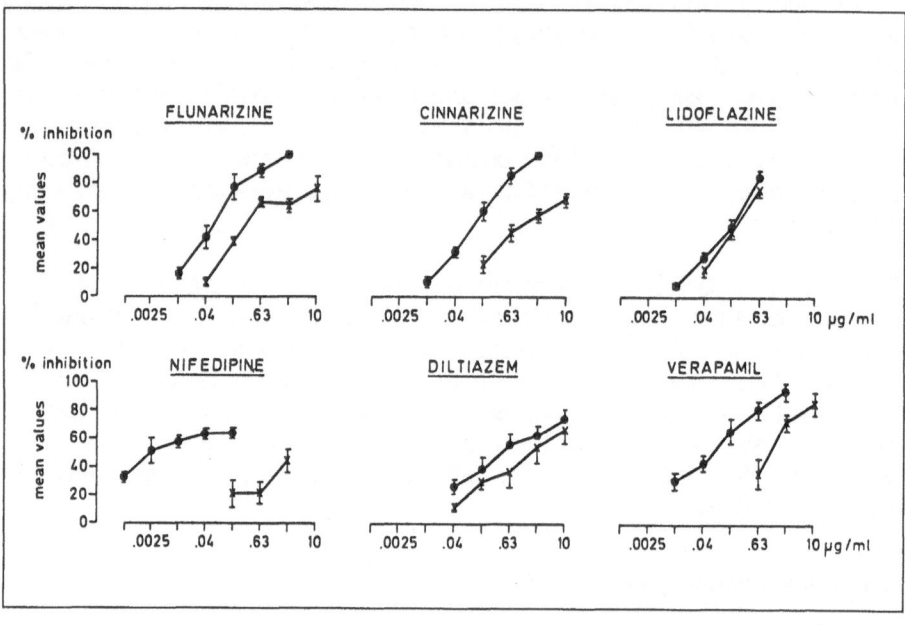

Figure 2 : Effect of calcium (•) and norepinephrine (x) induced submaximal contraction of the rat caudal artery suspended in depolarizing and normal physiological solutions respectively. Data shown as per cent inhibition. Means ± S.E.M. (n: 3-6).

Vasoconstriction can also be evoked by non-adrenergic endogenous substances. Upon stimulation (e.g. some hypoxic conditions) blood platelets release the vasoactive substance 5-hydroxytryptamine and synthetize the vasoactive prostaglandins thromboxane A_2, prostaglandins E_2 and $F_{2\alpha}$. As is the case for norepinephrine, vasoconstriction induced by these substances also depends upon the relative involvement of the different sources of Ca^{2+}. Thrombin-stimulated rat platelets, as well as platelets activated on the de-endothelialized blood vessel, induce a substantial contraction of the rat caudal artery preparation in vitro. Biochemical measurements of the various mediators involved, as well as pharmacological analysis showed 5-hydroxytryptamine and prostaglandins - in particular thromboxane A_2 - to be the principal mediators responsible for the platelet-mediated vasoconstriction, with predominance for 5-hydroxytryptamine in this particular preparation. The platelet-mediated vascular contraction is inhibited in a concentration-dependent way by flunarizine. The inhibition had a gradual onset and a prolonged duration of action after repeated wash-outs (Fig. 3). Specific measurements involving [^{14}C]-5-hydroxytryptamine, labelled platelets, malondialdehyde and thromboxane B_2 production from endogenous, thrombinliberated arachidonic acid show that flunarizine, in concentrations effective against vascular contractions, does not significantly affect the thrombin-induced release of 5-hydroxytryptamine from the platelets nor the production of the vasoconstrictive thromboxane A_2 by these blood cells; therefore its primary site of action is on the activation of the vascular smooth muscle cell rather than on the production/release of mediators by the platelets. The finding that flunarizine is effective both against 5-hydroxytryptamine- and thromboxane A_2-induced vasoconstriction, is in agreement with the inhibition by flunarizine of vascular contractions induced by 5-hydroxytryptamine and by prostaglandin F_{2a}; it supports the involvement of a transmembrane influx of Ca^{2+} in the activation of vascular smooth muscle contraction by the monoamine and by some prostaglandins (Bohr, 1964, 1973; Bohr et al., 1978; De Clerck and David, 1981; De Clerck and Van Nueten, 1982a,b; Ellis et al., 1976; Godfraind and Miller, 1981; Johansson, 1978; Van Breemen, 1977; Van Nueten and Vanhoutte, 1981b).

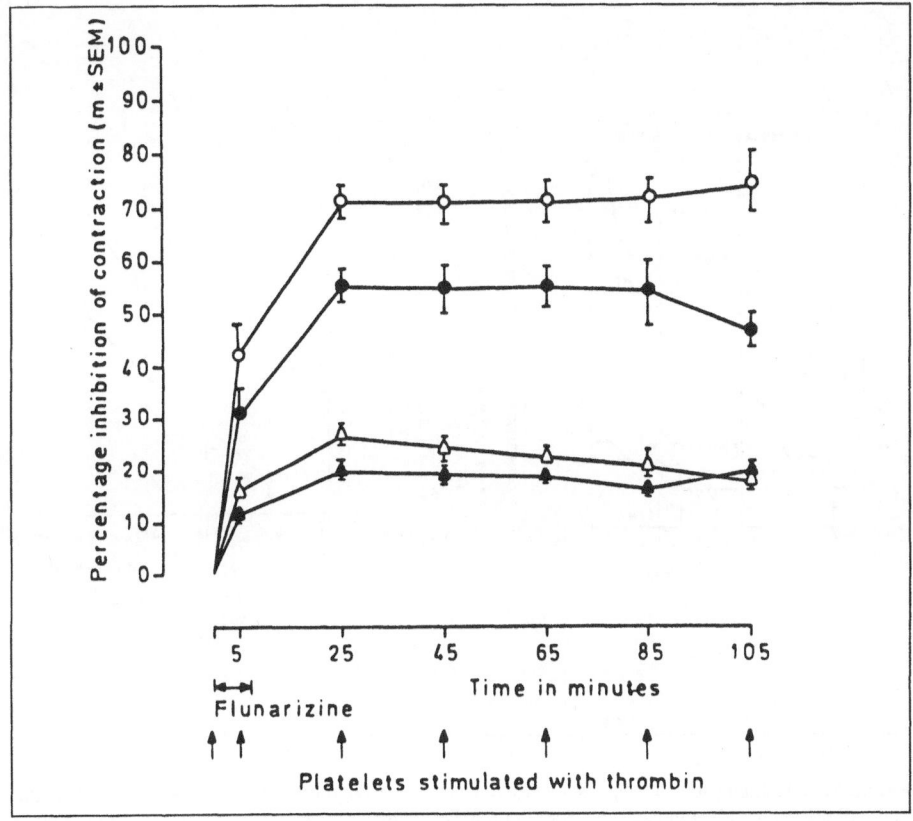

Figure 3: Concentration-dependent inhibition by flunarizine ($\blacktriangle$ = 3.1 x 10^{-7} M; $\triangle$ = 6.2 x 10^{-7} M, $\bullet$ = 1.25 x 10^{-6} M; o = 5 x 10^{-6} M; contact 8 min) of the rat caudal artery contractions induced by washed platelets (2.5 x 10^{10}/l) stimulated with thrombin (0.002 N.I.H. U/ml). Mean ± S.E.M. of 6 to 11 experiments on different artery preparations (De Clerck and Van Nueten, 1982b, with permission).

The responsiveness of the blood vessel wall to vasoconstrictor substances can be modulated by the local conditions to which the vascular smooth muscle cells are exposed. One example is the marked further increase in tension caused by acute hypoxia in canine blood vessels when these vessels are first exposed to a vasoconstrictor substance; these hypoxic contractions are inhibited by calcium entry blockers (e.g. bepridil, flunarizine, lidoflazine, verapamil). This is particularly evident in canine cerebral vasculature (e.g. basilar, middle cerebral, internal carotid artery, Fig. 4). These findings are corroborated by the observation that flunarizine possesses brain-protective properties in animal models related to cerebral damage (Campbell *et al.*, 1981; Vanhoutte, 1976, 1982a; Van Nueten and Vanhoutte, 1980b; Van Nueten and De Clerck, 1982; Van Nueten *et al.*, 1982; Van Reempts *et al.*, 1982; Wauquier *et al.*, 1982; White *et al.*, 1982).

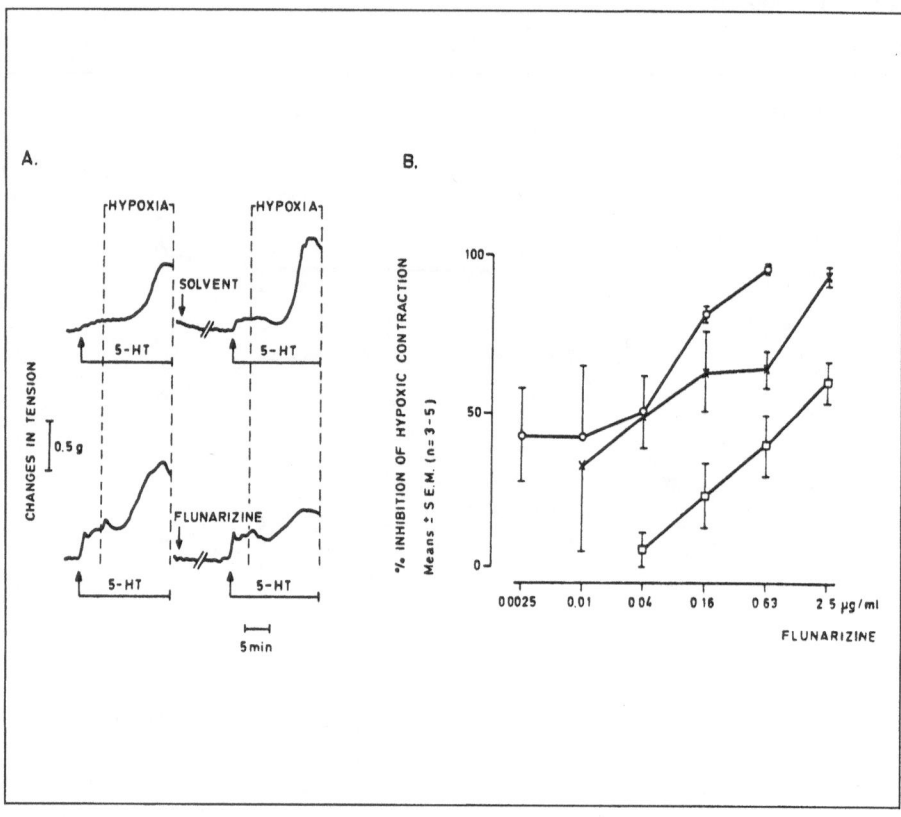

Figure 4: A: Isometric tension recordings in two basilar artery segments from te same dog, showing the effect of solvent (0.1% ethanol) and flunarizine (0.04 μg/ml, 90 min contact time) on the contractile response to hypoxia in the presence of 5-hydroxytryptamine (0.63 ng/ml; 5-HT). B: Inhibitory effect of flunarizine on hypoxia-induced contractions of canine basilar (o), middle cerebral (x) and internal carotid (□) arteries in the presence of 5-HT. The data are shown as means ± S.E.M. expressed as per cent inhibition of the contraction induced by hypoxia before the addition of the drug and corrected for control values. The incubation period for flunarizine or its solvent was 90 minutes (Van Nueten *et al.*, 1982, with permission).

2.2. Myogenic activity

Myogenic tone is characteristic of most arteriolar or small precapillary blood vessels; this phenomenon depends upon the influx of extracellular Ca^{2+}. A generalized, exaggerated constriction at the arteriolar level occurs in certain forms of hypertension. Myogenic activity is also developed by portal-mesenteric veins; this typical phasic activity also highly depends on the availability of extracellular Ca^{2+}. Hence it is not surprising that some calcium entry blockers (e.g. verapamil, D600, nifedipine, diltiazem) markedly inhibit myogenic activity in isolated portal-mesenteric veins and decrease arteriolar resistance. Calcium entry blockers that are particularly effective in inhibiting myogenic activity, such as nifedipine and verapamil, lower arterial blood pressure in hypertensive animals and hypertensive patients.

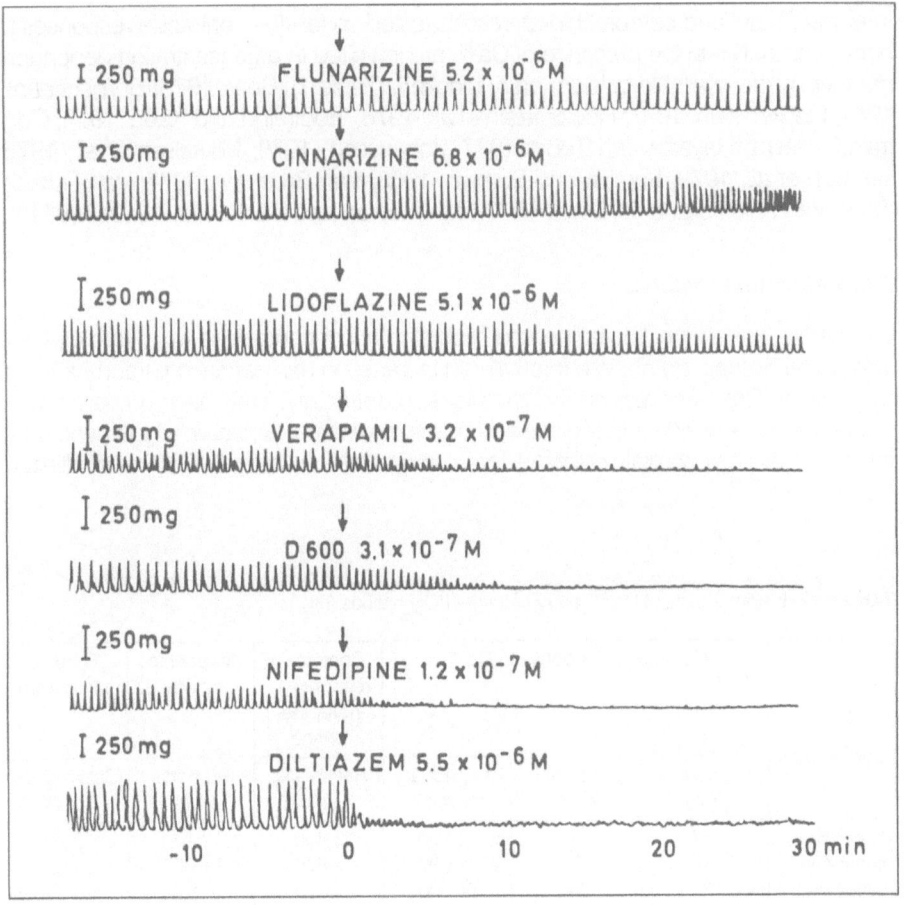

Figure 5: Isometric tension recordings in isolated portal-mesenteric veins of the rat. The influence of seven calcium-entry blockers on myogenic activity was studied at concentrations producing 80-100% inhibition of the response to Ca^{2+} in the depolarized rat caudal artery preparation (Modified from Van Nueten and Vanhoutte, 1981b).

A remarkable diversity exists among the available calcium entry blockers in their capacity to depress the rhythmicity of portal-mesenteric veins in that some calcium entry blockers (e.g. flunarizine, cinnarizine) have little effect on myogenic activity (Fig. 5) (Table 1). This could mean that the latter compounds interfere little with the regulation of blood flow at the arteriolar level. On the other hand, studied on the depolarized portal-mesenteric vein, all Ca^{2+}-entry blockers inhibit Ca^{2+}-induced contractions, as they do on other blood vessels (Bevan, 1979; Church and Zsotér, 1980; Golenhofen and Lammel, 1972; Johansson, 1978; Olivari et al., 1979; Rahwan et al., 1979; Robinson and Collier, 1979; Uchida and Bohr, 1969; Vanhoutte, 1978, 1982a; Vanhoutte and Van Nueten, 1980; Van Nueten, 1978; Van Nueten and Wellens, 1979; Van Nueten et al., 1978; Van Nueten and Vanhoutte, 1980a, 1981a,b).

2.3. Sustained depolarization of the cell membrane

In all peripheral and cerebral blood vessels tested so far, the contractile responses to high levels of K^+ in the presence of Ca^{2+} are inhibited in a concentration-dependent manner by the available calcium entry blockers (Table 1) (Bohr, 1973; Borgers et al., 1981; Fleckenstein, 1977; Fleckenstein et al., 1975; Godfraind and Kaba, 1972; Godfraind, 1981a; Hayashi and Toda, 1977; Johansson, 1978; Mikkelsen et al., 1978; Rahwan et al., 1979; Somlyo and Somlyo, 1968; Van Breemen, 1977; Van Nueten, 1969; Van Nueten and Janssen, 1973; Van Nueten and Vanhoutte, 1980a, 1981a).

2.4. Myocardial tissues

Cinnarizine, flunarizine, lidoflazine and nifedipine at concentrations which are effective in vascular tissues, do not interfere with an increase in myocardial contractile force in response to Ca^{2+} nor with normal myocardial contractility. They have no negative inotropic effects, except for lidoflazine and nifedipine, which, at relatively high concentrations, depress myocardial contractile force. In contrast, verapamil, D600 and diltiazem

Table 1: Inhibitory effects of Ca^{2+} entry blockers [IC_{50}-values (nM)]

Compounds	Contractile Response to Ca^{2+}			Contractile response to norepinephrine	Myogenic activity	Cardiac inotropism
	Rat caudal artery[a]	Rat portal vein[a]	Cat papillary muscle[b]	Rat caudal artery	Rat portal vein	Cat papillary muscle[b]
cinnarizine	370	—	> 22 000	3 400	2 700	> 22 000
flunarizine	100	77	≧ 21 000	670	≧ 21 000	> 21 000
lidoflazine	320	—	14 000	360	2 100	9 300
verapamil	100	27	320	1 600	40	610
D600	19	—	26	1 400	17	280
nifedipine	11	—	490	> 7 200	34	2 700
diltiazem	1 400	142	19 500	—	310	10 900

a: K^+-depolarized tissue;   b: Electrically stimulated tissue.   —: not tested.

have potent inhibitory effects on the Ca^{2+}-induced positive inotropic responses of myocardial tissue and have a direct negative inotropic effect at concentrations slightly higher than those which inhibit vasoconstriction; this indicates a relative lack of tissue selectivity (Table 1) (Van Nueten et al., 1978; Van Nueten and Wellens, 1979).

Acknowledgements

I thank Dr. P.M. Vanhoutte for valuable discussion.
The assistance of Mr. J. Van Beek in finalizing the manuscript is greatly acknowledged. Part of this study was supported by a grant from I.W.O.N.L.

References

Bevan, J.A. Some bases of differences in vascular response to sympathetic activity. Variations on a theme. Circ. Res., **45**, 161-171. (1979)

Bohr, D.F. Electrolytes and smooth muscle contraction. Pharmacol. Rev., **16**, 85-111. (1964)

Bohr, D.F. Vascular smooth muscle updated. Circ. Res., **32**, 665-672. (1973)

Bohr, D.F., Greenberg, S. and Bonaccorsi, A. Mechanisms of action of vasoactive agents. In 'Microcirculation' (Eds. G. Kaley and B.M. Altura), Vol. II, University Park Press, Baltimore, p. 311-348. (1978)

Bolton, T.B. Mechanisms of action of transmitters and other substances on smooth muscle. Physiol. Rev., **59**, 606-717. (1979)

Borgers, M., Thoné, F. and Van Nueten, J.M. The subcellular distribution of calcium and the effects of calcium-antagonists as evaluated with a combined oxalate-pyroantimonate technique. Acta Histochem., **Suppl. 24**, 327-332. (1981)

Borgers, M., Thoné, F., Van Reempts, J. and Verheyen, A. The role of calcium in cellular dysfunction. Proc. Int. Symp. on Cerebral Resuscitation (Ed. B. White), Detroit, July 7-8, 1982, American J. of Emergency Medicine, **1**, 154-161. (1983)

Campbell, J.K., Marshall, R.J. and Winslow, E. Comparative effects of bepridil and verapamil on isolated coronary and systemic arterial smooth muscle. Brit. J. Pharmacol., **74**, 832P-833P. (1981)

Casteels, R. and Van Breemen, C. Active and passive Ca^{2+} fluxes across cell membranes of the guinea-pig taenia coli. Pfluegers Arch., **359**, 197-207. (1975)

Casteels, R. Electro- and pharmacomechanical coupling in vascular smooth muscle. Chest, **78**, 150-156. (1980)

Church, J. and Zsotér, T.T. Calcium antagonistic drugs. Mechanisms of action. Can. J. Physiol. Pharmacol., **58**, 254-264. (1980)

De Clerck, F. and David, J.L. Pharmacological control of platelet and red blood cell function in the microcirculation. J. Cardiovasc. Pharmacol., **3**, 1388-1412. (1981)

De Clerck, F. and Van Nueten, J.M. Platelet-mediated vascular contractions: Inhibition of the serotonergic component by ketanserin. Thromb. Res., **27**, 713-727. (1982a)

De Clerck, F. and Van Nueten, J.M. Platelet-mediated vascular contractions: Inhibition by flunarizine, a Ca^{2+}-entry blocker. Biochem. Pharmacol., **32**, 765-771. (1983)

Droogmans, G., Raeymaekers, L. and Casteels, R. Electro- and pharmacomechanical coupling in the smooth muscle cells of the rabbit ear artery. J. Gen. Physiol., **70**, 129-148. (1977)

Ellis, E.F., Oelz, O., Jacson Roberts II, L., Payne, N.A., Sweetman, B.J., Nies, A.S. and Oates, J.A. Coronary arterial smooth muscle contraction by a substance released from platelets: Evidence that it is thromboxane A_2. *Science*, **193**, 1135-1137. (1976)

Fleckenstein, A., Nakayama, K., Fleckenstein-Grün, G. and Byon, Y.K. Interactions of vasoactive ions and drugs with Ca-dependent excitation contraction coupling of vascular smooth muscle. In 'Calcium Transport in Contraction and Secretion' (Eds. E. Carafoli and F. Clementi), North-Holland Publishing Company, Amsterdam, Oxford, 555-565. (1975)

Fleckenstein, A. Specific pharmacology of calcium in myocardium, cardiac pacemakers, and vascular smooth muscle. *Ann. Rev. Pharmacol. Toxicol.*, **17**, 149-166. (1977)

Godfraind, T. and Kaba, A. The role of calcium in the action of drugs on vascular smooth muscle. *Arch. Int. Pharmacodyn. Ther.*, **196**, 35-49. (1972)

Godfraind, T. and Morel, N. Inhibitors of calcium influx.
In 'Mechanisms of Vasodilatation' (Eds. P.M. Vanhoutte and I. Leusen), Basel, S. Karger, pp. 144-151. (1978)

Godfraind, T. Mechanisms of action of calcium entry blockers. *Fed. Proc.*, **40**, 2866-2871. (1981a)

Godfraind, T. Calcium influx and receptor-response coupling. In 'New Perspectives on Calcium Antagonists' (Ed. G.B. Weiss), Bethesda, Maryland, American Physiological Society, pp. 95-107. (1981b)

Godfraind, T. and Miller, R.C. Prostaglandin $F_{2\alpha}(PGF_{2\alpha})$-mediated contraction and $^{45}[Ca]$-influx into rat mesenteric arteries: inhibition by flunarizine, a calcium entry blocker. *Brit. J. Pharmacol.*, **73**, 252. (1981)

Golenhofen, K. and Lammel, E. Selective suppression of some components of spontaneous activity in various types of smooth muscle by iproveratril (verapamil). *Pfluegers Arch.*, **331**, 233-243. (1972)

Grün, G. and Fleckenstein, A. Die electromechanische Entkoppelung der glatten Gefässmuskulatur als Grundprinzip der Coronardilatation durch 4-(2-Nitrophenyl)-2,6-Dimethyl-1,4-Dihydropyridin-3,5-Dicarbonsäure-Dimethylester (BAY a 1040, Nifedipine). *Arzneim. Forsch.*, **22**, 334-344. (1972)

Hayashi, S. and Toda, N. Inhibition by Cd^{2+}, verapamil and papaverine of Ca^{2+}-induced contractions in isolated cerebral and peripheral arteries of the dog. *Brit. J. Pharmacol.*, **60**, 35-43. (1977)

Johansson, B. Processes involved in vascular smooth muscle contraction and relaxation. *Circ. Res.*, **34** (Suppl. 1), I-14-I-20. (1978)

Kazda, S., Hoffmeister, F., Garthoff, B. and Towart, R. Prevention of the postischaemic impaired reperfusion of the brain by nimodipine (BAY e 9736). *Acta Neurol. Scand.*, **72**, 302-303. (1979)

Kitamura, K. and Kuriyama, H. Effects of acetylcholine on the smooth muscle cell of isolated main coronary artery of the guinea-pig. *J. Physiol.*, **293**, 119-133. (1979)

Labrid, C., Grosset, A., Dureng, G., Mironneau, J. and Duchene-Marullaz, P. Some membrane interactions with bepridil, a new antianginal agent. *J. Pharm. Exp. Ther.*, **211**, 546-554. (1979)

Mikkelsen, E., Andersson, K.E. and Lederballe-Pedersen, O. The effect of nifedipine on isolated human peripheral vessels. *Acta Pharmacol. Toxicol.*, **43**, 291-298. (1978)

Olivari, M.T., Bartorelli, C., Polese, A., Fiorentini, C., Moruzzi, P. and Guazzi, M.D. Treatment of hypertension with nifedipine, a calcium antagonistic agent. *Circulation*, **59**, 1056-1062. (1979)

Rahwan, R.G., Piascik, M.F. and Witiak, D.T. The role of calcium antagonism in the therapeutic action of drugs. *Can. J. Physiol. Pharmacol.*, **57**, 443-460. (1979)

Robinson, B.F. and Collier, J.G. Vascular smooth muscle. Correlations between basic properties and responses of human blood vessels. *Brit. Med. Bull.*, **35**, 305-312. (1979)

Somlyo, A.P. and Somlyo, A.V. Vascular smooth muscle. I. Normal structure, pathology, biochemistry and biophysics. *Pharmacol. Rev.*, **20**, 197-272. (1968a)

Somlyo, A.P. and Somlyo, A.V. Electromechanical and pharmacomechanical coupling in vascular smooth muscle. *J. Pharm. Exp. Ther.*, **159**, 129-145. (1968b)

Somlyo, A.P. and Somlyo, A.V. Vascular smooth muscle. II. Pharmacology of normal and hypertensive vessels. *Pharmacol. Rev.*, **22**, 249-353. (1970)

Triggle, D.J. and Swamy, V.C. Pharmacology of agents that affect calcium: agonists and antagonists. *Chest*, **78**, 157-165. (1980)

Uchida, E. and Bohr, D.F. Myogenic tone in isolated perfused vessels: Occurrence among vascular beds and along vascular trees. *Circ. Res.*, **25**, 549-555. (1969)

Van Breemen, C. Calcium requirement for activation of intact aortic smooth muscle. *J. Physiol.*, **272**, 317-329. (1977)

Van Breemen, C., Aaronson, P., Loutzenhiser, R. and Meisheri, K. Ca^{2+} movements in smooth muscle. *Chest*, **78**, 157-165. (1980)

Vanhoutte, P.M. Effects of anoxia and glucose depletion on isolated veins of the dog. *Am. J. Physiol.*, **230**, 1261-1268. (1976)

Vanhoutte, P.M. Heterogeneity of vascular smooth muscle.
In 'Microcirculation' (Eds. G. Kaley and B.M. Altura), Vol. II, Baltimore, University Park Press, pp. 181-309. (1978)

Vanhoutte, P.M. and Van Nueten, J.M. The pharmacology of lidoflazine. *Proc. Royal Soc. Med., Congress and Symposia Series*, **29**, 61-77. (1980)

Vanhoutte, P.M., Verbeuren, T.J. and Van Nueten, J.M. Effect of lidoflazine on systemic arteries and veins. *Angiology*, **31**, 581-593. (1980)

Vanhoutte, P.M., Verbeuren, T.J. and Webb, R.C. Local modulation of the adrenergic neuroeffector interaction in the blood vessel wall. *Physiol. Rev.*, **61**, 151-247. (1981)

Vanhoutte, P.M. Differential effects of calcium entry blockers on vascular smooth muscle. In ''New Perspectives on Calcium Antagonists'' (Ed. G.B. Weiss), Clinical Physiology Series, The American Physiological Society, Washington, D.C., pp. 109-121. (1981)

Vanhoutte, P.M. Calcium entry blockers and vascular smooth muscle. *Circulation*, **65** (Suppl. I), I-11-I-19. (1982a)

Vanhoutte, P.M. Heterogeneity of postjunctional vascular α-adrenoceptors and handling of calcium. *J. Cardiovasc. Pharmacol.*, **4**, S91-S96. (1982b)

Van Nueten, J.M. Comparative bioassay of vasoactive drugs using isolated perfused rabbit arteries. *Eur. J. Pharmacol.*, **6**, 289-293. (1969)

Van Nueten, J.M. and Janssen, P.A.J. Comparative study of the effects of flunarizine and cinnarizine on smooth muscle and cardiac tissues. *Arch. Int. Pharmacodyn. Ther.*, **204**, 37-55. (1973)

Van Nueten, J.M. Vasodilatation or inhibition of vasoconstriction?
In 'Mechanisms of Vasodilatation' (Eds. P.M. Vanhoutte and I. Leusen), Basel, S. Karger, 137-143. (1978)

Van Nueten, J.M., Van Beek, J. and Janssen, P.A.J. Effect of flunarizine on calcium-induced responses of peripheral vascular smooth muscle. *Arch. Int. Pharmacodyn. Ther.*, **232**, 42-52. (1978)

Van Nueten, J.M. and Wellens, D. Mechanisms of vasodilatation and antivasoconstriction. *Angiology*, **30**, 440-446. (1979)

Van Nueten, J.M. and Vanhoutte, P.M. Improvement of tissue perfusion with inhibitors of calcium ion influx. *Biochem. Pharmacol.*, **29**, 479-481. (1980a)

Van Nueten, J.M. and Vanhoutte, P.M. Effect of the Ca^{2+} antagonist lidoflazine on normoxic and anoxic contractions of canine coronary arterial smooth muscle. *Eur. J. Pharmacol.*, **64**, 173-176. (1980b)

Van Nueten, J.M., Van Beek, J. and Vanhoutte, P.M. Inhibitory effect of lidoflazine on contractions of isolated canine coronary arteries caused by norepinephrine, 5-hydroxytryptamine, high potassium, anoxia and ergonovine maleate. *J. Pharmacol. Exp. Ther.*, **213**, 179-187. (1980)

Van Nueten, J.M. and Vanhoutte, P.M. Calcium entry blockers and vascular smooth muscle heterogeneity. *Fed. Proc.*, **40**, 2862-2865. (1981a)

Van Nueten, J.M. and Vanhoutte, P.M. Selectivity of calcium-antagonism and serotonin-antagonism with respect to venous and arterial tissues. *Angiology*, **32**, 476-484. (1981b)

Van Nueten, J.M. and De Clerck, F. Protection against hypoxia-induced decrease in tissue blood flow. In 'Cerebral Hypoxia in the Pathogenesis of Migraine (Eds. F. Clifford-Rose and W. Amery), Pitman Books Limited, London, p. 176-184. (1982)

Van Nueten, J.M., De Ridder, W. and Van Beek, J. Hypoxia and spasms in the cerebral vasculature. *J. Cer. Blood Flow Metab.*, **2**, S29-S31. (1982)

Van Nueten, J.M. Selectivity of calcium entry blockers. In 'Calcium Modulators (Eds. T. Godfraind, A. Albertini and R. Paoletti), Elsevier Biomedical Press, p. 199-208. (1982)

Van Reempts, J., Borgers, M., Van Dael, L., Van Eyndhoven, J. and Van de Ven, M. Protection with flunarizine against hypoxic-ischaemic damage of the rat cerebral cortex. A quantitative morphologic assessment. Arch. Pharmacodyn. Ther., **262**, 76-88. (1983)

Wauquier, A., Ashton, D., Clincke, G. and Van Reempts, J. Pharmacological protection against brain hypoxia; the efficacy of flunarizine, a calcium entry blocker. In 'Cerebral Hypoxia in the Pathogenesis of Migraine (Eds. F. Clifford-Rose and W. Amery), Pitman Books Limited, London p. 139-154. (1982)

Weiss, G.B. Sites of action of calcium antagonists in vascular smooth muscle. In 'New Perspectives on Calcium Antagonists' (Ed. G.B. Weiss), Bethesda, Maryland, American Physiological Society, pp. 83-94. (1981)

White, B.C., Gadzinski, D.S., Hoehner, P.J., Krome, C., Hoehner and White, J.D. Correction of canine cerebral cortical blood flow and vascular resistance after cardiac arrest using flunarizine, a calcium antagonist. *Ann. Emerg. Med.*, **22**, 118-127. (1982)

Calcium homeostasis in human red blood cells

H.J. Schatzmann

Summary

The human red cell plasma membrane is extremely tight to Ca^{2+} (the leak flux under the physiological gradient of 10'000 is 10 - 50 μmole/l cells.h at 37°C). The membrane contains an ATP dependent Ca^{2+} pump, whose maximal capacity is of the order of 10 mmole/l cells.h at 37°C. Consequently the steady state internal Ca^{2+} concentration is kept below $10^{-6}M$. The pump can cope with increased influx rates seen under mechanical strain or in certain (hereditary) pathological alterations. Failure of keeping intracellular Ca^{2+} low has several consequences: (1) Opening of the Ca^{2+} sensitive potassium channel, which leads to cell shrinking. (2) Shape change from discocyte to echinocyte, spherical echinocyte and ultimately spherocyte. (3) Inhibition of the Na-K pump at very high Ca^{2+} concentration.

The leak flux of Ca^{2+} is not a simple matter of diffusion but shows the characteristics of a saturable process. The Ca^{2+} pump is a well defined system, whose requirements and kinetics are partially known. Some data concerning the energetics are available. However, no mechanistic model bringing the ATP-ase reaction of the system together with the translocation of the Ca^{2+} can be proposed at the moment.

Résumé

La membrane plasmatique du globule rouge humain est extrêmement imperméable à Ca^{2+} (le flux d'infiltration sous le gradient physiologique de 10.000 est de 10 - 50 μmole/l de cellules.h à 37°C) La membrane contient une pompe de Ca^{2+} dépendant d'ATP, dont la capacité maximale est de l'ordre de 10 mmole/l de cellules.h à 37°C. Conséquemment, la concentration steady state interne de Ca^{2+} est maintenue en-dessous de $10^{-6}M$. La pompe peut venir à bout des taux accrus d'infiltration qu'on peut observer lors d'un effet mécanique ou dans le cas de certains troubles pathologiques (héréditaires). L'incapacité de maintenir le Ca^{2+} intracellulaire à un niveau très bas comporte plusieurs conséquences : (1) Ouverture du canal de potassium sensible à Ca^{2+}, ce qui entraîne l'effondrement cellulaire. (2) Passage de la forme discocyte à la forme échinocyte, échinocyte sphérique et enfin sphérocyte. (3) Inhibition de la pompe Na-K à une concentration de Ca^{2+} très élevée.
Le flux d'infiltration de Ca^{2+} n'est pas une simple question de diffusion. Il présente aussi les caractéristiques d'un processus saturable. La pompe de Ca^{2+} constitue un système bien déterminé dont les exigences et la cinétique sont connues partiellement. On dispose de certaines données relatives à l'énergétique. Toutefois, on ne peut actuellement proposer aucun modèle mécanique faisant le lien entre la réaction ATPase du système et le transfert de Ca^{2+}.

Resumen

La membrana del glóbulo rojo humano es muy poco traspasable por Ca^{2+} (el flujo bajo el gradiente fisiológico de 10.000 es 10 - 50 μmol/l células/hora a 37° Celsio). La membrana contiene una bomba Ca^{2+} dependiente de ATP, cuya máxima capacidad es del valor de 10 mmol/l células/hora a 37° Celsio. Como consecuencia, la concentración normal intracelular de Ca^{2+} está conservada bajo 10^{-6} M. La bomba puede dar abasto a velocidades crecientes de influjo observadas durante tensión mecánica o en ciertas alteraciones patológicas (hereditarias). El fallo de conservar bajo el Ca^{2+} intracelular tiene varias consecuencias : 1. Apertura del canal potasio sensible al Ca^{2+}, lo que conduce al encogimiento celular 2. Cambio de forma de discocito a equinocito, equinocito esférico y finalmente esferocito 3. Inhibición de la bomba Na-K a una concentración Ca^{2+} muy alta.
El flujo de pérdida de Ca^{2+} no es mera cuestión de difusión, sino que muestra los característicos de un proceso saturable. La bomba Ca^{2+} es un sistema bien definido, cuyos requisitos y cinética son parcialmente conocidos. Algunos datos, sobre la energética están disponibles. No obstante, no se puede proponer en este momento, un modelo de mecanismo que junte la reacción ATP-asa del sistema a la translocación del Ca^{2+}.

Zusammenfassung

Die Plasmamembran des menschlichen Erythrozyten ist für Ca^{2+} in hohem Masse undurchlässig (die Einstromquote unter dem physiologischen Gradienten von 10.000 ist 10-50 μmol/l Zellen.h bei 37°C). Die Membran enthält eine ATP-abhängige Ca^{2+}-Pumpe, mit einer Höchstkapazität in der Grössenordnung von 10 mmol/l Zellen.h bei 37°C. Demzufolge wird die innere Ca^{2+}-Steady-State-Konzentration unter $10^{-6}M$ gehalten. Die Pumpe ist imstande, der unter mechanischer Belastung bzw. bei bestimmten (vererbten) pathologischen Veränderungen erhöhten Einstromgeschwindigkeit erfolgreich zu begegnen. Kann das intrazelluläre Ca^{2+} nicht niedrig gehalten werden, so hat dies mehrere Folgen : (1) die Öffnung des Ca^{2+}-empfindlichen Kaliumkanals, mit der Folge einer zellulären Schrumpfung; (2) eine Formänderung vom Diskozyten zum Echinozyten, zum sphärischem Echinozyten und schliesslich zum Sphärozyten; (3) Hemmung der Na-K-Pumpe bei sehr hoher Ca^{2+}-Konzentration.
Der Einstrom des Ca^{2+} ist nicht nur einfach diffusionsabhängig, er zeigt auch die Charakteristika eines sättigungsfähigen Prozesses. Die Ca^{2+}-Pumpe ist ein gut umschriebenes System, dessen Erfordernisse und Kinetik teilweise bekannt sind. Über die energetischen Eigenschaften sind einige Daten verfügbar. Jedoch besteht derzeit noch kein mechanisches Modell, in dem das Verhältnis zwischen ATPase-Reaktion des Systems und Ca^{2+}-Transport dargestellt werden kann.

Introduction

The free internal Ca^{2+} concentration in human red cells is set according to the leak-and-pump principle: There is a finite passive Ca^{2+} influx at the physiological Ca^{2+}-gradient across the membrane which is compensated by Ca^{2+} pumping in the outward direction with a rate given by the degree of saturation of the ATP-fuelled Ca-pump at the steady-state internal Ca^{2+} concentration.

Simons (1982) recently devised a method allowing the measurement of the steady-state internal Ca^{2+} concentration. Cells are suspended in media of different Ca^{2+} content whose Ca^{2+} concentration is monitored by a Ca^{2+}-selective electrode. When the cells are lysed (by digitonin) there is an upward or downward deflection of the electrode signal. At the point of zero deflection, the cellular Ca^{2+} concentration equals that of the medium. The result is, that in fresh human red blood cells the Ca^{2+} concentration is $\leqq 0.4\ \mu M$ (this is an upper estimate; the true value may be considerably lower).

The calcium leak

The net influx of Ca^{2+} measured in cells metabolically depleted by incubation for 1 - 2 h in the presence of iodo-acetamide and inositol, is some 10 μmoles/l cells.h at the physiological Ca^{2+}-gradient (Ferreira & Lew, 1977). This is a very low rate of penetration, but it is obvious that it is not a diffusional flow for the following reasons. Ferreira and Lew (1977) have shown that the process obeys saturation kinetics. In their experiments net influx saturated at about 5 mM Ca_0^{2+} concentration and a large part of the efflux was dependent on external Ca^{2+} concentration and saturated at about 1 mM Ca_0^{2+} concentration. This not only implies that the transmembrane Ca^{2+} movement is via a "carrier", but that the carrier allows of some exchange of Ca_i^{2+} for Ca_0^{2+}. As a matter of fact, the exchange flux is several times the unidirectional non-exchange flux (or net flux).

Interestingly, the authors found that the saturating internal concentrations for both the exchange and non-exchange efflux are 20 - 30 μM. This different affinity on the cis and trans side is not exceptional, but is encountered also in other passive transport systems, e.g. in the red cell glucose transport system. The system remains truly passive in spite of the affinity change from outside to inside, because the rate constant of the transfer from the low affinity side is by necessity that much larger than in the opposite direction as the affinity is lower (for a lucid discussion see Widdas, 1980).

Lew et al. (1982) very recently showed that in non-starved red cells in plasma at low $[Ca_i^{2+}]$ (10 - 50 nM) net passive Ca^{2+}-influx is larger (40 - 50 μmole/l cells.h). Passive transport thus seems to depend on metabolism and to be reduced by internal Ca^{2+}. It is quite easily conceivable that internal Ca^{2+} changes the permeability to Ca^{2+} because Ca^{2+} has profound effects on the membrane chemistry, for instance by activating phospholipases and kinases. These experiments also suggest that the physiological $[Ca_i^{2+}]$ is substantially lower than the upper estimate by Simons (1982).

The calcium pump

Human red cells are unique in having only one Ca^{2+}-extrusion mechanism, namely the ATP-fuelled Ca^{2+}-pump (Schatzmann, 1982, 1983), whereas the Na-Ca-exchange encountered in many other animal cells is absent. At saturating Ca^{2+} concentration the rate of the pump is more than 10 mmoles/l cells.h, that is 500 - 1000 times faster than the inward leak.

This pump is an integral membrane protein of 130 - 140 kD molecular weight (Knauf et al., 1974; Niggli et al., 1979; Gietzen et al., 1980) and is an ATPase, requiring Ca^{2+} + Mg^{2+} for its function. The apparent K_{Ca} on the internal surface is 1 μM or less in EGTA-buffered solutions. ATP has to be present on the internal surface. There are two sites for ATP, the enzyme site proper with a K_m of 1 - 3 μM and a "regulatory" site with a K_{ATP} of 100 - 300 μM (Richards et al., 1978; Muallem & Karlish, 1979). The role of Mg^{2+} is discussed below. The protein undergoes cyclic phosphorylation-dephosporylation from ATP during the transport cycle, whereby inorganic phosphate is liberated inside the cells. For phosphorylation Ca^{2+} is an absolute requirement at concentrations corresponding to K_{Ca} in the ATPase function. There is good evidence that the phosphoprotein undergoes a conformation-change ($E_1 \sim P \blacktriangleright E_2 \sim P$) and that Mg^{2+} is necessary for this (Garrahan & Rega, 1978). Dephosphorylation requires high ATP concentration (at the regulatory site) (Garrahan & Rega, 1978). Muallem and Karlish (1981) have presented evidence for Mg-ATP being the active agent at this step (at 37°C and in the presence of calmodulin). Other observations (Enyedi et al., 1982 point in the same direction.

The pump is calmodulin dependent (Larsen & Vincenzi, 1979), and calmodulin is found in the cytosol of the human red cell at a concentration of $\sim$ 5 μM which is in excess over the number of pump sites in the membrane (Foder & Scharff, 1981). Calmodulin binds to the pump only in a Ca-form (possibly that with 3 Ca and 1 Mg (Scharff, 1980)). Foder and Scharff (1981) have demonstrated that the pump-calmodulin stoichiometry is 1 : 1. The affinity of the pump protein for Ca-calmodulin is of the order of 10 nM. Physiological conditions are such that calmodulin is normally detached from the pump (Foder & Scharff, 1981). The effect of calmodulin consists of an increase in Ca^{2+} affinity of the pump (K_{Ca} is 1 μM with and somewhere near 30 μM without calmodulin) and possibly an increase in the V_{max} (i.e. the turnover rate of the pump).

Au (1978) has pointed out that the cytosol also contains an inhibitor protein of the (Ca^{2+} + Mg^{2+})-ATPase. Sarkadi et al. (1980, b) have demonstrated that crude and partially purified membrane free haemolysate stimulates at low and inhibits at higher concentration the Ca^{2+} transport in inside-out vesicles. Wütrich (1982) has recently isolated a 20 kD protein which is inhibitory on (Ca^{2+} + Mg^{2+})-ATPase and Ca^{2+}-pump activity and whose action has kinetics which are the mirror image of those of calmodulin. However, it is not a simple competitor with calmodulin, nor seems to bind to calmodulin.

The action of calmodulin can be mimicked by acidic lipids (Niggli et al., 1981a; Stieger & Luterbacher, 1981) and interestingly by controlled cleavage of the main protein by trypsin (Taverna & Hanahan, 1980; Sarkadi et al., 1980a; Niggli et al., 1981a; Stieger & Schatzmann, 1981). The latter point can be interpreted by assuming that the pump protein contains a peptide sequence which is inhibitory and whose attenuating effect is relieved by calmodulin-binding. The activating effect of trypsin treatment is only obtained when Ca^{2+} is present in the medium at concentrations similar to those required in transport activation (Rossi & Schatzmann, 1982).

The pump protein has been isolated by calmodulin affinity chromatography (Niggli et al., 1979; Gietzen et al., 1980). With respect to ATPase activity the pure protein shows most of the characteristics described so far for the membrane-bound system (Stieger & Luterbacher, 1981; Stieger, 1982). The pure protein has been incorporated into artificial lipid vesicles whereby it could be demonstrated to retain the Ca^{2+}-transporting property (Niggli et al., 1981 b; Stieger, 1982).

Inhibitors of the Ca-pump

Many artificial inhibitors have been described, none of which seems to be very specific. La^{3+} is interesting in that it seems to block in moderate concentrations (0.1 - 0.2 mM) the Mg^{2+}-sensitive conformational change (Luterbacher & Schatzmann, 1983). The kinetics of the inhibition by vanadate are such as to suggest an action on the back reaction of $E_2 \blacktriangleright E_1$ which is compatible with its similarity to the phosphate anion (Barrabin et al., 1980). Phenotiazine neuroleptics have been claimed to block the pump because of their affinity to calmodulin. In fact, the calmodulin-elicited activity is about 5 times more sensitive to trifluoperazine than the basal activity (Hinds et al., 1981). However, the specificity for calmodulin must seriously be doubted in view of the fact that the system deinhibited by trypsin-treatment and the calmodulin activated system are nearly equally sensitive to trifluoperazine (Stieger, 1982). A novel compound which is very potent on the Ca-pump and very ineffective on the Na-K-pump has recently been described (Gietzen et al., 1981).

Significance of low internal Ca²⁺ concentration

Failure to keep the Ca^{2+} concentration inside the cells low leads to K^+ loss (Gardos, 1958; Blum & Hoffman, 1971), to echinocyte formation (Szasz et al., 1978) ending in smooth spherocytes with impaired filterability of the cells (Kirkpatrick et al., 1975) and (at very high internal Ca^{2+} concentration) to blockade of the Na-K-pump.

Red cells abnormally leaky to Ca^{2+} occur in sickle cell anaemia (Eaton et al., 1973), microcytic haemolytic anaemia (Wiley & Gill, 1976) and in high PC/PE anaemia (an extremely rare disease characterized by an increase in the phosphatidylcholine to phosphatidylethanolamine ratio among the membrane lipids and a moderate Na-K leak) (Bucher et al., 1978). In addition to the enormous leak in sickle cells there is a defect in the Ca-pump. Under conditions of sickling Bookchin and Lew (1980) have described a progressive decline of the Ca-pump activity.

References

Au, K.S. An endogenous inhibitor of erythrocyte membrane (Ca^{2+} + Mg^{2+})-ATPase. *Int. J. Biochem.*, **9**, 477-480. (1978)

Barrabin, H., Garrahan, P.J. and Rega, A.F. Vanadate inhibition of the Ca^{2+}-ATPase from human red cell membranes. *Biochim. Biophys. Acta*, **600**, 796-804. (1980)

Blum, R.M. and Hoffman, J.F. The membrane locus of Ca-stimulated K-transport in energy depleted human red blood cells. *J. membrane Biol.*, **6**, 315-328. (1971)

Bookchin, R.M. and Lew, V.. Progressive inhibition of the Ca-pump and Ca: Ca exchange in sickle red cells. *Nature*, **284**, 561-563. (1980)

Bucher, U., Coninx, S., Furlan, M., Bürgin, H., Schatzmann, H.J. and Zahler, P. Hereditary nonsphaerocytic haemolytic disorder associated with increased membrane permeability. 17th Congress int. Soc. Hematol. Abstr. p. 61. (1978)

Eaton, J.W., Skelton, T.D., Swofford, H.S. and Jacob, H.S. Elevated erythrocyte calcium in sickle cell disease. *Nature*, **246**, 105-106. (1973)

Enyedi, A., Sarkadi, B. and Gardos, G. On the substrate specificity of the red cell calcium pump. *Biochim. Biophys. Acta*, **687**, 109-112. (1982)

Ferreira, H.G. and Lew, V.L. Passive Ca transport and cytoplasmic Ca buffering in intact red cells. In: Membrane Transport in Red Cells. J.C. Ellory, V.L. Lew ed. Acad. Press, p. 53-100. (1977)

Foder, B., and Scharff, O.. Decrease of apparent calmodulin affinity of erythrocyte (Ca^{2+} + Mg^{2+})-ATPase at low Ca^{2+} concentrations. *Biochim. Biophys. Acta*, **649**, 367-376. (1981)

Gardos, G. The function of calcium in the potassium permeability of human red cells. *Biochim. Biophys. Acta*, **30**, 653-654. (1958)

Garrahan, P.J. and Rega, A.F. Activation of partial reactions of the Ca^{2+}-ATPase from human red cells by Mg^{2+} and ATP. *Biochim. Biophys. Acta*, **513**, 59-65. (1978)

Gietzen, K., Tejcka, M. and Wolf, H.U. Calmodulin affinity chromatography yields a functional purified erythrocyte (Ca^{2+} + Mg^{2+})-dependent ATPase. *Biochem. J.*, **189**, 81-88. (1980)

Gietzen, K., Wütrich, A. and Bader, H. A new powerful inhibitor of red blood cell Ca^{2+} transport ATPase and of calmodulin in regulated functions. *Biochem. Biophys. Res. Comm.*, **101**, 418-425. (1981)

Hinds, Th. R., Raess, B.U. and Vincenzi, F.F. Plasma membrane Ca^{2+} transport: Antagonism by several potential inhibitors. *J. membrane Biol.*, **58**, 57-65. (1981)

Kirkpatrick, F.H., Hillman, D.G. and La Celle, P.L. A 23187 and red cells: changes in deformability, K^+, Mg^{2+}, Ca^{2+} and ATP. *Experientia*, **31**, 653-654. (1975)

Knauf, P.A., Proverbio, F. and Hoffman, J.F. Electrophoretic separation of different phosphoproteins associated with Ca-ATPase and Na, K-ATPase in human red cell ghosts. *J. Gen. Physiol.*, **63**, 324-336. (1974)

Larsen, F.L. and Vincenzi, F.F. Calcium transport across the plasma membrane: Stimulation by calmodulin. *Science*, **204**, 306-308. (1979)

Lew, V.L., Tsien, R.Y. and Miner, C. The physiological $[Ca^{2+}]_i$-level and pump-leak turnover in intact red cells measured with the use of an incorporated Ca-chelator. *Nature*, **298**, 478-481. (1982)

Luterbacher, S. and Schatzmann, H.J. The site of action of Ca^{2+} in the reaction cycle of the human red cell membrane. *Experientia*, **39**, 311-312. (1983)

Muallem, S. and Karlish, S.J.D. Is the red cell calcium pump regulated by ATP? *Nature*, **277**, 238-240. (1979)

Muallem, S. and Karlish, S.J.D. Studies on the mechanism of regulation of the red cell Ca^{2+}-pump by calmodulin and ATP. *Biochim.. Biophys. Acta*, **647**, 73-86. (1981)

Niggli, V., Adunyah, E.S. and Carafoli, E. Acidic phospholipids, unsaturated fatty acid and limited proteolysis mimic the effect of calmodulin on the purified erythrocyte Ca^{2+}-ATPase. *J. Biol. Chem.*, **256**, 8588-8592. (1981a)

Niggli, V., Adunyah, E.S., Penniston, J.F. and Carafoli, E. Purified $(Ca^{2+} + Mg^{2+})$-ATPase of the erythrocyte membrane: Reconstitution and effect of calmodulin and phospholipids. *J. Biol. Chem.*, **256**, 395-401. (1981b)

Niggli, V., Penniston, J.T. and Carafoli, E. Purification of the $(Ca^{2+} + Mg^{2+})$-ATPase from human erythrocyte membranes using a calmodulin affinity column. *J. Biol. Chem.*, **254**, 9955-9958. (1979)

Richards, D.R., Rega, A.F., and Garrahan, P.J. Two classes of sites for ATP in the Ca^{2+}-ATPase from human red cell membranes. *Biochim. Biophys. Acta*, **511**, 194-201. (1978)

Rossi, J.P.F.C. and Schatzmann, H.J. Trypsin activation of the red cell Ca^{2+}-pump is calcium sensitive. *Cell Calcium*, **3**, 583-590. (1982)

Sarkadi, B., Enyedi, A. and Gardos, G. Molecular properties of the red cell calcium pump. I. Effects of calmodulin, proteolytic digestion and drugs on the kinetics of the active calcium uptake in inside-out red cell membrane vesicles. *Cell Calcium*, **1**, 287-297. (1980a)

Sarkadi, B., Szasz, I. and Gardos, G. Characteristics and regulation of active calcium transport in inside-out red cell membrane vesicles. *Biochim. Biophys. Acta*, **598**, 326-338. (1980b)

Scharff, O. Kinetics of calcium-dependent membrane ATPase in human erythrocytes. In: Membrane Transport in Erythrocytes. U.V. Lassen, H.H. Ussing, J.O. Wieth ed. Munksgaard, Copenhagen, p. 236-254. (1980)

Schatzmann, H.J. The plasma membrane calcium pump of erythrocytes and other animal cells. In: Membrane Transport of Calcium, E. Carafoli ed. Acad. Press, p. 41-108. (1982)

Schatzmann, H.J. The red cell calcium pump. *Ann. Rev. Physiol.*, **45**, 303-312. (1983)

Simons, T.J.B. A method for estimating free Ca within human red blood cells with an application to the study of their Ca-dependent K permeability. *J. membrane Biol.*, **66**, 235-247. (1982)

Stieger, J. Charakterisierung und Rekonstitution der isolierten $(Ca^{2+} + Mg^{2+})$-ATPase aus Erythrocytenmembranen. Doctoral Thesis, University of Bern. (1982)

Stieger, J. and Luterbacher, S. Some properties of the purified $(Ca^{2+} + Mg^{2+})$-ATPase from human red blood cell membranes. *Biochim. Biophys. Acta*, **641**, 270-275. (1981)

Stieger, J. and Schatzmann, H.J. Metal requirement of the isolated red cell Ca-pump ATPase after elimination of calmodulin-dependence by trypsin attack. *Cell Calcium*, **2**, 601-616. (1981)

Szasz, I., Sarkadı, B., Schubert, A. and Gardos, G. Effects of lanthanum on calcium dependent phenomena in human red cells. *Biochim. Biophysics Acta*, **512**, 331-340. (1978)

Taverna, R.D. and Hanahan, D.J. Modulation of human erythrocyte $(Ca^{2+} + Mg^{2+})$-ATPase activity by phospholipase A and proteases. A comparison with calmodulin. *Biochem. Biophys. Res. Comm.*, **94**, 652-659. (1980)

Widdas, W.F. The asymmetry of the hexose transfer system in the human red cell membrane. *Current Topics membr. transp.*, **14**, 165-223. (1980)

Wiley, J.S. and Gill, F.M. Red cell calcium leak in congenital hemolytic anaemia with extreme microcytosis. *Blood*, **47**, 197-210. (1976)

Wütrich, A. Isolation from haemolysate of a proteinaceous inhibitor of the red cell Ca^{2+}-pump ATPase. Its action on the kinetics of the enzyme. *Cell Calcium*, **3**, 201-214. (1982)

Impact of Ca^{2+} entry blockers on Ca^{2+}-dependent mechanisms in red blood cells, platelets and endothelial cells

F. De Clerck and J. Hladovec

Summary

At the level of the red blood cell excessive Ca^{2+}-influx as induced experimentally by the ionophore A23187 induces loss of functional deformability and eventually shape changes. The order of potency for inhibition of these Ca^{2+}-induced changes by Ca^{2+}-entry blockers was flunarizine > cinnarizine > lidoflazine > D600 > verapamil; nifedipine, niludipine and prenylamine were inactive. At the level of the vascular endothelium Ca^{2+}-entry blockers provide protection against damage subsequent to distur- bance of the Ca^{2+}-homeostasis, the order of potency on a mg/kg basis in the rat being nifedipine > flunarizine > prenylamine > carbochromen > verapamil = cinnarizine > lidoflazine. At the level of the blood platelets verapamil, nifedipine, nisoldipine and lidoflazine inhibit certain aspects of platelet activa- tion; their effect is difficult to explain on the basis of Ca^{2+}-channel blockade only.

Résumé

Au niveau du globule rouge, l'influx excessif de Ca^{2+} provoqué expérimentalement par l'ionophore A23187 entraîne une perte de déformabilité fonctionnelle et éventuellement des changements de forme. L'inhibition effectuée par les agents bloqueurs de l'entrée de Ca^{2+} sur ces changements induits par le Ca^{2+}, se présente dans l'ordre de puissance suivant: la flunarizine > la cinnarizinne > la lidoflazine > le D600 > le vérapamil. La nifédipine, la niludipine et la prénylamine se sont montrées inefficaces. Au niveau de l'endothélium vasculaire, les agents bloqueurs de l'entrée de Ca^{2+} fournissent une protection contre l'endommagement résultant d'une perturbation de l'homéostasie du Ca^{2+}, avec un ordre de puissance (sur base de mg/kg chez le rat) se présentant comme suit: la nifédipine > la flunarizine > la prénylamine > le carbocromène > le vérapamil = la cinnarizine > la lidoflazine. Au niveau des plaquettes sanguines, le vérapamil, la nifédipine, la nisoldipine et la lidoflazine inhibent certains aspects de l'activité plaquettaire. Leur effet est difficile à expliquer sur base d'un simple blocage du canal de Ca^{2+}.

Resumen

A nivel del eritrocito, el influjo excesivo de Ca^{2+}, al ser provocado experimentalmente con ionóforo A 23187, causa pérdida de deformabilidad funcional y hasta cambio de forma. El orden de la potencia de los inhibidores de estas alteraciones provocadas por Ca^{2+} fue el siguiente: flunarizina > cinnarizina > lidoflazina > D 600 > verapamil; nifedipino, niludipina y prenilamina eran inactivos.
A nivel del endotelio vascular, los inhibidores de Ca^{2+} proveen protección contra el perjuicio causado por la perturbación de la homeostasia Ca^{2+}; el orden de potencia, a base de mg/kg en la rata es nifedipino > flunarizina > prenilamina > carbocromeno > verapamil = cinnarizina > lidoflazina.
A nivel de las plaquetas sanguíneas, verapamil, nifedipino, nisoldipino y lidoflazina, inhiben ciertos aspectos de la actividad de las plaquetas; es difícil explicar estos efectos exclusivamente a base de un bloqueo de los canales Ca^{2+}.

Zusammenfassung

Bei Erythrozyten erzeugt ein durch das Ionophor A23187 experimentell hervorgerufener, übermässiger Ca^{2+}-Einstrom einen Verlust an funktioneller Verformbarkeit und schliesslich Formveränderungen. Folgende Ca^{2+}-Einstromhemmer sind nach fallender Wirksamheit, in der sie die durch Ca^{2+} verursachten Änderungen blockieren, geordnet: Flunarizin > Cinnarizin > Lidoflazin > D600 > Verapamil; Nifedipin, Niludipin und Prenylamin waren dabei unwirksam. Am Gefässendothel bieten Ca^{2+}-Einstromhemmer Schutz gegen Schäden infolge einer gestörten Ca^{2+}-Homöostase, mit der folgenden, nach fallender Potenz geordneten Wirksamkeit (Ratte, mg/kg): Nifedipin > Flunarizin > Prenylamin > Carbochromen > Verapamil und gleichwirksam, Cinnarizin > Lidoflazin. An Thrombozyten hemmen Verapamil, Nifedipin, Nisoldipin und Lidoflazin bestimmte Schritte in der Aktivierung; aufgrund einer Blockierung des Ca^{2+}-Kanals allein ist diese Wirkung nicht ganz zu erklären.

Apart from cardiovascular control, the behaviour of the formed elements of the blood contributes to the maintenance or disturbance of adequate tissue perfusion and of vascular integrity (De Clerck and David, 1981). The present study will focus on the role of Ca^{2+}-balance in the function of red blood cells (RBC), the platelets and the endothelial cells with emphasis on the effect of Ca^{2+}-entry blockers on this process.

1. Red blood cells

Recently changes in blood viscosity, including a reduction of red blood cell (RBC) deformability have been related to the occurrence of arterial disease and may promote ischemia (Lowe et al. 1981).

Clinical trials have shown that the Ca^{2+}-entry blocker cinnarizine reduces the whole blood viscosity of patients with peripheral arterial disease (Di Perri et al., 1979; De Cree et al., 1979). For the parent compound flunarizine it was demonstrated specifically that impaired RBC deformability of patients with atherosclerosis, post-myocardial infarction conditions, diabetes mellitus and pregnancies at risk is improved by the treatment (De Cree et al., 1979; Heilman, 1980).
A similar effect on RBC deformability has been reported in patients with vascular disease treated with nifedipine (Slonim et al., 1981). Red blood cell deformability is mainly dependent upon the cellular geometry, its internal viscosity and the intrinsic membrane viscosity (Wells, 1964).

From the initiating work of Weed and La Celle (Weed et al., 1969) it is known that the intrinsic membrane deformability, at least in aging stored blood in vitro, depends upon the interplay between Ca^{2+} and energy metabolism reflected by ATP-levels. Normal cells can maintain their low intracellular Ca^{2+}-level against a gradient up to 10,000 by a low membrane permeability to Ca^{2+} and by an outward directed "Ca^{2+}-pump", the activity of which is reflected by (Ca^{2+} + Mg^{2+})-activated membrane ATP-ase (Schatzmann and Vincenzi, 1969). This "Ca^{2+}-pump" is directly dependent upon ATP-hydrolysis as an energy source and is regulated by calmodulin which enhances both the velocity and Ca^{2+}-affinity of the (Ca^{2+} + Mg^{2+}) ATP-ase (Roufogalis, 1979).

The biochemical consequences of increased membrane Ca^{2+} relating to RBC flexibility and/or shape changes in model systems include direct effects on membrane lipids (phosphatidylserine, phosphatidylinositol) and proteins (polymerized spectrin-actin) and metabolic effects such as formation of diacylglycerol and accumulation of phosphatidate, inhibition of spectrin phosphorylation and abnormal protein interactions by a Ca^{2+}-activated transaminase (Szasz et al., 1978; Kirkpatrick et al., 1975). The exact biochemical background responsible for reduced RBC deformability in peripheral occlusive disease remains to be elucidated. Nevertheless a number of possible contributing factors have been characterized. RBC's from claudication patients with increased whole blood viscosity show an increased lipid peroxidation potential (Dormandy et al., 1973). In diabetes patients RBC 2,3-diphosphoglycerate, bearing on ATP-resynthesis, would be reduced (Alberti et al., 1972) in relation to reduced deformability (Le Devehat et al., 1979).

Environmental changes such as hypercapnia (Kikuchi, 1979; Foulhaux et al., 1977), lactacidosis (Murphy, 1967; Schmid-Schönbein et al., 1972) and hyperosmolarity (Rand et al., 1964), simulating an ischemic condition (Weed et al., 1969) reduce deformability. In ischemic blood stored for various time periods, the (passive) uptake of ^{45}Ca was found to be higher and faster than in normal blood (Scott and Chasin, 1978). Even physiological shear stresses enhance the passive membrane permeability of human RBC and enhance the Ca^{2+}-stimulated ATP-ase activity (Larsen et al., 1981). Increased uptake of Ca^{2+} by RBC thus may be a cause for their deteriorated rheological behaviour.

In order to verify this Ca^{2+}-hypothesis in relation to the mechanism of action of Ca^{2+}-entry blockers on the RBC, their effects on RBC changes induced by the ionophore A 23187 were examined. The divalent cation ionophore A 23187 selectively and rapidly transports divalent cations, including Ca^{2+}, across the membrane resulting in decreased filtrability and shape changes (or crenation) of the RBC (Kirkpatrick et al., 1975; Kuettner et al., 1977; White, 1974) thus providing a useful tool for pharmacological experiments on stimulated Ca^{2+}-fluxes (De Clerck et al., 1981). In these experiments (De Clerck et al., 1981) flunarizine produced a concentration-dependent inhibition of the shape changes of RBC induced by their exposure to A 23 187 in the presence of Ca^{2+}. At a constant concentration of ionophore this inhibition increased as the Ca^{2+}-concentration in the medium was lowered. A comparison of flunarizine with a number of other Ca^{2+}-entry blockers in this test (Table 1) revealed the former compound to be the most potent drug, D 600, verapamil and nifedipine being weakly or not active. These experiments corroborate the hypothesis that some compounds, in particular flunarizine may improve RBC deformability by blocking excessive Ca^{2+}-influx and/or its biochemical consequences at the level of the RBC membrane.

Table 1 : Effect of Ca^{2+}-entry blockers on the human RBC shape change induced by A 23 187 in the presence of Ca^{2+}.

Compound	Inhibition of RBC shape change[1]
flunarizine	81.7 ± 4.6[2]
cinnarizine	30.4 ± 13.1[2]
lidoflazine	29.2 ± 3.0[2]
D 600	17.1 ± 7.3[2]
verapamil	5 ± 1.5[2]
nifedipine	6.6 ± 10.4
niludipine	0 ± 0
prenylamine	0 ± 0

[1]Percentage inhibition of crenation versus solvent. Mean ± S.E.M. of 3-7 experiments washed human RBC incubated for 20 min at 37° C with A 23 187 5 x 10^{-7} M and Ca^{2+} 5 x 10^{-5} M. Compounds tested at 1 x 10^{-5} M.
[2]P ≤ 0.05 versus solvent. Student t-test. Enlarged from ref. De Clerck et al., 1981.

2. Endothelial cells

The integrity of the vascular endothelium is essential for blood-tissue homeostasis (Zweifach, 1980): acute disturbances of functional and/or structural integrity of the endothelium, e.g. produce activation of platelets and increase vascular permeability;

steady state endothelial injury may contribute to atherogenesis (see Hladovec and De Clerck, 1981; Harker et al., 1978).

The stability of the endothelial lining is probably mainly regulated by the concentration of available Ca^{2+}-ions at the endothelial membrane level. Calcium has been shown to have a major role in maintaining membrane permeability to ions as well as cell reactivity to many agonists (Zweifach, 1980). Recently it was shown that the contraction of endothelial cells stimulated with thrombin in vitro strictly requires the presence of ionized Ca^{2+} (De CLerck et al., 1981). The increase of vascular permeability associated with Ca^{2+}-chelation on the other hand suggests a weakening of the cell-to cell functional complexes (Clementi and Pallade, 1969) or changes in the glycocalix of the endothelial cells (Bridwell, 1978).

In vivo the injection of, e.g. citrate in rats results in damage of the endothelial cells and detachment or desquamation. The endothelial damage can be quantified by counting the detached endothelial cells in peripheral blood (Hladovec and De Clerck, 1981). Oral pretreatment of the animals with Ca^{2+}-entry blockers results in significant protection of the endothelial lining against the desquamating effect of citrate as summarized in Table 2 (Hladovec and De Clerck, 1981; Hladovec, 1979).

Table 2: Optimal oral doses for protection against the endothelial desquamation induced by citrate I.V. in rats.

Compound	Optimal dose (mg/kg orally)
flunarizine	0.1
cinnarizine	1
lidoflazine	3
nifedipine	0.09
prenylamine	0.25
carbochromen	0.5
verapamil	1

From ref. Hladovec and De Clerck, 1981; Hladovec, 1979.

Figure 1: Schematic representation of the possible mechanism of action of agonists (I) and antagonists (II) on Ca^{2+}-dependent endothelial stability. From ref. Hladovec and De Clerck, 1981.

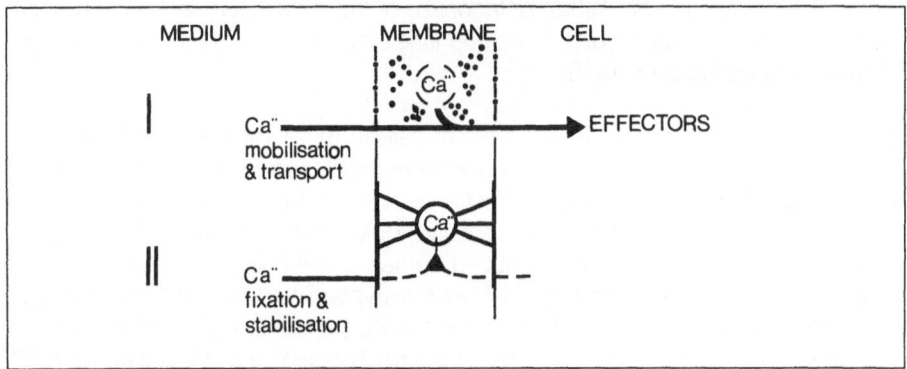

The possible mechanism of action of these compounds probably consists of an interference with a Ca^{2+}-exchange at the level of the endothelial cells (Fig. 1). Normally Ca^{2+}-ions are bound to membrane components "stabilizing" them when present in suitable concentrations. Agonists may interfere with the binding of Ca^{2+} either to glycoproteins of the endothelial cement or to other membrane structures producing destabilization, increased membrane permeability and passage of membrane-bound and external Ca^{2+} to deeper target structures. Protective Ca^{2+}-entry blockers may either "fix" calcium to the intercellular glycoproteins or to the cellular glycocalix thus stabilizing the membrane, thereby preventing membrane permeability for ions to occur and consequently decreasing the external Ca^{2+}-influx causing a noxious reaction. One such reaction could implicate an endothelial cell contraction through Ca^{2+}-activation of its actin-myosin system, a mechanism which, at least *in vitro* is partly reduced both with flunarizine and verapamil (De Clerck et al., 1981).

3. Platelets

Platelets respond to various stimuli, except epinephrine, with a uniform sequence of events including the shape change, reversible aggregation and the release reaction (De Clerck and David, 1981).

Convincing evidence suggests that a rise of free Ca^{2+}-ions in the cytoplasm mediates the platelet functional changes. However, Ca^{2+} from an internally releasable pool, rather than external Ca^{2+} entering through the plasma membrane would serve to initiate the activation by most agonists. The divalent cation ionophore A 23 187 induces shape change and secretion in the presence, but also in the absence of extracellular Ca^{2+} (Feinstein and Fraser, 1975). Primary aggregation induced by ADP, although requiring the presence of extracellular ionized Ca^{2+}, is not associated with a transmembrane uptake of the cation, but with a redistribution from intracellular pools, probably the dense tubular system (see De Clerck and David, 1981; Massini and Luscher, 1976). During the release reaction induced by thrombin, ADP, and collagen the permeability of the human platelet membrane for Ca^{2+} increases, but this change was proven to be the consequence rather than the cause of granule secretion (Massini and Luscher, 1976; Robbles et al., 1973). One exception is human platelet aggregation induced by epinephrine: human platelets isolated from the plasma take up Ca^{2+} during epinephrine-induced primary aggregation but not during ADP reactions (Owen and Le Breton, 1980; Owen et al., 1980). Antagonism of the platelet a-receptors with phentolamine results in inhibition of both epinephrine-induced Ca^{2+}-uptake and aggregation (Massini and Luscher, 1976).

Inhibition by several Ca^{2+}-entry blockers of platelet functional changes induced by epinephrine, and by other agonists as well, have been reported to occur both *in vitro* and *in vivo*. A number of these effects are difficult to explain on the basis of Ca^{2+}-channel blockade only. At comparatively high concentrations (20-500 $\mu g/ml$) verapamil inhibits the epinephrine-induced human platelet aggregation, formation of thromboxane B_2 and release of $[^{14}C]$-5-hydroxytryptamine, but is ineffective against ADP- or thrombin-induced platelet activation, a similar pattern being found for nifedipine (Addonizio et al., 1980); the inhibition by verapamil of epinephrine-induced and of ADP-amplified reactions to epinephrine can be overcome by the addition of ionized Ca^{2+} (Owen and Le Breton, 1980; Owen et al., 1980). On the contrary, in cat platelet-rich plasma verapamil and nisoldipine (50 μg/ml) but not nifedipine and nimodipine inhibit ADP-induced aggregation, verapamil only reducing arachidonic acid-induced aggregation as well; again the inhibition could be overridden by the addition of Ca^{2+} (Addonizio et al., 1980). Also in rat, dog and rabbit platelet-rich plasma verapamil (300-600 μg/ml) inhibits ADP-induced platelet aggregation (Kreiskott and Hofman, 1973; Ribeiro et al., 1982).

In another study on human platelet-rich plasma nifedipine (8-25 μg/ml) in vitro inhibits both the primary and secondary aggregation induced by ADP, arachidonic acid, collagen and epinephrine; oral administration of the compound would reduce ADP-, arachidonic acid- and collagen-induced aggregation, but paradoxically does not affect epinephrine-induced reactions (Johnsson, 1981).

Lidoflazine (50-250 μg/ml) in vitro also inhibits primary and secondary human platelet aggregation in plasma induced by ADP and collagen and reduces (5-25 μg/ml) the aggregation and secretion of [^{14}C]-5-hydroxytryptamine induced by collagen and thrombin in washed human platelet suspensions (De Clerck, 1972); on the contrary flunarizine both in vitro and after oral administration to man does not affect aggregation induced by ADP, Thrombofax*, collagen, epinephrine nor epinephrine reactions amplified by other agents in platelet-rich plasma (unpublished observation).

Apart from Ca^{2+}-entry blockers, several compounds that interfere with the intracellular movements of Ca^{2+} in muscle cells, including 8-(N,N-diethylamino-octyl 3,4,5-trimethoxybenzoate, HCl (TMB-8), TMB-6, 2-propyl-3-dimethylamino-5,6-methylenedioxyindene, HCl (2-PIA), chlortetracycline and deuterium oxide affect several aspects of Ca^{2+}-dependent mechanisms in platelets (see De Clerck and David, 1981; Mürer et al., 1981). The relevance of the observed effects of both types of Ca^{2+}-blockers for strictly Ca^{2+}-dependent mechanisms in platelets remains limited. Indeed these pharmacological experiments measure only a summation of all the actions of these compounds on all platelet events involved, whether calcium-dependent or calcium-independent; furthermore calcium-dependent processes may be influenced secondary only to primary calcium-independent processes induced by agonists or the compounds themselves (Mürer et al., 1981).

Critical experiments by Mürer et al. (Mürer et al., 1981) indeed show that TMB-8, 2-PIA and chlortetracycline either produce platelet metabolic depression or membrane effects expressed by leakage of [^{14}C]-adenine nucleotides and/or [^{14}C]-5-hydroxytryptamine as well as morphological changes of the platelets. A similar sphering of platelets and loss of ^{14}C-5-hydroxytryptamine occurs with active concentrations of lidoflazine (De Clerck, 1972); at lower concentrations both lidoflazine and verapamil inhibit the active uptake of 5-hydroxytryptamine which is largely unrelated to Ca^{2+}-fluxes (Addonizio et al., 1980; De Clerck and Reneman, 1973). In addition, some Ca^{2+}-entry blockers, in particular verapamil, inhibit the formation of thromboxane B_2 from platelets, stimulated with epinephrine or arachidonic acid (Addonizio et al., 1980; Okamutsu et al., 1981). The exact mechanism of action of Ca^{2+}-entry blockers on blood platelet function therefore remains unknown.

Acknowledgements

This study was partly supported by a grant from the I.W.O.N.L.

References

Addonizio, V.P , Fischer, C.A and Edmunds, L.H. Effects of verapamil and nifedipine on platelet activation. *Circulation*, **62**, Suppl. III, III-326, Abstract 1258 (1980)

Alberti, K., Emerson, P.M , Darly, J.M. and Hockaday, T. Red cell 2-3 diphosphoglycerate and diabetes. *Lancet*, I, 843-845 (1972)

Bridwell, C R. Identification and role of fibronectin in cultured bovine endothelial cells. *Proc. Natl. Acad. Sci. USA*, **75**, 3273 (1978).

Clementi, F. and Pallade, G. Intestinal capillaries. II Structural effects of EDTA and histamine. *J. Cell Biol.*, **42**, 706 (1969).

De Clerck, F Effect of lidoflazine (R 7904) in human platelet function *in vitro*. *Thromb. Diathes. Haemorrh.*, **28**, 228-236 (1972).

De Clerck, F. and Reneman, R.S. Effect of lidoflazine (R 7904) on uptake and release of serotonin by human platelets *in vitro*. *Naunyn-Schmiedeberg's Arch. Pharmacol.*, **278**, 261-269 (1973).

De Clerck, F., Beerens, M , Thoné, F. and Borgers, M The effect of flunarizine and other vasoactive compounds on the human RBC crenation and on the calcium-deposition induced by ionophore A 23 187. *Thromb Res.*, **24**, 1-12 (1981).

De Clerck, F., De Brabander, M , Neels, H. and Van de Velde, V. Direct evidence for the contractile capacity of endothelial cells *Thrombos. Res.*, **23**, 505-520 (1981).

De Clerck, F. and David, J L. Pharmacological control of platelet and red blood cell function in the microcirculation. *J Cardiovasc Pharmacol* , **3**, 1388-1412 (1981).

De Cree, J , De Cock, W , Geukens, H , De Clerck, F., Beerens, M. and Verhaegen, H. The rheological effects of cinnarizine and flunarizine in normal and pathological conditions *Angiology*, **31**, 505-515 (1979).

Di Perri, T., Forconi, S and Maurizio, G. Action of cinnarizine on the hyperviscosity of blood in patients with peripheral obliterative arterial disease. *Angiology*, **30**, 13-20 (1979).

Dormandy, J.A , Hoare, E., Colley, J , Arrowsmith, D.E and Dormandy, T L Clinical, haemodynamic, rheological and biochemical findings in 126 patients with intermittent claudication. *Brit. Med. J* , **4**, 576-581 (1973).

Feinstein, M.B and Fraser, C Human platelet secretion and aggregation induced by calcium ionophores *J. Gen Physiol.*, **66**, 561-581 (1975)

Foulhaux, P., Voisin, D. and Normier, G Influence de la tension CO_2 et de O_2 sur le comportement des érythrocytes dans les filtres de porosité 5 μ *Comp. Rend. Soc. Biol.*, **171**, 27-33 (1977).

Harker, L.A., Ross, R. and Glomset, J A. The role of endothelial cell injury and platelet response in atherogenesis *Thrombos Haemostas. (Stuttg.)*, **39**, 312-321 (1978).

Heilman, L Hamorheologische Veränderungen bei Risikoschwangerschaften unter der Therapie mit Flunarizin *Vasa*, **9**, 388-394 (1980)

Hladovec, J The influence of calcium antagonists on endothelium. *Arzneim.-Forsch. (Drug Res.)*, **29**, 1101-1103 (1979)

Hladovec, J. and De Clerck, F. Protection by flunarizine against endothelial cell injury *in vivo* *Angiology*, **32**, 448-462 (1981).

Johnsson, H. Effects of nifedipine (ADALAT) on platelet function *in vitro* and *in vivo*. *Thromb. Res.*, **21**, 523-528 (1981).

Kikuchi, Y., Horimoto, M. and Koyuma, T. Reduced deformability of erythrocytes exposed to hypercapnia. *Experientia*, **35**, 343-344 (1979)

Kirkpatrick, F.H., Hillman, D G. and La Celle, P.L. A 23 187 and red cells: changes in deformability, K^+, Mg^{2+}, Ca^{2+} and ATP. *Experientia*, **31**, 653-654 (1975).

Kreiskott, H and Hofman, H P. Tierexperimentelle Untersuchungen zur Hemmung der Thrombocytenaggregation durch Verapamil *in vitro* und *in vivo* *Arzneim.-Forsch. (Drug Res.)*, **23**, 1555-1560 (1973).

Kuettner, J , Dreher, K.L., Rao, G.H.R., Eaton, J.W., Blackshear, P.L. and White, J.G. Influence of the ionophore A 23 187 on the plastic behaviour of normal erythrocytes. *Am. J. Pathol.*, **88**, 81 (1977).

Larsen, F.L., Katz, S., Raefogalis, B S and Brooks, D.E. Physiological shear stresses enhance the Ca^{2+} permeability of human erythrocytes. *Nature*, **294**, 667-668 (1981)

Le Devehat, C., Lemoine, A., Cirette, B. and Ramet, M. Filtration érythrocytaire et 2-3 DPG. Etude de corrélation chez le sujet diabétique avec complications vasculaires périphériques (artériopathie chronique des membres inférieures). IVème séminaire 1979, p. 99. Imprimeries Mont-Louis et Presse Réunies, Clermont-Ferrand (1979).

Lowe, G.D.O., Drummond, M.M., Forbes, C.D and Barbenel, J.L. Occlusive arterial disease and blood rheology. In: Clinical Aspects of Blood Viscosity and Cell Deformability, Lowe, G.D.O., Barsenel, J.L. and Forbes, C.D (Eds.), Springer-Verlag, Berlin, pp. 133-148 (1981).

Massini, P and Luscher, E F On the significance of influx of Ca^{2+}-ions into stimulated human blood platelets. *Biochem. Biophys. Acta*, **436**, 652-663 (1976).

Murphy, J.R The influence of pH and temperature on some physical properties of normal erythrocytes and erythrocytes from patients with hereditary spherocytosis. *J. Lab. Clin. Med.*, **69**, 758-775 (1967).

Mürer, E H , Stewart, G J., Davenport, K., Sigo, E., Rahwan, R.G. and Witiak, D.T Effect of three calcium antagonists on platelet secretion and metabolism. *Biochem. Pharmacol.*, **30**, 523-530 (1981).

Okamutsu, S , Peck, R.C. and Lefer, A.M Effects of calcium channel blockers on arachidonate-induced sudden death in rabbits *Proc Soc. Exp. Biol. Med.*, **166**, 551-555 (1981)

Owen, N E., Funberg, H. and Le Breton, G C Epinephrine induces Ca^{2+} uptake in human platelets. *Am. J. Physiol.*, **239**, H483-H488 (1980).

Owen, N E and Le Breton, G C. The involvement of calcium in epinephrine or ADP potentiation of human platelet aggregation *Thromb Res* , **17**, 855-863 (1980)

Rand, P.W and Lacombe, E Hemodilution, tonicity and blood viscosity. *J. Clin. Invest.*, **43**, 2214-2226 (1964).

Ribeiro, L.G T , Branden, T.A , Horak, J K., Ware, J.A., Miller, R.R. and Solis, R.T Inhibition of platelet aggregation by verapamil· quantification by *in vivo* and *in vitro* techniques *J. Cardiovasc. Pharmacol.*, **4**, 170-173 (1982).

Robblee, L.A., Shepro, D , Belaramich, F.A and Towle, C. Platelet Ca^{2+} flux and the release reaction *Ser Haematol* , **6**, 311-316 (1973)

Roufogalis, B.P Regulation of calcium translocation across the red cell membrane. *Can. J. Physiol. Pharmac.*, **57**, 1331-1349 (1979)

Schatzmann, H.J. and Vincenzi, F.F Calcium movements across the membrane of human red cells. *J. Physiol.*, **201**, 369-395 (1969)

Schmid-Schönbein, H , Volger, E , Klose, H.J. and Weiss, J. Blood microrheology and the development of stasis in the microvasculation after injury. *Adv Exp Med Biol.*, **33**, 65-73 (1972).

Scott, C.K and Chasin, M. Effects of flunarizine on red blood cells *The Pharmacologist*, **20**, 204 (1978).

Slonim, A., Cristal, W., Erez, R. and Shainkin-Kestenbaum, R. The effect of nifedipine, a calcium antagonist on red blood cell filtrability (RCF). Abstract: 2nd Eur. Conf. Clin. Haemorheology, 30 Sept.-2 Oct., London (1981).

Szasz, I., Hasitz, M., Breuer, J.H., Sarkadi, B. and Gardos, G. Biconcave shape and its transformation in human red cells. *Acta Biol. Acad. Sci. Hung.*, **29**, 1-17 (1978).

Weed, R.J., La Celle, P. and Merrill, E.W. Metabolic dependence of red blood cell deformability. *J. Clin. Invest.*, **48**, 795-809 (1969).

Wells, R.E. Rheology of blood in the microvasculature. *N. Eng. J. Med.*, **270**, 832-839 (1964).

White, J.G. Effects of an ionophore, A 23 187, on the surface morphology of normal erythrocytes. *Am. J. Pathol.*, **77**, 507 (1974).

Zweifach, B.W. Integrity of vascular endothelium. In: Vascular Endothelium and Basement Membranes, Altura, B.M. (Ed.), S. Karger, Basel, Adv. Microcirc., **9**, 206 (1980).

90

Red blood cell microrheology and calcium antagonists

J.F. Stoltz

Summary

In peripheral vascular diseases, it might be assumed that the calcium antagonists operate on two levels:
- by opposing vasospasm
- by reducing intracellular calcium concentration in the red blood cell
Regarding the first aspect, a certain number of substances such as cinnarizine, flunarizine, verapamil, lidoflazine, perhexiline and bepridil inhibit calcium penetration in the vascular smooth muscle cells and oppose their contraction caused by anoxia. In pathological conditions where vasospactic episodes contribute to the tissue ischemia, inhibitors of Ca^{2+} influx must have a beneficial effect.
As concerns the action on blood rheology and more particularly on red blood cell micro-rheology, numerous studies emphasize the important part played by calcium penetration on red cell deformability. Although the action mechanisms have not yet been fully determined, the change in flow conditions, a local increase in shear rates, and hypoxia are all factors that are likely to encourage calcium accumulation in the red blood cells resulting in a reduction in deformability. This aggravates the rheological problems by feed-back. The decreased deformability, combined with the reduced blood flow favors the occurrence of "rouleaux formation", which further increases blood viscosity and peripheral resistance.
It is therefore reasonable to suppose that calcium entry blockers will have a favourable and regulating effect. The action of these drugs would be better understood and appreciated if more complete microrheological studies were carried out with the main calcium entry blockers used in cardiology. It would also be preferable if a precise rheological study procedure was designed in order to facilitate comparison.
There is no doubt, that the bioclinical approach to the microrheological action of calcium antagonists should supply a more accurate definition of the potential value of this type of therapy for correcting the reductions in erythrocyte deformability generally observed during ischemic diseases.

Résumé

On peut supposer, dans les maladies vasculaires périphériques, que les antagonistes de calcium opèrent à deux niveaux:
- en arrêtant le vasospasme
- en réduisant la concentration calcique intracellulaire dans le globule rouge
En ce qui concerne le premier point, un certain nombre de substances telles que la cinnarizine, la flunarizine, le vérapamil, la lidoflazine, la perhexiline et le bépridil inhibent la pénétration du calcium dans les cellules du muscle lisse vasculaire et empêchent leur contraction due à l'anoxie. Dans les états pathologiques lors desquels les épisodes angiospastiques contribuent à susciter une ischémie tissulaire, les inhibiteurs de l'influx de Ca^{2+} doivent avoir un effet bénéfique.
En ce qui concerne l'action exercée sur la rhéologie sanguine et plus particulièrement sur la microrhéologie du globule rouge, de nombreuses études soulignent le rôle important que joue la pénétration du calcium dans la déformabilité du globule rouge. Bien que les mécanismes d'action n'aient pas été déterminés complètement, la modification du flux, une augmentation locale des taux de cisaillement ainsi que l'hypoxie constituent tous des facteurs susceptibles d'encourager l'accumulation de calcium dans les globules rouges, réduisant ainsi la déformabilité de ceux-ci. Ceci aggrave les problèmes rhéologiques par feed-back. La diminution de la déformabilité combinée à la réduction du flux sanguin favorise l'apparition de formations en rouleaux, lesquelles augmentent à leur tour la viscosité sanguine et la résistance périphérique.
Il apparaît dès lors raisonnable de présumer que les bloqueurs d'entrée de calcium auront un effet favorable et régulateur. Des études microrhéologiques plus complètes sur les principaux bloqueurs d'entrée de calcium en cardiologie devraient permettre d'acquérir une meilleure compréhension et appréciation de l'action de ces substances. De même la mise au point d'une procédure d'étude rhéologique précise permettrait de faciliter la comparaison.
Il ne fait aucun doute que l'analyse bioclinique de l'action microrhéologique des antagonistes de calcium fournirait une définition plus précise de la valeur potentielle de ce type de traitement quant à la correction des réductions de déformabilité de l'érythrocyte, observées généralement lors de maladies ischémiques.

Resumen

En enfermedades vasculares periféricas, se prodría suponer que los inhibidores de la penetración intracelular de calcio funcionan en dos niveles:
- oponiendo los vasoespasmos
- reduciendo la concentración cálcica intracelular en el glóbulo rojo.
En cuanto al primer aspecto, cierto número de sustancias, tales como cinarizina, flunarizina, verapamil, lidoflazina, perhexilina y bepridil, inhiben la penetración cálcica en las células musculares lisas vasculares y se oponen a su contracción causada por anoxia. En condiciones patológicas, en las cuales episodios vasoespásticos contribuyen a la isquemia de tejido, inhibidores de Ca^{2+} deben de tener un efecto beneficial.
Refiriéndose a la acción en la reología sanguínea, y más específicamente en la micro-reología del glóbulo rojo, numerosos estudios hacen hincapié en el importante papel de la penetración cálcica en la deformabilidad del glóbulo rojo. Aunque los mecanismos de acción todavía no han sido determinados, el cambio en las condiciones del flujo, el incremento local en la tasa de cizallamiento e hipoxia, son todos factores que pueden aumentar la acumulación de calcio en los glóbulos rojos, resultando en una reducción de su deformabilidad. Esto agrava los problemas reológicos por retroalimentación. La deformabilidad disminuida, combinada con el flujo sanguíneo reducido, favorece la formación de rollos, y ello, aumenta todavía más la viscosidad sanguínea y la resistencia periférica.
Por eso, es razonable suponer que los inhibidores de la penetración intracelular de calcio tengan un efecto favorable y regulador. La acción de estas drogas se entendería y se apreciaría mejor si se efectuaran más completos estudios microrreológicos con los principales inhibidores de la penetración intracelular de calcio, empleados en la cardiología. También sería preferible si se proyectara un preciso procedimiento de estudio reológico para facilitar una comparación.
No cabe duda de que el enfoque bioclínico de la acción microrreológica de los antagonistas de calcio proporcionará una definición más precisa del valor potencial de este tipo de terapia para corregir las reducciones en la deformabilidad del eritrocito, generalmente observada durante enfermedades isquémicas.

Zusammenfassung

Bei peripheren Gefässkrankheiten ist anzunehmen, dass die Kalziumantagonisten auf zwei Ebenen wirksam sind:
- indem sie Vasospasmen aufheben;
- indem sie die intrazelluläre Kalziumkonzentration in den Erythrozyten herabsetzen.

In Anbetracht des ersten Faktors ist festzustellen, dass eine Anzahl von Substanzen, wie Cinnarizin, Flunarizin, Verapamil, Lidoflazin, Perhexilin und Bepridil, den Kalziumeintritt in die Gefässzellen der glatten Muskeln hemmen, und die durch Anoxie verursachte Kontraktion dieser Zellen aufheben. Unter pathologischen Umständen, wo vasospastische Perioden zur Gewebe-Ischämie beitragen, haben Inhibitorenen des Ca^{2+}-Einstroms sicherlich eine günstige Wirkung.

In zahlreichen Studien wird, in Anbetracht der Wirkung auf die Blutrheologie, oder, genauer, auf die Mikrorheologie der Erythrozyten, die wichtige Rolle der Kalziumpenetration auf die Verformbarkeit der Erythrozyten betont. Obwohl die Wirkungsmechanismen noch nicht völlig aufgeklärt sind, weiss man, dass geänderte Strömungsverhältnisse eine lokale Erhöhung der Schubgeschwindigkeit, und Hypoxie wahrscheinlich eine Kalziumanhäufung in den Erythrozyten fördern, was zu einer niedrigeren Verformbarkeit führt. Durch Feedback werden die rheologischen Probleme noch erschwert. Die herabgesetzte Verformbarkeit, zusammen mit dem erniedrigten Blutstrom, fördert das Entstehen von Geldrollenaggregaten, wodurch die Blutviskosität und der periphere Widerstand weiter steigen.

Man kann daraus logisch ableiten, dass Kalziumantagonisten eine günstige und regulierende Wirkung haben sollten. Die Wirkung dieser Arzneimittel wäre besser zu verstehen und einzuschätzen, wenn umfangreichere mikrorheologische Untersuchungen mit den wichtigsten in der Kardiologie verwendeten Kalziumantagonisten durchgeführt würden. Um einen Vergleich einfacher zu machen, ist auch die Erarbeitung eines präzisen rheologischen Untersuchungsverfahrens wünschenswert.

Ohne Zweifel wird die bioklinische Betrachtung zur mikrorheologischen Wirkung von Kalziumantagonisten eine genauere Definition der potentiellen Bedeutung dieser Behandlungsart herbeiführen, d.h. ihrer korrigierenden Rolle für die bei ischämischen Erkrankungen allgemein auftretende Verminderung der Erythrozytenverformbarkeit.

In addition to the control mechanisms of the cardiovascular system, the behavior of blood cells plays its part in maintaining correct tissue perfusion. Among the factors likely to influence the metabolism and regulation mechanisms, calcium plays a decisive role. However, at present, the relationships between calcium and the rheological properties of blood or blood cells are relatively unknown. Since the main determining factors regarding blood viscosity are now well defined (hematocrit, plasma viscosity, rouleaux formation, erythrocyte deformability), there is no doubt that calcium/blood rheology interferences will mainly be found on the microrheological level.

It is for this reason that we shall view, in turn, a reminder of the main determinants of red cell rheology, the influence of calcium on these properties and, finally, the pharmacological consequences by means of a study on some molecules known for their calcium antagonist effect and likely to operate on the microrheological level.

1. Main determinants of the red blood cell rheological properties

The degree of erythrocyte deformation is a function of the external forces acting on the cell as well as the intrinsic deformability. The deforming stress varies with the external fluid viscosity and the shear rates at the cell surface. The intrinsic deformability is determined by three main parameters: internal fluid viscosity, viscoelastic and molecular rheological properties of the membrane and the geometric relationships between membrane surface area and cell volume (shape) (Stoltz, 1981).

1.1. Internal viscosity

The mean corpuscular hemoglobin concentration (MCHC) is normally 33 g/100 ml ($\simeq$ 5 mMol/l). The viscosity of such a highly concentrated macromolecular solution is approximately 7 mPa.s. However, the internal viscosity of the erythrocyte, when measured by spectroscopic methods (particularly EPR) is found to be only 4 to 5 mPa.s. This viscosity is affected by the physicochemical state of hemoglobin. Setting aside the pathological modifications, we should point out that pH and partial oxygen pressure are important parameters. According to La Celle greater rigidity is observed when PO_2 is less than 12 mm Hg. It is also the case for a decrease in pH. This last factor is expected to enhance splenic strapping of old erythrocytes.

1.2. Modification of the geometric relationships between membrane surface area and cell volume

A large number of theoretical and experimental investigations have been carried out on the origin of the very characteristic shape of the red blood cell. It appears likely that the shape is the net result of the equilibrium between surface tension, ratio of cell radius to membrane thickness, extensional stiffness of the membrane, structure of the cytoskeleton, and differential pressure across the membrane.

Normal red cells have a mean membrane surface area of approximately 140 μm^2 and a mean volume of approximately 90 μm^3 thus making possible deformations at constant area. The relationships between the cell volume (V) and the surface area (A) can be expressed in terms of a sphericity index S_i. Thus the value of S_i is 1 for spheres and is approximately equal to 0.7 in the case of normal erythrocytes. Any change in the area to volume ratio, and therefore in the sphericity index, will result in an alteration in cell deformability.

1.3. Rheological properties of the erythrocyte membrane

Elastic behavior of the membrane: the general elastic behavior observed in the case of the erythrocyte may be attributed to its membrane properties. But a survey of the published results reveals wide variations in assessment of this parameter. In fact, this scatter is only apparent and may be attributed to the membrane non-linear behaviour and to differences in the types of deformation involved. Three main types of elastic deformation can thus be discerned:
- deformation at constant area
- deformation with increase of area
- deformation which changes the curvature of the cell.

Viscosity of the red cell membrane: there is no doubt that a viscosity modulus can be associated with each of the three types of elastic deformation described above. Concerning the viscosity modulus related to a change in area, no assessment has been made, but its value is probably low. The viscosity associated with shear deformation is estimated to be 10^{-3} dyn/sec/cm. Finally, the viscosity associated with bending is still completely unknown.

The tank tread motion: one of the remarkable properties of the red blood cell is the existence of a continuous tank-tread rotation around the fluid cell content. This type of movement has been visualized experimentally *in vitro* by Fischer and Schmid-Schönbein.

2. Calcium and red blood cell

2.1. Calcium and R.B.C. physiology

The role of Ca^{2+} in the physiological properties of the erythrocyte has been emphasized many times. General reviews have been recently published which cover a considerable amount of work concerning this very complex problem (Sarkardi, 1980). We want only to summarize the essential facts.

The Ca^{2+} content in the human red blood cell is very low ($\simeq$ 0.1 μmol/l of cells), 90 % of this ion is membrane bound. The external side of the membrane has a low affinity for Ca^{2+} and three types of sites have been identified: proteins, sialic acid and phospholipids.

The use of liquid phase electrophoresis has, via the study of surface charge changes in the presence of calcium, supplied a means of assessing the number of membrane fixation sites for calcium, which was found to be in the vicinity of $7.6.10^6$ sites per erythrocyte. (Seaman, Vassar and Kendall 1969; Stoltz et al. 1971). On the internal side, at least two types of sites seem to exist.

The membrane passive permeability for Ca^{2+} is very low (1-10 μmol/L of cells per hour), and this ion is continuously extruded from the cell by the Calcium ATPase. The rate of Ca^{2+} extrusion by the enzyme is 85 μmol/L of cells per min. at 37° and pH 7.4. The normal substrate for the Ca^{2+} ATPase is Ca-ATP (Graf and Penningston 1981) but the enzyme must be phosphorylated by Mg ATP with a complex concentration dependence.

Ca^{2+} ATPase is regulated by a low molecular weight protein (16500 daltons) named calmodulin. It is well established now that calmodulin contains four calcium binding sites. Upon Ca^{2+} binding calmodulin undergoes a conformational change which is necessary for its biological activity. (Soclet, 1981). A Mg^{2+} dependent activator of Ca^{2+}-ATPase, distinct from calmodulin has been identified recently.

A considerable amount of work has been done concerning the perturbations induced by Ca^{2+} on the erythrocyte. The principal effects observed when Ca^{2+} enters the red blood cell, are the following: the cell loses its discoid form and becomes echinocytic or spheroechinocytic, K^+ is extruded (The Gardos effect) with a simultaneous penetration of Na^+, numerous enzymatic systems are either activated or inhibited, inducing perturbations in the conformation of membrane proteins and in the repartition of phospholipids.

The mechanism of the increase in passive permeability to K^+ is not well understood. It implies the existence of specific membrane sites with high affinity for Ca^{2+}. However, this effect on K^+ permeability seems to be of low physiological importance in normal RBC, since it is observed only when considerable internal Ca^{2+} concentration variations are experimentally induced. More recently a model of regulation has been given, which supposes the existence of different configurations of the Ca^{2+} ATPase, themselves induced by the binding of Ca^{2+}.

2.2. R.B.C. deformability and calcium

Although there is no denying the importance of calcium in red blood cell deformability phenomena, there is still considerable debate concerning the nature of the rheological modifications. Accordingly, two main types of rheological modifications have been put forward. The first concerns a change in the internal viscosity of the red blood cell, whilst the second relates to a change in membrane rheology.

Consequently, according to Clark et al. (1981) and Mohandas et al. (1981) the analysis of the influence that the osmolarity of the suspension medium has on deformability, reveals that there are two independent processes. The first process which is calcium independent produces a reduction in the surface-volume ratio as a result of the formation of sphero-erythrocytes, whilst the second process, which is calcium dependent, results in an increase in internal viscosity due to leakage of potassium and intra-cellular liquid. According to the above authors, the loss of deformability caused by an increase in internal viscosity is also observed in cells that are depleted in ATP where calcium is present and in red blood cells treated with the ionophore A 23 187 and calcium with no previous reduction in ATP. This theory has been confirmed by Smith et al. (1981) who observed no significant change in the membrane's elasticity modulus.

In parallel with this hypothesis, the possibility of rheological changes in the membrane has also been put forward (Anderson, Davis, Carraway, 1977). Two main types of arguments have been given. The first imply a modification of the spectrin network, the second give the principal role to a modification of the phospholipidic part of the membrane.

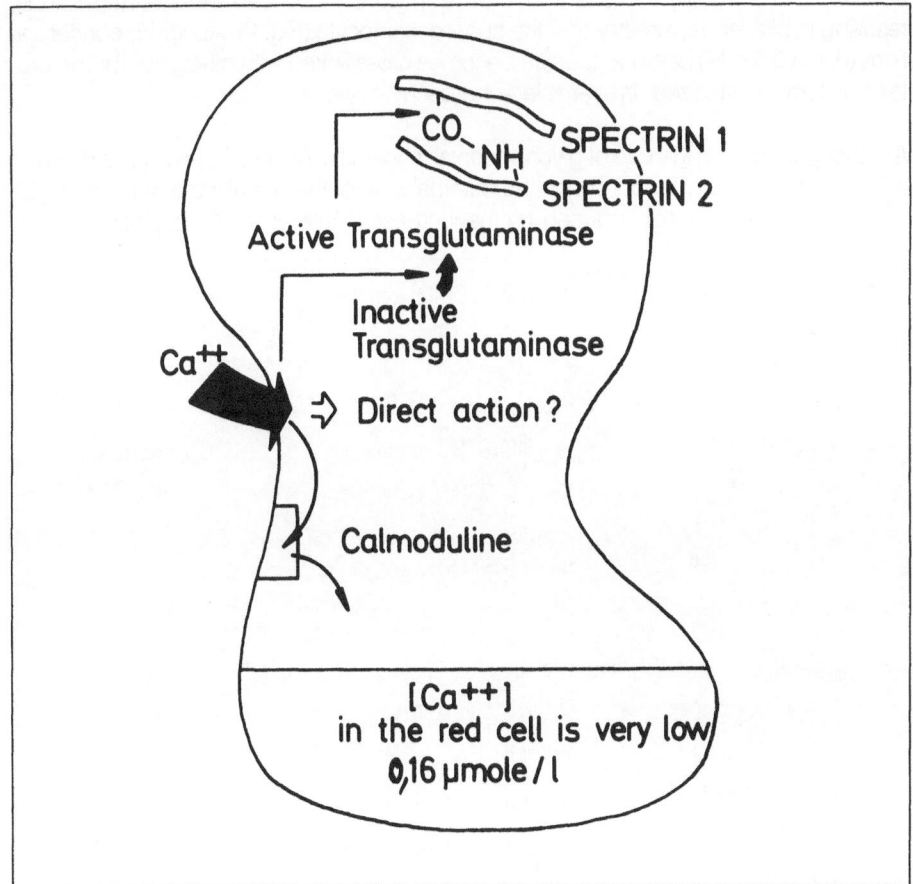

Figure 1: The role of Ca^{2+} on R.B.C. derformability

Palek et al. (1977) observed that the shape transformation induced by Ca²⁺ or Ca²⁺ + ATP was not observed on cell ghosts incubated with N.ethyl maleimide or cell ghosts washed many times in hypotonic buffer, thus spectrin depleted. Purified spectrin has a low affinity for Ca²⁺, although its flexibility and deformability are reduced by the presence of divalent ions in the millimolar range. At low concentration, Ca²⁺ introduced in the red cell induces a diminution of the spectrin extractability. The viscosity of the combined extract of spectrin and actin solution shows a strong Ca²⁺ concentration dependency: (a maximum is observed around 5.10⁻⁷M calcium); this observation indicates that the complex associations of the internal membrane proteins play a fundamental role in the regulation of the erythrocyte shape. Spectrin itself has been found to regulate the activity of Ca²⁺-ATPase and as previously indicated, Ca²⁺ acts on the mechanism of spectrin phosphorylation; but the role of this phenomenon in the regulation of the RBC shape is controversial (Fig. 1). For Kretchman and Rogers (1981) calcium induced shape transformation is a result of spectrin moving into closer contact thus producing a contraction of the inner half of the lipid bilayer. For low Ca²⁺ concentrations (1 to 2.10⁻⁶M) there is a decrease in space between the spectrin bands, resulting in bilayer asymmetry and the spheroechinocyte (Fig. 2). At higher concentrations (0.1 to 0.5 mM) calcium-spectrin becomes cross linked with other membrane proteins to form a stabilized, irreversible spheroechinocyte.

Another possibility is the role of glycophorin as shown by Anderson et al. (1977), when a lectin is bound to glycophorin on the external side of the membrane, the discocyte-echinocyte transformation induced by the increase in internal Ca²⁺ is blocked.

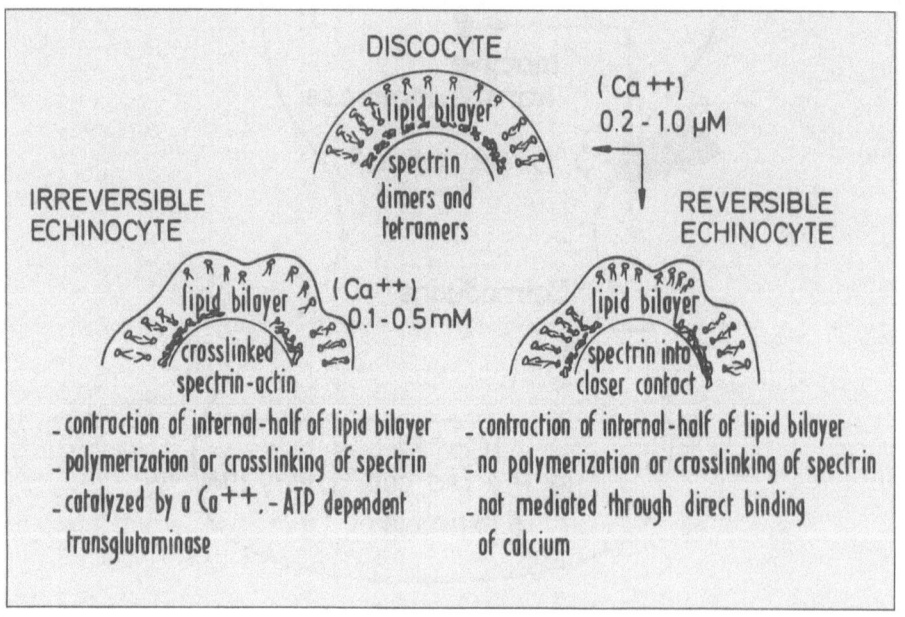

Figure 2: Calcium induced shape transformation is a result of spectrin moving into closer contact, producing a contraction of the inner half of the lipid bilayer (from Kretchman et al.)

Other enzymes are activated by Ca^{2+} in red blood cells. Allen and Cadman have observed the activation of endogeneous proteases, and the adsorption of Hb, catalase and band 8 is increased on the membrane of red blood cells loaded with calcium.

The activation of phospholipases has been reviewed previously in the study of the microvesicle formation. At low Ca^{2+} concentration a marked activation of the phosphatidyl-lysolecithine acylation is observed. Since lysoderivatives are strong modifiers of the membrane fluidity, this mechanism could explain in part the observed shape changes in the light of the bilayer couple theory of Sheetz and Singer. Ca^{2+} ion induces phase changes and fusion phenomena in the membrane.

It must also be noted that apart from possible changes in the rheological properties of the red blood cells, flow conditions also alter the calcium/membrane relationships of the erythrocytes. Accordingly, Larsen et $al.$ (1981) have revealed that membrane permeability to calcium increases with the shear rate applied and that the lower the ATP level in the erythrocytes, the bigger the increase (for example 20 vs. 3 μmol Ca^{2+} uptake per cell/per h for $\dot{\gamma} = 10^2 sec^{-1}$ and 100 vs. 5 μmol Ca^{2+} uptake per cell/per h for $\dot{\gamma} = 10^3 sec^{-1}$).

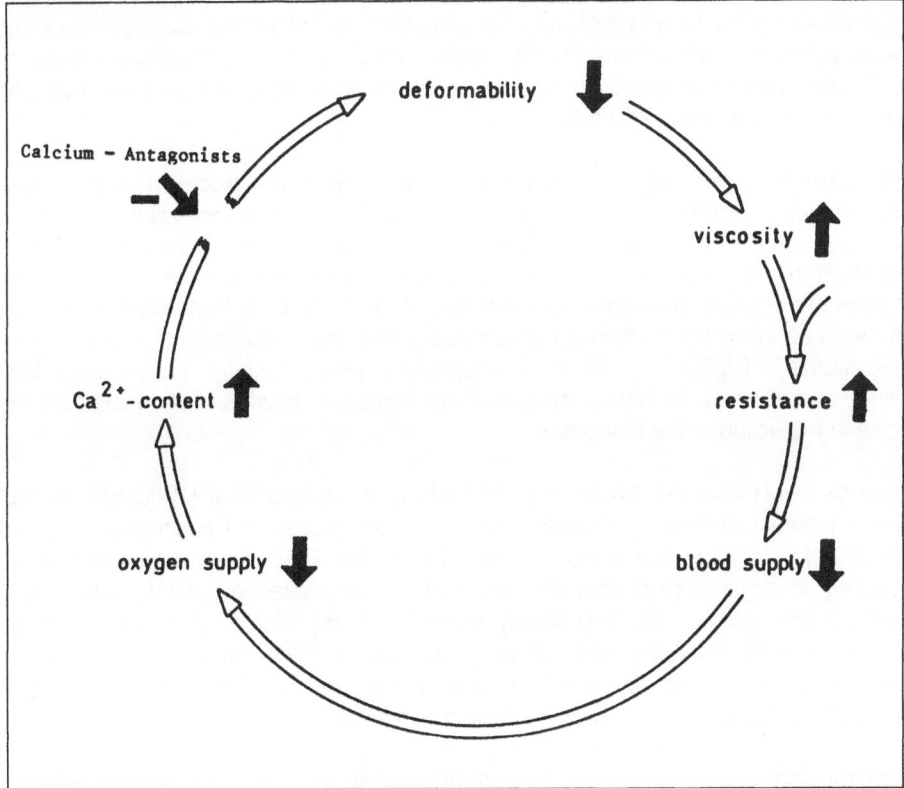

Figure 3: Calcium-antagonists: common mechanism of action on erythrocyte deformability and hemodynamics.

3. Hemorheology, tissue perfusion and calcium antagonists

Although calcium antagonists are used regularly in coronary pathology (Fleckenstein, 1977), few studies have been undertaken regarding erythrocyte microrheology and the available results are not easy to interpret. It would appear, however, that changes in calcium kinetics or content in the erythrocyte have been observed during various pathological conditions. Palek (1977), for example, observed an excessive accumulation of calcium during hemoglobinosis S and various hemolytic anemias (Bernard, Bournier, Boivin, 1975), and Scott et al. (1980) reported faster and greater erythrocyte calcium adsorption during ischemic diseases compared with the values for normal cells (increase of more than 150% for ischemic patients after 12 hours).

The effect of this disorder would therefore appear to increase ischemia by reduced erythrocyte deformability. Moreover, according to Van Nueten et al. (1978; 1980), the increase in intracellular calcium concentration may either be due to increased penetration of the ion caused by a pharmacological agent (vaso-active substance, for example), or, under certain pathological conditions with hypoxia, due to inhibition of the normal removal process. It can be appreciated therefore that calcium inhibitors that reduce the membrane penetration flow of this ion may be valuable pharmacological agents used with a view to achieving the return to normal of red blood cell deformability and avoiding the possibility of a vicious circle setting in and, via hyperviscosity, leading to hypoxia and subsequently to an increase in intra-erythrocyte calcium level, thus emphasizing the phenomenon (Fig. 3).

Regarding pharmacological research, most of the present-day studies have been carried out either using ATP depleted erythrocytes or by artificially increasing calcium inflow by means of the ionophore A 23 187, which is an antibiotic that encourages this reaction in the presence of calcium, and without ATP reduction. Accordingly, De Clerck et al. (1980), via a comparative study, were able to classify in vitro the action of 10 vaso-active compounds in decreasing order of activity (flunarizine > butenizine > cinnarizine > lidoflazine > D600 > verapamil > pentoxifylline = naftidrofuryl). This study also revealed that two of the compounds studied, dipyridamol and suloctidil, increase the action of the ionophore.

The results of this study have been confirmed, in part, by Scott et al. (1980) who revealed an increase in calcium adsorption inhibition in the presence of flunarizine (inhibition of 25% for 10^{-6}M of flunarizine and 60% for 10^{-4}M). They also revealed that blood viscosity in ischemia patients is reduced in vitro in the presence of 10^{-4}M of the pharmacological agent. As far as pentoxifylline is concerned, mention should be made of the work undertaken by Porsche and Stefanovich (1981) who suggest that the microrheological effect usually described for this agent might be partly related to the control of ATPase activity which is inhibited by calcium.

The rheological effect of another calcium antagonist, nifedipine, was also revealed in vivo by Slonim et al. (1981) in 12 patients with ischemic heart diseases. According to their results, the increase in erythrocyte filterability is directly related to the observed clinical effect.

In parallel with calcium antagonists it should be remembered that other pharmacological agents are likely to affect the calcium/red blood cell relationship. Thus, chlorpromazine and papaverine reduce the viscosity of ATP depleted red blood cell suspension (Rogausch, 1978). In this case both drugs are known to displace membrane-bound calcium.

Acknowledgement

This work was partly supported by DRET (Biological Department)

References

1. Anderson, D.R., Davis, J.L. and Carraway, K.L.: Calcium-promoted changes of the human erythrocyte membrane. *J. of Biological Chemistry*, **252**, 6617-6623, (1977).

2. Bernard, J.F., Bournier, O. and Boivin, P.: Human erythrocyte calcium concentration in hemolytic anemia. *Biomedicine*, **23**, 431-433, (1975).

3. Clark, M.R., Mohandas, N., Feo, C. and Jacobs, M.S.: Separate mechanisms of deformability loss in ATP-depleted and Ca-loaded erythrocytes. *J. Clin. Invest.*, **67**, 531-539, (1981).

4. De Clerck, F. and David, J.L.: Pharmacological control of platelet and red blood cell function in the microcirculation. *J. of Cardiovasc. Pharmacol.*, **3**, 1388-1412, (1980).

5. De Clerck, F., Beerens, M., Thone, F., Borgers, M. and Verheyen, A.: The effect of flunarizine on the human cell shape changes and calcium deposition induced by A 23 187. In: Hemorheology and diseases. Proceedings of the First European Conference on clinical hemorheology, Nancy, October 1979. J.F. Stoltz and P. Drouin publ. (Paris), 669-676, (1980).

6. Fleckenstein, A.: Specific pharmacology of calcium in myocardium, cardiac pacemakers, and vascular smooth muscle. *Ann. Rev. Pharmacol., Toxicol.*, **17**, 149-166, (1977).

7 Graf, E. and Penningston, J.J.: Ca-ATP: the substrate at low concentration of Ca^{2+} ATPase from human erythrocyte membranes. *J. Biol. Chem.*, **256**, 1587-1592, (1981).

8. Kirkpatrick, G.H., Hillman, D.G. and La Celle, P.L.: A 23 187 and red cells: changes in deformability, K^+, Mg^{++}, Ca^{2+}, and ATP. *Experientia*, **31**, 653-654, (1975).

9. Kretchman, E.M. and Rogers, B.S.: Erythrocyte shape transformation associated with calcium accumulation. *Am. J. Med. Technicol.*, **47**, 561-566, (1981).

10. Kuettner, J.F., Dreher, K.L., Rao, G.H.R., Eaton, J.W., Blackshear, P.L. and White, J.G.: Influence of the ionophore A 23 187 on the plastic behavior of normal erythrocytes. *Amer. J. Pathol.*, **88**, 81-94, (1977).

11. Larsen, F.L., Katz, S., Roufogalis, B.D. and Brooks, D.E.: Physiological shear stresses enhance the Ca^{2+} permeability of human erythrocytes. *Nature*, **294**, 667-668, (1981).

12. Mohandas, N., Clark, R., Feo, C., Jacobs, M.S. and Shotet, B.: Factors that limit whole cell deformability in erythrocytes after calcium loading and ATP depletion. *Prog. Clin. Res.*, **55**, 423-437.

13. Palek, J.: Red cell calcium content and transmembrane calcium movements in sickle cell anemia. *J. Lab. Clin. Med.*, **89**, 1365-1374, (1977).

14. Palek, J., Liu, A., Liu, D., Snyder, L.M., Fortier, N.L., Njoku, G., Kiernan, F., Funk, D., Crusberg, T.: Effect of procaine HCl on ATP/calcium dependent alterations in red cell shape and deformability. *Blood*, **50**, 155-164, (1977).

15. Porsche, E. and Stefanovich, V.: Die Wirkung von Pentoxifyllin auf den Ca^{2+} induzierten Kalium-Ausstrom und auf die ATP-ase-Aktivität von Erythrozyten. *Arzneim. Forsch.*, **31**, 825-828, (1981).

16. Rogausch, H.: Influence of Ca^{2+} on red cell deformability and adaptation to sphering agents. *Pflügers Arch.*, **373**, 43-47, (1978).

17. Sarkardi, B.: Active calcium transport in human red cells. *Biochim. Biophys. Acta*, **604**, 159-160, (1980).

18. Scott, C.K., Persico, F.J., Carpentier, K. and Chasin, M.: The effects of flunarizine, a new calcium antagonist, on human red blood cells in vitro. *Angiology*, **31**, 320-330, (1980).

19. Seaman, G.V.F., Vassar, P.S. and Kendall, M.J.: Calcium ion binding to blood cell surfaces. *Experientia*, **25**, 1259, (1969).

20. Slonim, A., Cristal, N., Erez, R., Shainkin-Kestenbaum, R.: The effect of nifedipine, a calcium antagonist on red blood cell filterability (RCF). Second European conference on clinical hemorheology, London (1981) (abstract 176)

21. Smith, B.D., La Celle, P.L., Siefring, G.E., Lowe-Krentz, L. and Lorand, L.: Effects of the calcium mediated enzymatic cross linking of membrane proteins on cellular deformability. *J. Memb. Biol.*, **61**, 75-80, (1981).

22. Stoclet, J.C.: An ubiquitous protein which regulates calcium dependent cellular functions and calcium movements. *Biochem. Pharmacol.*, **30**, 1723-1729, (1981).

23. Stoltz, J.F., Streiff, F., Larcan, A. and Niclause, M.: Mise en évidence de la fixation des ions calcium sur la membrane des globules rouges humains à l'aide de l'électrophorèse en phase liquide. *J. de Chimie Physique*, **10**, 1555-1556, (1971).

24. Stoltz, J.F.: Main determinants of red blood cell deformability. Clinical and pharmacological approaches. In: Recent advances in cardiovascular disease, 2 (suppl.), 1-20 (1981)

25. Van Nueten, J.M., Van Beek, J. and Janssen, P.A.J.: The vascular effects of flunarizine as compared with those of other clinically used vasoactive substances. *Arzneim. Forsch.*, **28**, 2082-2087, (1978).

26. Van Nueten, J.M. and Vanhoutte, P.M.: Improvement of tissue perfusion with inhibitors of calcium ion influx. *Biochem. Pharmacol.*, **29**, 479-481, (1980).

Calcium entry blockers in the treatment of peripheral obliterative arterial disease

T. Di Perri, F. Laghi Pasini, M. Guerrini

Summary

Important pharmaco-clinical criteria for selecting calcium entry blockers useful in the treatment of peripheral obliterative arterial disease (POAD) seem to be:
1. potent antivasoconstrictor activity, which does not mean generalized vasodilator activity;
2. antagonism of blood hyperviscosity;
3. potentiation of vascular defense mechanisms such as reactive hyperemia.
The clinical results with selective calcium entry blockers in terms of relief of symptoms and particularly in terms of increase of walking distance are worthwhile.

Résumé

On peut distinguer plusieurs critères pharmaco-cliniques importants dans le choix de bloqueurs de l'entrée de calcium utilisables pour le traitement de troubles de la circulation périphérique:
1. action antivasoconstrictrice puissante, ce qui ne veut pas dire vasodilatation générale;
2. antagonisme de l'hyperviscosité sanguine;
3. potentialisation de mécanismes de défense vasculaires, tels que l'hyperémie réactionnelle.
Les résultats cliniques obtenus avec les inhibiteurs de l'entrée de calcium sont très valables en ce qui concerne la diminution des symptômes, et en particulier en ce qui concerne l'augmentation du périmètre de marche.

Resumen

Los criterios siguientes parecen ser importantes para seleccionar distintos inhibidores de la penetración intracelular de Ca^{2+} por el tratamiento de trastornos obliterativos de la circulación periférica:
1. una fuerte actividad antivasoconstrictora, pero nó una vasodilatación general excesiva;
2. un antagonismo de hiperviscosidad de la sangre;
3. una mejoración de mecanismos vasculares defensivas como la hiperemía reactiva.
Los resultados clínicos obtenidos con inhibidores selectivos de la penetración intracelular del calcio son positivos en cuanto a la disminución de los síntomas y a la aumentación del trecho de marcha de los pacientes.

Zusammenfassung

Für die Selektion von Kalziumeintritthemmern bei der Behandlung von peripheren obliterativen Durchblutungsstörungen sind die folgenden Eigenschaften offensichtlich anzustreben:
1. Ausgeprägte antivasokonstriktorische Wirkung, was nicht bedeutet, dass eine allgemeine Vasodilatation erwünscht wäre;
2. Hemmung der Hyperviskosität des Blutes;
3. Verbesserung von vaskulären Adaptationsmechanismen, z.B. der reaktiven Hyperämie.
Die klinischen Resultaten mit selektiven Kalziumeinstromhemmern sind beachtlich, sowohl vom Standpunkt der Verbesserung von Symptomen als auch der Verlängerung der Gehstrecke bei den Patienten.

Introduction

Peripheral obliterative arterial disease (POAD) is mainly the consequence of atherosclerotic lesions which are slowly developing. The time interval between the beginning of the atherosclerotic changes and the clinical signs of circulatory insufficiency is quite variable. In combating the development and/or consequences of POAD calcium entry blockers may be useful in several respects.

Firstly, there are experimental findings showing that calcium entry blockers protect the vascular endothelium (Hladovec and De Clerck, 1981). Consequently they may prevent the genesis of a number of atherosclerotic lesions or they may refrain the atherosclerotic processes. The clinical relevance of these findings may be very important but remains speculative.

Secondly, clinical observations have shown that, in many instances, POAD is associated with vasospasms and/or with hyperviscosity (Di Perri, 1979). It has been proven that selective calcium entry blockers can antagonize these phenomena very efficiently and thus improve the circulation in the jeopardized area (Emanuel, 1979; Di Perri et al., 1979a). Through their selectivity of action these drugs are devoid of the risks of a "steal effect" as described for many peripheral vasodilators (Gillespie, 1959) and of the risks of a negative influence on the myocardial pump function.

Thirdly, selective calcium entry blockers can markedly improve the peripheral circulatory defense mechanisms, such as reactive hyperemia. This is also proven in patients with POAD (Verhaegen et al., 1974; Jageneau and Haag, 1977).

In this respect, we made a comparative study of flunarizine, which is known as a selective calcium entry blocker, and nifedipine, which has also an important general vasodilator action. The results are described further on.

Last but not least, it is the clinical improvement of patients which matters. Although the above mentioned activities strongly suggest that calcium entry blockers provide new approaches in treating POAD, the clinical relevance should be established e.g. in double blind studies measuring the influence of treatment on the walking distance of POAD-patients. The second part of this contribution will deal with such a study.

Effect of calcium entry blockers on the reactive hyperemia

In patients with POAD the reactive hyperemia appears to be modified as follows:
- in a first stage the amplitude of the hyperemic reaction, i.e. the peak flow, diminishes (type I);
- with progression of POAD the hyperemic reaction is slowed down and there is a marked delay of the peak flow (type II);
- finally the hyperemic reaction after arterial occlusion may be absent or there may even be a paradoxical reduction of blood flow (type III).

It is reported in various studies that oral treatment with selective calcium entry blockers, such as cinnarizine and flunarizine, improves the vascular defense mechanisms and, particularly, the reactive hyperemia (Verhaegen et al., 1974; Emmanuel, 1979).

We have tested the effect of a single infusion of flunarizine (10 mg i.v. in 2 min.) and of a single infusion of nifedipine (1 mg i.v. in 2 min.) on the rest flow of lower limbs as well as on the peak flow during reactive hyperemia.

Measurements were done with a **Periflow*** venous occlusion plethysmograph (Di Perri et al., 1979b; Forconi, 1983). The results are shown in figures 1 to 4. The rest flow in normal subjects (Fig. 1) and in POAD patients (Fig. 3) is markedly increased by nifedipine over a period of approximately 15 minutes whereas there is only a small increase of rest flow after flunarizine. On the other hand there is a marked impairment of the reactive hyperemia for more than 15 minutes after nifedipine infusion since the peak flow is markedly decreased during the whole period of peripheral vasodilatation in normal subjects (Fig. 2) as well as in POAD patients (Fig. 4). In clear contrast with the effect of nifedipine, the infusion of flunarizine potentiated the reactive hyperemia since the peak flow was increased over a period of more than 60 min. in normal subjects (Fig. 2) and even more than 6 hours in POAD patients (Fig. 4).

The acute vasodilator effect of nifedipine was associated with a reduction of arterial blood pressure and with an increase of heart rate. Blood pressure and heart rate were not affected by flunarizine.

These clinical pharmacological findings thus show:
1. that the vasodilator effect of nifedipine goes along with an impairment of the reactive hyperemia as was also described by Lorentsen and Landmark (1983);
2. that the intravenous infusion of flunarizine potentiates the reactive hyperemia in normal subjects and in POAD patients, as has previously been reported during oral treatment;
3. that there are important qualitative differences between calcium entry blockers to be considered when used for the treatment of POAD.

It is clear that not all calcium entry blockers are indicated for the treatment of POAD. A marked degree of "selectivity" is required to ascertain that the positive hemokinetic actions prevail over the myocardial depressant effects (Wellens et al., 1980). Moreover, calcium entry blockers which also provoke potent peripheral vasodilation, can be liable for undesired effects. Our study showed that vascular defense mechanisms can be hampered after nifedipine. In addition potent vasodilators may induce steal effects in the jeopardized tissues and they may also provoke an increase of intra-capillary pressure and oedema, as has been repeatedly reported in the literature. Therefore, only some "selective" calcium entry blockers have gained widespread recognition in the treatment of POAD.

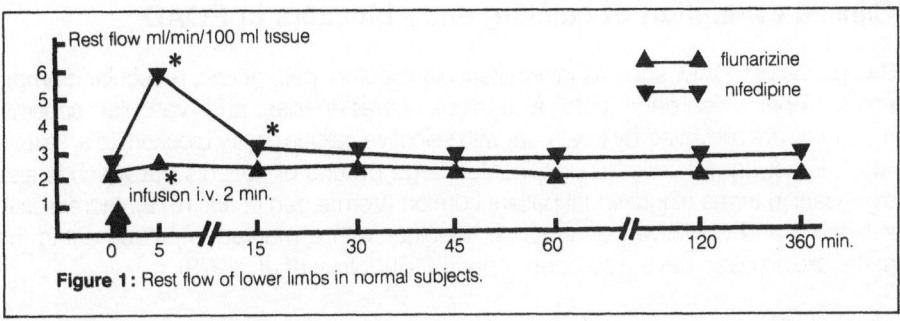

Figure 1: Rest flow of lower limbs in normal subjects.

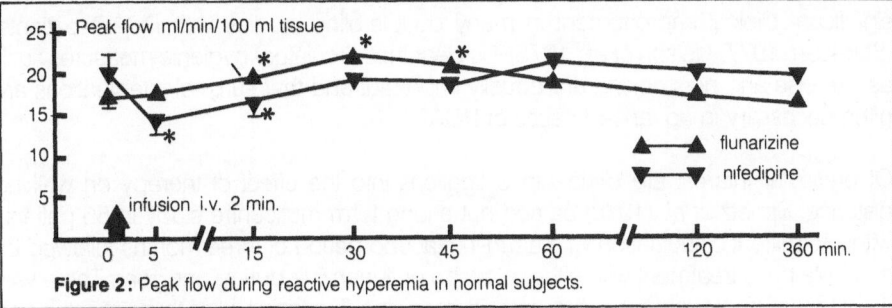

Figure 2: Peak flow during reactive hyperemia in normal subjects.

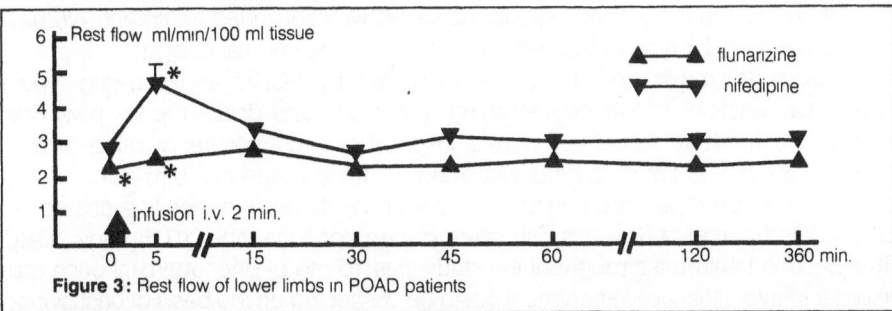

Figure 3: Rest flow of lower limbs in POAD patients

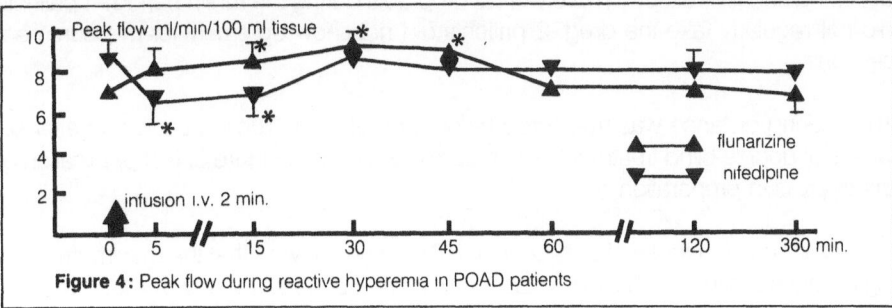

Figure 4: Peak flow during reactive hyperemia in POAD patients

Figure 1 to 4: Effect of a single i.v. infusion (2 minutes) of flunarizine 10 mg or nifedipine 1 mg.
Mean values (n = 20); SE indicated when exceeding the symbol. ✳p ≦ 0.05

Clinical evaluation of calcium entry blockers in POAD

Symptoms of POAD, such as intermittent claudicaton, pain at rest, muscular cramps, some trophic disorders, cold extremities, paraesthesias and vascular spasms, reportedly are alleviated by treatment with selective calcium entry blockers to an extent which is not only statistically significant in large groups of patients but which is also significant in terms of individual patient comfort (Verhaegen et al., 1979). Increases in subjective and objective performance, together with a marked improvement in the metabolic situation have also been reported (Rudofsky et al., 1979).

Although there is no doubt that drugs such as cinnarizine and flunarizine elicited a significant clinical improvement in many double-blind studies with POAD patients, (Staessen, 1977; Nelson et al., 1978) it is clear that circulatory hygienic measures such as exercise and no-smoking are equally important and that surgical interventions are often necessary in advanced cases of POAD.

Of particular interest are clinical investigations into the effect of therapy on walking distance. Schetz et al. (1978) carried out a long term muticentre study in 56 patients with intermittent claudication with a run-in placebo period of three months followed by a double-blind treatment with either placebo or flunarizine during one year. There was a significant improvement in the patients receiving flunarizine after three months and the difference with the placebo group increased with continued treatment. We have carried out a similar type of trial with the following experimental design:
Outpatients (26 males and 10 females) affected by POAD and showing type II hyperemic reactions in Periflow-recordings (decrease and delay of peak flow) were selected for the study. All of them were smokers; they had a painfree walking distance between 50 and 300 m on a horizontal treadmill at the speed of 3,5 miles/hour. After a run-in single-blind placebo period of 6 weeks patients were randomly allocated in a double-blind period of 6 weeks with either placebo or flunarizine (10 mg/day, orally). The placebo treatment throughout the study was 15 mg of phenobarbital once daily in order to avoid that active treatment could be suspected on the basis of occasionally occurring sedative effects. There were 6 drop-outs during the run-in period: 4 patients did not regularly take the drug, 2 patients did not show up timely for measurement sessions.

The walking distance was measured before and after the run-in period and after six weeks of double-blind treatment. The results are shown in Figure 5. Full publication of the study is in preparation.

Our results confirm those of Schetz et al. (1978) who showed that the maximum walking distance of smokers had increased from some 300 to some 650 m after 3 months of flunarizine treatment. We noted an increase of the painfree walking distance from 194 ± 19.1 m to 276.3 ± 24.6 after 6 weeks of flunarizine treatment.

It may be concluded that the clinical results obtained with selective calcium entry blockers mark a substantial progress in the pharmacological treatment of POAD.

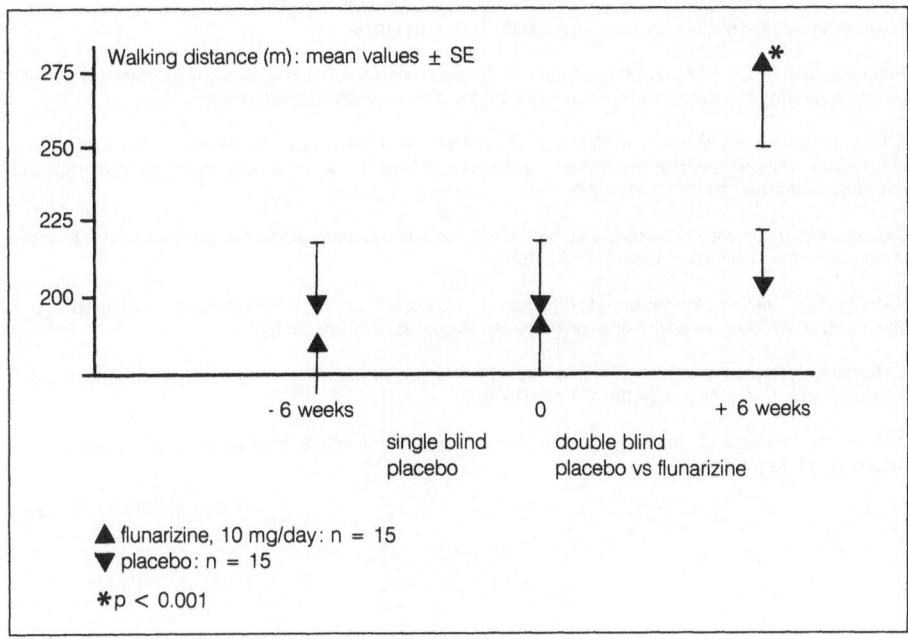

Figure 5: Painfree walking distance in patients with POAD

References

Di Perri, T. Rheological factors in circulatory disorders. *Angiology*, **30**, 480-486 (1979).

Di Perri, T., Forconi, S., Guerrini, M., Laghi Pasini, F., Del Cipolla, R., Rossi, C. and Agnusdei, D. Action of cinnarizine on the hyperviscosity of blood in patients with peripheral obliterative arterial disease. *Angiology*, **30**, 13 (1979a).

Di Perri, T., Forconi, S., Guerrini, M., Pecchi, S., Cappelli, R. and Bruni, F. The post-ischemic hyperemia: a strain gauge plethysmographic study in normal subjects and in vascular disease. In: Haemodynamique des Membres, P. Puel, H. Boccalon, A. Enjalbert Eds., 159, Toulouse-France (1979b).

Di Perri, T., Forconi, S., Guerrini, M., Pecchi, S., Cappelli, R. Modificazioni emoreoliche nelle arteriopatie. *Giorn. Geront.*, **29**, 487 (1981).

Emanuel, M.B. Specific calcium antagonists in the treatment of peripheral vascular disease. *Angiology*, **30**, 454-469 (1979).

Forconi, S. Continuous measurement of peripheral blood flow by venous occlusion strain gauge plethysmography. Atherosclerosis Reviews, 10, Hegyeli, R.J., Ed., Raven Press, 143, New York (1983).

Gillespie, J.A. The case against vasodilator drugs in occlusive vascular disease of the legs. *Lancet*, **3**, 995 (1959).

Hladovec, J. and De Clerck, F. Protection by flunarizine against endothelial cell injury *in vivo*. *Angiology*, **32**, 448-462 (1981).

Jageneau, A. and Haag, F. Flunarizin bei Patienten mit Durchblutungsstörungen den unteren Extremitäten: Doppelblindstudie. *Med. Welt.*, **28**, 1050-1055 (1977).

Lorentsen, E. and Landmark, K. The acute effect of nifedipine on calf and forefoot blood flow in patients with peripheral arterial insufficiency. *Angiology*, **34**, 46-52 (1983).

Nelson, M., Dewitz, G., Dom, J. and Hörig, Ch. Trial of the activity of **Sibelium** (flunarizine) in circulatory disorders. A multicentre double blind study. *Med. Welt*, **29/30**, 1175-1181 (1978).

Rudofsky, G., Brock, F.E., Elrich, M. and Nobbe, F. Clinical evaluation of flunarizine: walking distance, ergometric performance and hemodynamic and biochemical effects. *Angiology*, **30**, 470-479 (1979).

Schetz, J., Bostoen, H., Clement, D., Fornhoff, M., Haerens, A., Roekaerts, P. and Staessen, A.J. Flunarizine in chronic obstructive peripheral arterial disease: a placebo-controlled, double-blind, randomized multicentre trial. *Current Therapeutic Res.*, **23**, 121-130 (1978).

Staessen, A.J. Treatment of circulatory disturbances with flunarizine and cinnarizine. A multicentre, double-blind and placebo-controlled evaluation. *Vasa*, **6**, 59-71 (1977).

Verhaegen, H., Roels, V., Adriaensen, H., Brugmans, J., De Cock, W., Dony, J., Jageneau, A. and Schuermans, V. The arteriolar effects of cinnarizine and flunarizine. *Angiology*, **25**, 261-278 (1974).

Verhaegen, H., Reyntjens, A., Hörig, Ch. and Pötsch, W. Responsiveness of various symptoms of vascular disorders to calcium antagonists. *Angiology*, **30**, 447-453 (1979).

Wellens, D., Goossens, T. and Reyntjens, A. Positive hemokinetic effects after selective calcum-antagonism. *Angiology*, **31**, 821-827 (1980).

Chapter III:

Calcium entry blockers and myocardial function

Pharmacology of calcium entry blockers in animal and human coronary arteries

T. Godfraind, R.C. Miller

Summary

The difference of sensitivity of agonists in different types of blood vessels to inhibition by calcium entry blockers suggest that it is possible to selectively inhibit calcium channels associated with a particular agonist, or with a particular vascular bed, leaving the responses of other vascular beds relatively unchanged.

The present value of calcium entry blockers in the treatment of coronary vascular disorders stems from their ability to inhibit a final common pathway of contraction, namely, the stimulated entry of extracellular calcium into the vascular smooth muscle cell.

A feature of older human isolated coronary arteries is the presence of spontaneous rhythmic activity. This activity and contractions evoked by possible mediators of coronary vasospasm, depolarization, noradrenaline, serotonin and some products of cyclo-oxygenase activity such as $PGF_{2\alpha}$ are sensitive to inhibition by calcium entry blockers. The role of various other possible mediators of arterial spasm is unknown.

Coronary artery sensitivity to the contractile effect of histamine and noradrenaline as well as to the effects of some of the calcium entry blockers, may increase with age or with pathologic changes.

Résumé

La différence de sensibilité des agonistes vis-à-vis de l'inhibition produite par les agents bloqueurs de l'entrée de calcium dans les différents types de vaisseaux sanguins, suggère qu'il est possible d'inhiber sélectivement les canaux de calcium associés à un agoniste particulier, ou à un lit vasculaire particulier, tout en maintenant les réactions des autres lits vasculaires relativement inchangées.

La valeur actuelle des agents bloqueurs de l'entrée de calcium dans le traitement de troubles vasculaires coronaires provient de leur capacité d'inhiber une voie commune finale de contraction, c'est-à-dire l'entrée activée de calcium extracellulaire dans la cellule vasculaire de muscle lisse.

Une caractéristique des artères coronaires humaines plus âgées prises séparément est la présence d'une activité rythmique spontanée. Cette activité et ces contractions suscitées par des médiateurs possibles de vasospasme coronaire, soit la dépolarisation, la noradrénaline, la sérotonine et certains produits provenant de l'activité cyclo-oxygénase tels le $PGF_{2\alpha}$, sont sensibles à l'inhibition des agents bloqueurs de l'entrée de calcium. Plusieurs autres médiateurs possibles de vasospasme ont un rôle inconnu.

La sensibilité de l'artère coronaire vis-à-vis de l'effet contractile de l'histamine et de la noradrénaline ainsi que vis-à-vis de l'effet des bloqueurs de l'entrée de calcium peut augmenter avec l'âge ou avec des changements pathologiques.

Resumen

La diferencia de sensibilidad de agonistas en distintos vasos sanguíneos, en cuanto a su inhibición por inhibidores de la penetración intracelular de Ca^{2+}, sugiere que sea posible inhibir selectivamente los canales cálcicos asociados con un agonista particular, o con un lecho vascular particular, dejando las reacciones de otros lechos vasculares relativamente incambiados.

El valor actual de los inhibidores de la penetración intracelular de Ca^{2+} en el tratamiento de trastornos coronarios vasculares, proviene de su habilidad de inhibir un común camino final de contracción, es decir, la entrada estimulada de Ca^{2+} extracelular en la célula vascular del músculo liso.

Una característica de las arterias coronarias aisladas de hombres mayores, es la presencia de espontánea actividad rítmica. Esta actividad y contracciones, provocadas por mediadores posibles de vasoespasmo coronario, depolarización, noradrenalina, serotonina y algunos productos de actividad ciclo-oxigenasis, tales como $PGF_{2\alpha}$ son antagonisadas por inhibidores de la entrada de Ca^{2+}. El papel de muchos otros mediadores de espasmos arteriales posibles es desconocido.

La sensibilidad de las arterias coronarias, en cuanto al efecto contráctil de histamina y noradrenalina y también en cuanto a los efectos de algunos de los inhibidores de la penetración intracelular de Ca^{2+} puede aumentar con los años o con cambios patológicos.

Zusammenfassung

Die unterschiedliche Empfindlichkeit der sich in verschiedenen Blutgefäßen befindlichen Agonisten für Hemmung durch Kalziumantagonisten deutet auf die Möglichkeit hin, mit einem bestimmten Agonisten bzw. mit einem bestimmten Gefäßbett verknüpfte Kalziumkanäle selektiv zu hemmen, ohne daß andere Gefäßbetten in ihrem Verhalten wesentlich beeinflußt werden.

Der heutige Wert der Kalziumeinstromhemmer bei der Behandlung von Koronargefäßstörungen ist darauf zurückzuführen, daß sie imstande sind, einen endgültigen gemeinsamen Kontraktionsweg, nämlich den stimulierten Eintritt extrazellulären Kalziums in die glatte Gefäßmuskelzelle, zu hemmen.

Isolierte Koronararterien älterer Menschen zeigen eine spontane rhythmische Aktivität. Diese Erscheinung, zusammen mit Kontraktionen, die durch mögliche Mediatoren vom Koronargefäßkrampf ausgelöst werden, sowie Depolarisation, Noradrenalin, Serotonin und einige Produkte der Zyklooxygenasewirkung wie $PGF_{2\alpha}$, sind für Hemmung durch Kalziumantagonisten empfindlich. Die Rolle verschiedener sonstiger Mediatoren des Arterienkrampfes ist noch unbekannt.

Die Empfindlichkeit von Koronararterien für die kontraktile Wirkung von Histamin und Noradrenalin kann beim Alterwerden oder nach pathologischen Veränderungen zunehmen. Dies geht mit einer zunehmenden Empfindlichkeit für die Wirkungen bestimmter Kalziumeinstromhemmer einher.

Prinzmetal et al., (1959) first described a variant form of angina which occurred in patients at rest and proposed that this syndrome was the result of coronary artery spasm. Coronary arteriography performed in patients experiencing an attack of variant angina confirmed the occurrence of vasospasm of large epicardial vessels (Oliva et al., 1973), and in recent years evidence has accumulated to suggest an important role of coronary vasospasm in the etiology of angina pectoris and myocardial infarction (see for example Maseri et al., 1978).

Many spasmogens have been suggested as possible mediators of vasospasm but it may reasonably be assumed that whatever the initiating event or events are, the contractile response is dependent on a rise in the intracellular level of free calcium (Bolton, 1979). Therefore the pharmacology of possible mediators of coronary vasoconstrictor effects in human coronary arteries and animal models, in relation to the pharmacology of compounds known to alter the relative permeability of cell membranes to calcium, is of some interest. A group of compounds in this latter category are the calcium entry blockers which can be defined as compounds which specifically inhibit the stimulated influx of extracellular calcium into cells. Examples such as nifedipine, verapamil and lidoflazine have been introduced into clinical use as an adjunct to the treatment of such conditions as hypertension, cardiac arrhythmias and peripheral vascular disease as well as variant angina and angina pectoris.

Little is known of the ability of possible mediators of coronary vasospasm to mobilize calcium from extracellular or intracellular sources, or both, in coronary arteries. This review is an attempt to summarize available data obtained in isolated coronary arteries with reference to more detailed information obtained in isolated vessels from other vascular beds.

Depolarization

Depolarization of vascular smooth muscle by exposure to physiological solutions enriched in potassium produces contractions which are totally dependent on the availability of extracellular calcium (Godfraind and Kaba, 1969). Agonists, interacting with specific membrane receptors, can also increase smooth muscle membrane permeability to calcium and produce a contraction. It has been assumed that under these different circumstances separate mechanisms or channels for the admission of calcium are activated (see Bolton, 1979).

Concentrations of nifedipine producing 50% of the maximal reduction of contractile responses dependent on extracellular calcium (IC_{50} values) in the rat aorta and mesenteric artery are similar, being about $3 \times 10^{-9}M$ when the contraction is induced by depolarization and $2 \times 10^{-8}M$ when the contraction is induced by noradrenaline respectively. However, flunarizine is 10 times more potent as an antagonist of depolarization-induced contractions in the mesenteric artery (IC_{50} $2 \times 10^{-9}M$) than in the aorta (IC_{50} $1.9 \times 10^{-8}M$). These results indicate that while the interaction of nifedipine with the membrane potential sensitive calcium channels could occur at a common membrane site related to these channels in the two tissues the results with flunarizine might indicate differences between these channels in different tissues (Godfraind and Miller, 1983a; Hagiwara and Byerly, 1981).

Contractions induced by particular agonists in the coronary vascular bed of different species also exhibit different sensitivities to the depressant effects of some calcium entry blockers, for example lidoflazine is more potent at inhibiting serotonin and depolarization induced contractions in human than in dog coronary arteries and diltiazem is more potent in pig than in human coronaries.

Depolarization of dog, pig, cattle and human coronary arteries produces a stable contraction which can be completely inhibited by diltiazem, nifedipine, verapamil, D 600, SKF 525A and FR 7534 (Ginsburg et al., 1980a; Gross et al., 1981; Watson, 1978; Fleckenstein et al., 1977; Van Breemen and Siegel, 1980; Pieper and Schmidt, 1972). Godfraind and Miller (1983a) found that while nifedipine, lidoflazine and flunarizine completely inhibited such contractions in older coronaries, contractions of younger arteries were partially resistant to the calcium entry blocking compounds. The difference was most marked in the case of nifedipine which was 100 times more potent in older arteries. Flunarizine potency increased by about 10 times and that of lidoflazine by about 4 times (Table 1).

Table 1 : Concentrations of calcium entry blockers (M) producing a 50% inhibition of depolarization and serotonin induced contractions and of serotonin induced rhythmic activity (IC_{50} values), in human coronary arteries of different ages (< 40 YRS AND > 40 yrs)

	Lidoflazine	Flunarizine	Nifedipine
Depolarization < 40	4.3×10^{-7}	3.8×10^{-6}	1.1×10^{-8}
Depolarization > 40	1.1×10^{-7}	5.0×10^{-7}	0.9×10^{-10}
Serotonin < 40			$> 1 \times 10^{-8}$
Serotonin > 40		7.2×10^{-8}	$1\text{-}5 \times 10^{-8}$
Serotonin (Rhythmic) > 40		8.3×10^{-8}	0.3×10^{-8}

This may indicate a change in reactivity with increasing age or pathological condition. A nifedipine resistant component of depolarization induced contraction of rabbit, pig and human coronary arteries, which was however dependent on extracellular calcium, has also been described (Golenhofen, 1978; Golenhofen et al., 1977), Fleckenstein (1977), however, described depolarization induced contractions of pig coronary arteries which were completely inhibited by nifedipine and verapamil, while about 15% of the contracture seemed to be resistant to diltiazem. Lidoflazine, when added to dog coronary arteries already contracted by depolarization only inhibited the contractions by about 86.5% (Van Nueten et al., 1980), although it inhibited completely the contractions of pig coronary arteries (Godfraind and Polster, 1968).

In dog arteries depolarization induced contractions were depressed by lidoflazine, nifedipine, verapamil and tiapamil (Van Nueten et al., 1980; Watson, 1978; Eigenmann et al., 1981) and abolished by D 600 and SKF 525A (Van Breemen and Siegel, 1980).

Such observations indicate a degree of variability in the efficacy of calcium entry blocking drugs in the coronary vasculature similar to that seen in other vascular beds and probably indicates the heterogenous nature of potential sensitive calcium channels (Hagiwara and Byerly, 1981).

Calcium

Calcium in concentrations up to about 8 mM, in the absence of depolarization, induced contractions of cattle and pig coronary arteries which were antagonized by verapamil, D 600, prenylamine and nifedipine (Grün *et al.*, 1974). In dog coronary arteries calcium dependent action potentials could be elicited in the presence of tetra-ethyl ammonium and these were inhibited by bepridil and verapamil (Belardinelli *et al.*, 1979; Harder and Sperelakis, 1981).

Spontaneous activity

Various types of spontaneous rythmic activity in isolated human coronary artery preparations have been described but such phenomena are not always apparent. Godfraind and Miller (1983a) only noted spontaneous activity in some arterial segments from older hearts in which the arteries contained visible atherosclerotic plaques, figure 1 shows examples of such spontaneous activity. In nonactive segments, taken from the same arteries rhythmic activity could sometimes, but not always, be induced by histamine or serotonin. These spontaneous fluctuations in tone were inhibited in calcium free physiological solution and by nifedipine (Golenhofen, 1978; Godfraind and Miller, unpublished observations); induced rythmic tone changes were also inhibited (see below).

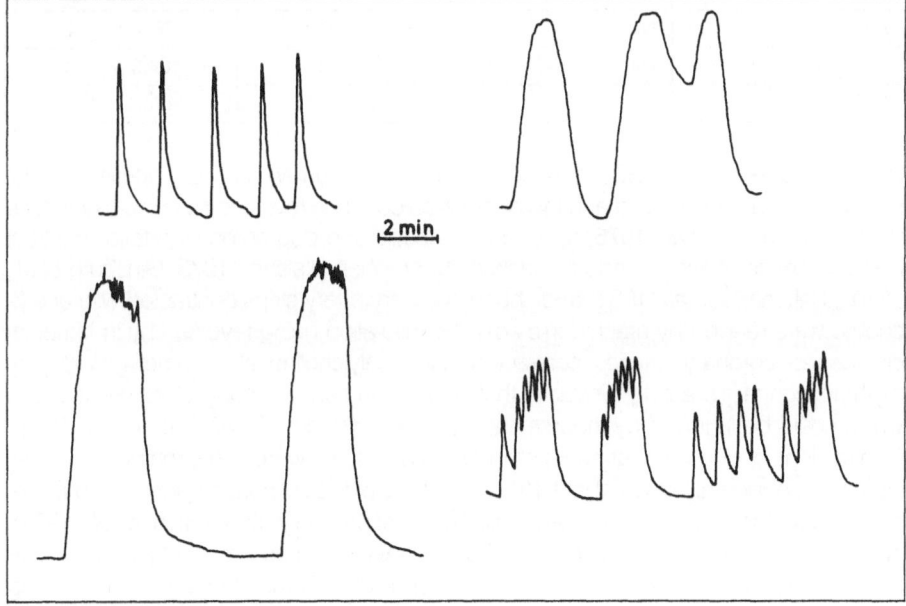

Figure 1: Examples of spontaneous activity in various segments of human coronary arteries. From Godfraind and Miller, 1983 a, with permission.

The cause of spontaneous contractile activity in human coronary arteries, which could be a prelude to spasmodic activity, is unknown.

Prostaglandins

Some prostaglandins are known to contract isolated human coronary arteries (Kulkarni et al., 1976, a, b; Ginsburg et al., 1980a). Godfraind and Miller (1983a) found that $PGF_{2\alpha}$ was about equipotent to acetylcholine and noradrenaline (in the presence of propranolol) in contracting human coronary arteries. However, the maximal contraction achieved by $PGF_{2\alpha}$ was about 75% greater than the one elicited by either acetylcholine, serotonin or depolarization and about 4 times greater than the one elicited by noradrenaline (Table 2). These $PGF_{2\alpha}$ induced contractions were totally inhibited by nifedipine 3 μM.

Table 2: Relative potencies of some contractile agents on human coronary arteries ($IC_{50} \pm$ s.e.m.). Maximal contractions induced by each agonist are expressed as a percentage of that produced by depolarization in 100 mM K^+ containing physiological solution ($\pm$ s.e.m.). All pretreatment concentrations were 1 μM.

Contractile agent	Pretreatment	$EC_{50}(x\ 10^{-8}M)$	Maximal contraction
100 mM K^+	NIL	-	100
Noradrenaline	NIL	-	0 - 6
Noradrenaline	Propranolol	24.4 $\pm$ 2.8	41.7 $\pm$ 5.9
Noradrenaline	Propranolol, Cocaine, Metanephrine	7.8 $\pm$ 0.9	46.8 $\pm$ 11.9
Acetylcholine	NIL	52.0 $\pm$ 6.2	96.4 $\pm$ 16.4
Serotonin	NIL	2.2 $\pm$ 0.8	104.3 $\pm$ 17.1
$PGF_{2\alpha}$	NIL	42.0 $\pm$ 5.4	175.1 $\pm$ 6.4

Both spontaneous and PGE_2 induced contractions of human coronary arteries are depressed by arachidonic acid and this depression could be reversed by cyclo-oxygenase inhibitors (Kulkarni et al., 1976, a, b). Human, cattle and dog coronary arteries contract in the presence of aspirin, indomethacin or ibuprophen (Kalsner, 1975; Ginsburg et al., 1980a; Sakanashi et al., 1981) and sheep coronary artery strips contracted with acetylcholine were relaxed by arachidonic acid, the relaxation being reversed by indomethacin. Sheep coronary arteries contracted with acetylcholine also sometimes display rhythmic contractile activity similar to that seen in human coronary artery preparations which could be inhibited by indomethacin (Cornish, Goldie, Krstew and Miller, 1983). Contractions of dog coronary arteries induced by aspirin were totally inhibited in a calcium free solution although about 16% and 27% of the response appeared to be resistant to inhibition by diltiazem and nifedipine respectively. (Sakanashi et al., 1981). This effect of aspirin was reversible. Cat coronary arteries are contracted by carbocyclic thromboxane A_2 (a stable analogue of thromboxane), the contractions being depressed by nifedipine but not completely inhibited, about 25% of the response being resistant. These nifedipine depressed contractions were potentiated when the calcium concentration of the medium was raised (Smith et al., 1981). A nifedipine resistant component of some agonist induced contractions has also been observed by others and there is some indication that this resistant component is also dependent on extracellular calcium (Golenhofen, 1978; Golenhofen et al., 1977).

118

There is evidence that prostacyclin is the major prostaglandin released spontaneously from rabbit, rat and guinea-pig hearts (De Deckere et al., 1977; Needleman et al., 1978; Wennmalm, 1979) or released from human, dog, rat and guinea-pig hearts following injections of arachidonic acid (Nowak et al., 1980, Mullane et al., 1979; Rosen and Schror, 1979; Schror et al., 1978). Low concentrations (less than 1 μM) relax human coronary arteries (Ginsburg et al., 1980a) and it is suggested that a continuous production of prostacyclin may actively lower cytosolic free calcium levels in the smooth muscle cells of healthy coronary arteries. Alterations in the rate of production of prostacyclin or another product of cyclo-oxygenase activity might precipitate changes in tone of the coronary vasculature and perhaps also alter its reactivity to other contractile substances. These changes might be partially resistant to the effects of some calcium entry blockers.

Noradrenaline

In man α-adrenergic mediated vasoconstriction may contribute significantly to myocardial ischemia in patients with coronary artery disease (Mudge et al., 1979). Noradrenaline contracts human and dog coronary arteries (Van Breemen and Siegel, 1980; Golenhofen, 1978).

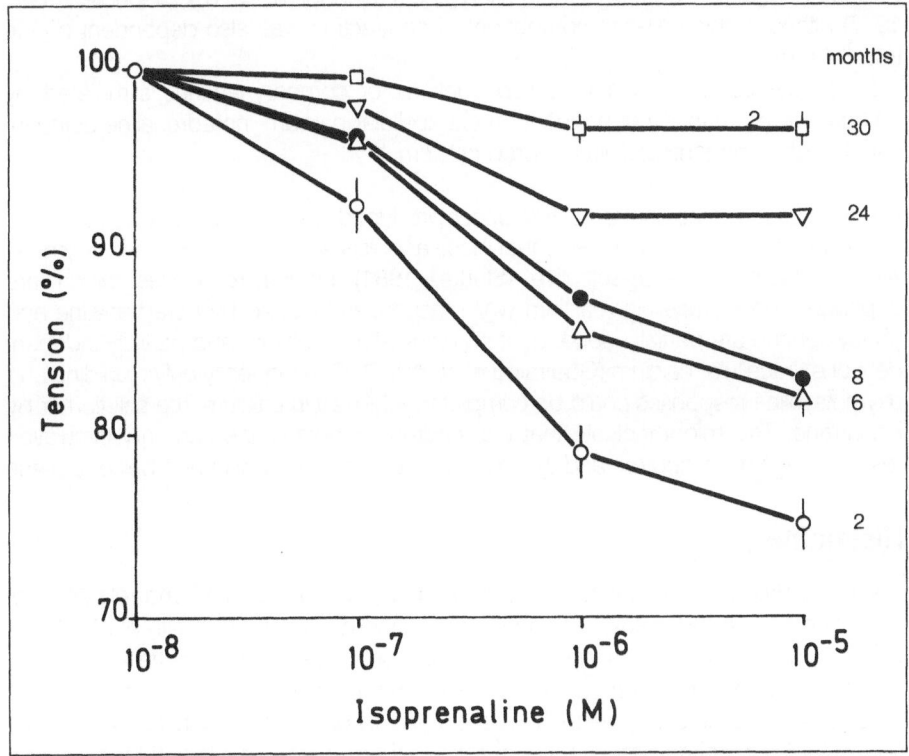

Figure 2: Concentration-relaxation curves elicited by isoprenaline in segments of rat aorta of varying ages (indicated in months), contracted by depolarization (100 mM K+). Vertical bars indicate s.e.m. From Godfraind, 1979, with permission.

119

Godfraind and Miller (1983a) could only elicit noradrenaline contractions in human coronary arteries in the presence of propranolol. Noradrenaline had a similar potency in human coronary arteries to acetylcholine and $PGF_{2\alpha}$ but produced a maximal contraction equal to about one half of that stimulated by depolarization, serotonin and acetylcholine and about one quarter of that stimulated by $PFG_{2\alpha}$ (Table 2). It was concluded that α-adrenoceptors were probably not of great importance in young healthy coronary arteries, β-adrenoceptor effects being predominant. However, it is known that β-adrenoceptor mediated relaxation of vascular tissue declines with age (Fleisch and Hooker, 1976; Godfraind, 1979) (Fig. 2) and while isoprenaline relaxes younger human coronary arteries contracted by depolarization it has no effect on older arteries (Godfraind and Miller, 1983a).

In dog coronary arteries it has been shown that noradrenaline induced contractions are almost completely abolished in calcium free solutions or in the presence of lanthanum 10 mM. Furthermore, these noradrenaline induced contractions were completely inhibited by the calcium entry blockers lidoflazine, D 600 and SKF 525A (Van Breemen and Siegel, 1980; Van Nueten and Vanhoutte, 1980). In human coronary arteries the contractions were depressed by diltiazem and D 600 (Ginsburg et al., 1980a). In dog, rabbit, pig and human coronaries about 20-40% of the noradrenaline induced contraction was resistant to nifedipine (Golenhofen, 1978; Golenhofen et al., 1977) although this resistant component of contraction was also dependent on extracellular calcium.
From these results it seems that contractions of coronary arteries stimulated by noradrenaline are totally dependent on extracellular calcium, noradrenaline being incapable of utilizing intracellularly stored calcium.

An investigation of the contractile responses produced by various α-adrenoceptor agonists in the rat aorta has suggested that those agonists such as clonidine and oxymetazoline, described as α_2-selective (Starke, 1981) induce responses which are dependent on extracellular calcium while responses induced by noradrenaline and phenylephrine are partially dependent on extracellular calcium and partially independent of extracellular calcium (Godfraind et al., 1982). Consequently only clonidine and oxymetazoline responses could be completely inhibited in calcium free solution or by cinnarizine. This might indicate that the α-adrenoceptors of the coronary circulation resemble α_2-adrenoceptors and that α_1-adrenoceptors are few in number or absent.

Histamine

Histamine produces contraction of larger human coronary arteries and relaxation of small arteries (Kountz, 1932), or simply contraction (Smith, 1950; Smith et al., 1951). Godfraind and Miller (1983 a, b) reported contraction, relaxation or no effect in different human coronary arterial preparations, not seemingly related to vessel size and also noted a decrease in sensitivity to the relaxant effects of histamine with increasing age. Many studies in animal tissues have described the presence of H_1 and H_2 receptors in coronary vessels, the different receptors subserving different functions (e.g. Broadley, 1975; Giles et al., 1977) and similar observations have been made in human coronary segments (Ginsburg et al., 1980 a, b; Godfraind and Miller, 1983 b).

Serotonin

Serotonin contracts human, pig, rabbit, sheep and larger dog coronary arteries (Takenaka, 1959; De La Lande et al., 1974; Brine et al., 1979; Van Nueten and Vanhoutte, 1980; Godfraind and Miller, 1983 a) but not smaller arteries of the dog (Porquet et al., 1982). In human arteries serotonin was more potent than acetylcholine, noradrenaline or $PGF_{2\alpha}$ (Table 2) and more potent than noradrenaline (variously about 2 or 100-300 fold) in larger dog arteries. In both human and dog vessels the magnitude of the serotonin contraction was about twice that induced by noradrenaline.

Serotonin contractions of dog coronaries were not completely inhibited by lidoflazine (about 21% resistant) although the IC_{50} concentration was similar to that obtained against noradrenaline (Van Nueten and Vanhoutte, 1980).

Serotonin (10 μM) induced an increase in basal tension and the appearance of rhythmic contractions in some but not all human coronary arteries of various ages. In very young arteries (9 and 15 years old) serotonin induced contractions without inducing rhythmic activity and these contractions were not readily inhibited by nifedipine 10^{-9} or 10^{-8}M. In older arteries (about 45 years old) serotonin induced an increase in basal tone and the appearance of rhythmic contractions in some preparations. Nifedipine abolished both of these effects but had a 10-fold greater potency against the rhythmic contractions, with an IC_{50} of about 3.3×10^{-9}M, while the IC_{50} value against basal tone was about $1-5 \times 10^{-8}$M (Table 1). Flunarizine also inhibited both tone and rhythmic activity induced by serotonin in arteries taken from a 45-year-old heart but had about equal potency in each instance (IC_{50} values of 7.2 and 8.3×10^{-8}M respectively).

Acetylcholine

Acetylcholine contracts human (Smith et al., 1951; Godfraind and Millers, 1983 a) (Table 2) and pig isolated coronary arteries being about equipotent with histamine and more potent than adrenaline (Smith, 1950) without producing a change in membrane potential (Ito et al., 1979). These acetylcholine contractions are still present after prolonged exposure to calcium free physiological solution. In guinea-pig coronary artery acetylcholine produces contractions associated with membrane hyperpolarization and is thought to increase membrane permeability to calcium and potassium and to liberate intracellularly stored calcium (Kitamura and Kuriyuma, 1979). These results imply that acetylcholine induced coronary contractions should be at least partially resistant to the effects of calcium entry blockers but direct information is lacking.

Anoxia

In dog coronary arteries anoxia induced in the presence of depolarization or serotonin contractions elicited a further contraction which could be completely inhibited by lidoflazine. In the presence of a noradrenaline induced contraction, the contraction elicited by anoxia was also depressed by lidoflazine, the IC_{50} concentration being of similar magnitude (3×10^{-6}M). However, in these circumstances, about 40% of the contraction was resistant to the effects of lidoflazine.

References

Belardinelli, L., Harder, D., Sperelakis, N., Rubio, R. and Berne, R.M. Cardiac glycoside stimulation of inward Ca^{2+} current in vascular smooth muscle of canine coronary artery (1979).*J. Pharmacol. Exp. Therp.*, **209**, 62. (1979)

Bolton, T.B. Mechanisms of action of transmitters and other substances on smooth muscle. *Physiol. Rev.*, **59**, 606. (1979)

Brine, F., Cornish, E.J. and Miller, R.C. Effects of uptake inhibitors on responses of sheep coronary arteries to catecholamines and sympathetic nerve stimulation. *Br. J. Pharmacol.*, **67**, 553. (1979)

Broadley, K.J. The role of H_1 and H_2 receptors in the coronary response to histamine of isolated perfused hearts of guinea-pigs and rabbits. *Br. J. Pharmacol.*, **54**, 511. (1975)

Cornish, E.J., Goldie, R.G., Krstew, E.V. and Miller, R.C. Effect of indomethacin on responses of sheep isolated coronary artery to arachidonic acid. *J. Clin. Exp. Pharmacol. Physiol.*, **10**, 171. (1983)

De Deckere, E.A.M., Nugteren, D.A. and Ten Hoor, F. Prostacyclin is the major prostaglandin released from the isolated perfused rabbit and cat hearts. *Nature* (Lond.), **268**, 160. (1977)

De La Lande, I.S., Harvey, J.A. and Holt, S. Response of the rabbit coronary arteries to autonomic agents. *Blood Vessels*, **11**, 319. (1974)

Fleckenstein, A. Specific pharmacology of calcium in myocardium, cardiac pacemakers, and vascular smooth muscle. *Ann. Rev. Pharmacol. Toxicol.*, **17**, 149. (1977)

Fleckenstein, A., Fleckenstein-Grün, G. and Byon, Y.K. Cardiovascular effects of the Ca^{2+} antagonist coronary drug fendiline (Sensit). *Arzneim. Forsch*, **27**, 562. (1977)

Fleisch, S.A. and Hooker, C.S. The relationship between age and relaxation of the vascular smooth muscle in the rabbit and rat. *Circulation*, **38**, 243. (1976)

Giles, R.W., Heiss, G. and Wilcken, D.E.L. Histamine receptors in the coronary circulation of the dog: Effects of mepyramine and metiamide on responses to histamine infusions. *Circulation Res.*, **40**, 541. (1977)

Ginsburg, R., Bristow, M.R., Harrison, D.C. and Stinson, E.B. Studies with isolated human coronary arteries. *Chest* (Suppl.), **78**, 180. (1980a)

Ginsburg, R., Bristow, M.R., Stinson, E.B. and Harrison, D.C. Histamine receptors in the human heart. *Life Sci.*, **26**, 2245. (1980b)

Godfraind, T. Alternative mechanisms for the potentiation of the relaxation evoked by isoprenaline in aorta from young and aged rats. *Eur. J. Pharmacol.*, **53**, 273. (1979)

Godfraind, T. and Kaba, A. Blockade or reversal of the contraction induced by calcium and noradrenaline in depolarized arterial smooth muscle. *Br. J. Pharmacol.*, **36**, 549. (1969)

Godfraind, T. and Miller, R.C. Specificity of action of Ca entry blockers, a comparison of their actions in rat arteries and in human coronary arteries. *Circulation Res.*, **52** (Suppl. 1), 81. (1983a)

Godfraind, T. and Miller, R.C. Effects of histamine and histamine antagonists mepyramine and cimetidine on human coronary arteries. *Br. J. Pharmacol.*, **79**, 979. (1983b)

Godfraind, T., Miller, R.C. and Socrates Lima, J. Selective a_{-1} and a_{-2}-adrenoceptor agonist induced contractions and ^{45}Ca fluxes in the rat isolated aorta. *Br. J. Pharmacol.*, **77**, 597. (1982)

Godfraind, T. and Polster, P. Etude comparative de médicaments inhibant la réponse contractile de vaisseaux isolés d'origine humaine ou animale. *Thérapie*, **23**, 1209-1220. (1968)

Golenhofen, K. Activation mechanisms in smooth muscle of human coronary arteries and their selective inhibition. *Naunyn Schmiedeberg's Arch. Pharmacol.*, **302**, Suppl. R36. (1978)

Golenhofen, K., Neuser, G. and Golenhofen, R. Inhibition of calcium activation in coronary arteries. *Naunyn Schmiedeberg's Arch. Pharmacol.*, **297** (Suppl. 11), **R30**. (1977)

Gross, G.J., Diemer, M.J., Warltier, D.C. and Hardman, H.F. Relaxation of potassium-depolarized canine, bovine and porcine large coronary arteries by nitroglycerin, chromonar and two dihydropyridine calcium antagonists. *Gen. Pharmacol.*, **12**, 199. (1981)

Grün, G., Fleckenstein, A. and Wader, U. Changes in coronary smooth muscle tone produced by Ca, cardiac glycosides and Ca antagonistic compounds (verapamil, D 600, prenylamine etc.), *Pflügers Arch.*, **374** (Suppl.), R1. (1974)

Hagiwara, S. and Byerly, L. Calcium channel. *Ann. Rev. Neurosci.*, **4**, 69. (1981)

Harder, D.R. and Sperelakis, N. Bepridil blockade of Ca^{2+}-dependent action potentials in vascular smooth muscle of dog coronary artery. *J. Cardiovasc. Pharmacol.*, **3**, 906. (1981)

Ito, Y., Kitamura, K. and Kuriyama, H. Effects of acetylcholine and catecholamines on the smooth muscle cell of the porcine coronary artery. *J. Physiol.*, **294**, 595. (1979)

Kalsner, S. Endogenous prostaglandin release contributes directly to coronary artery tone. *Can. J. Physiol.*, **53**, 560. (1975)

Kitamura, K. and Kuriyama, H. Effects of acetylcholine on the smooth muscle cell of isolated main coronary artery of the guinea-pig. *J; Physiol.*, **293**, 119. (1979)

Kountz, W.B. Studies on the coronary arteries of the human heart. *J. Pharmacol. Exp. Ther.*, **45**, 65. (1932)

Kulkarni, P.S., Roberts, R. and Needleman, P. Paradoxical endogenous synthesis of a coronary dilating substance from arachidonate. *Prostaglandins*, **12**, 337. (1976a)

Kulkarni, P.S., Roberts, R. and Needleman, P. Endogenous synthesis of a labile coronary dilatory substance from arachidonic acid. *Fed. Proc.*, **35**, 298. (1976b)

Maseri, A., L'Abbate, A., Baroldi, G., Chierchia, S., Marzilli, M., Ballestra, A.M., Severi, S., Parodi, O., Biagini, A., Distante, A. and Pesola, A. Coronary vasospasm as a possible cause of myocardial infarction. *New Eng. J. Med.*, **299**, 1271. (1978)

Mudge, G.H., Goldberg, S., Gunther, S., Mann, T. and Grossman, W. Comparison of metabolic and vasoconstrictor stimuli on coronary vascular resistance in man. *Circulation*, **59**, 544. (1979)

Mullane, K.M., Dusting, G.J., Salmon, J.A., Mocada, S. and Vane, J.R. Biotransformation and cardiovascular effects of arachidonic acid in the dog. *Eur. J. Pharmacol.*, **54**, 217. (1979)

Needleman, P., Bronson, S.D., Wyche, A., Sivakoff, M. and Nicolaou, K.C. Cardiac and renal prostaglandin I_2. *J. Clin. Invest.*, **61**, 839. (1978)

Nowak, J., Kaijser, L. and Wennmalm, A. Cardiac synthesis of prostaglandins from arachidonic acid in man *Prostaglandins Med.*, **4**, 205. (1980)

Oliva, P.B., Potts, D.E. and Pluss, R.G Coronary arterial spasm in Prinzmetals angina: documentation by coronary arteriography. *New Eng. J. Med.*, **288**, 745. (1973)

Pieper, V and Schmidt, E. Relaxation of coronary arteries by electro-mechanical decoupling or adrenergic stimulation *Pflügers Arch.*, **337**, 107. (1972)

Porquet, M.F., Pourrias, B. and Santamaria, R Effects of 5-hydroxytryptamine on canine isolated coronary arteries. *Br. J. Pharmacol.R*, **75**, 305. (1982)

Prinzmetal, M., Kennamer, R., Merliss, R., Wada, T. and Bor, N. Angina pectoris. I. A variant form of angina pectoris: preliminary report. *Am. J. Med.*, **27**, 375. (1959)

Rösen, P. and Schrör, K. Arachidonic acid-induced release of PGI_2 and PGE_2 from the diabetic heart. *Naunyn Schmiedeberg's Arch. Pharmac.*, **307** (Suppl. 124), R31. (1979)

Sakanashi, M., Araki, H., Furukawa, T, Rokutanda, M. and Yonemura, K. A study on constrictor responses of dog coronary arteries to acetylsalicylic acid *Arch. Int. Pharmacodyn. Ther.*, **252**, 86. (1981)

Schrör, K, Moncada, S., Ubatuba, F.B. and Vane, J.R. Transformation of arachidonic acid and prostaglandin endoperoxides by the guinea-pig heart. Formation of RCS and prostacyclin. *Eur. J. Pharmacol.*, **47**, 103. (1978)

123

Smith, D.J. Reactions of isolated surviving coronary artery to epinephrine, acetylcholine and histamine. *Proc. Soc. Exp. Biol.*, **73**, 449. (1950)

Smith, D.J., Syverton, J.T. and Coxe, J.W. In vitro studies of the coronary arteries of man and swine as demonstrated by a new techniwue, angioplethysmokyography. *Circulation*, **4**, 890. (1951)

Smith, E.F., Lefer, A.M. and Nicolaou, K.C. Mechanisms of coronary vasoconstriction induced by carboxyclic thromboxane A_2. *Am. J. Physiol.*, **240**, H493. (1981)

Starke, K. α-adrenoceptor subclassification. *Rev. Physiol. Biochem. Pharmacol.*, **88**, 199. (1981)

Takenaka, F. Response of coronary strips to acetylcholine, histamine, 5-hydroxytryptamine and adrenaline. *Jap. J. Pharmacol.*, **9**, 55. (1959)

Van Breemen, C. and Siegel, B. The mechanism of α-adrenergic activation of the dog coronary artery. *Circulation Res.*, **46**, 426. (1980)

Van Nueten, J.M., Van Beek, J. and Vanhoutte, P.M. Inhibitory effect of lidoflazine on contractions of isolated canine coronary arteries caused by norepinephrine, 5-hydroxytryptamine, high potassium, anoxia and ergonovine maleate. *J. Pharmacol. Exp. Ther.*, **213**, 179. (1980)

Van Nueten, J.M. and Vanhoutte, P.M. Effect of the Ca^{2+} antagonist lidoflazine on normoxic and anoxic contractions of canine coronary arterial smooth muscle. *Eur. J. Pharmacol.*, **64**, 173. (1980)

Watson, E.L. Effects of ionophores A23187 and X537A on vascular smooth muscle activity. *Eur. J. Pharmacol.*, **52**, 171. (1978)

Wennmalm, A. Prostacyclin-dependent coronary vasodilatation in rabbit and guinea-pig hearts. *Acta physiol. Scand.*, **106**, 47. (1979)

Calcium paradox and calcium entry blockers

T.J.C. Ruigrok, A.M. Slade, W.G.Nayler and F.L. Meijler

Summary

Reperfusion of isolated hearts with calcium-containing solution after a short period of calcium-free perfusion results in irreversible cell damage (calcium paradox). This phenomenon is characterized by an excessive influx of calcium into the cells, the rapid onset of myocardial contracture, exhaustion of tissue high-energy phosphates, massive release of cell constituents, and extensive ultrastructural damage. The calcium paradox can be regarded as the most severe form of myocardial necrosis that can be produced experimentally.

Under the experimental conditions described in this study, the calcium entry blockers verapamil, nifedipine, diltiazem and lidoflazine failed to reduce the massive release of enzymes that occurs in the severe form of the calcium paradox. Calcium entry blockers, however, may alter the time course of the events that occur during the development of the calcium paradox.

Calcium entry blockers may have a protective effect in a mild form of the calcium paradox. This is of interest for cardiac surgery where calcium-free cardioplegic solutions are widely used. Calcium entry blockers may decrease the potential hazard of the use of these solutions.

Résumé

Une reperfusion des coeurs isolés au moyen d'une solution contenant du calcium après une courte période de perfusion exempte de calcium entraîne une détérioration irréversible de la cellule (paradoxe de calcium). Ce phénomène est caractérisé par une pénétration excessive de calcium à l'intérieur des cellules, l'apparition d'une contracture myocardique, l'épuisement des phosphates tissulaires à haute énergie, une libération massive de constituants cellulaires et une détérioration ultrastructurale étendue. On peut considérer le paradoxe de calcium comme étant la manifestation la plus sévère de la nécrose myocardique susceptible de se produire sur le plan expérimental.

Dans les conditions expérimentales décrites dans cette étude, les bloqueurs de l'entrée de calcium vérapamil, nifédipine, diltiazem et lidoflazine ont échoué à réduire la libération massive des enzymes se produisant sous la forme sévère du paradoxe de calcium.

Les bloqueurs de l'entrée de calcium ont un effet protecteur dans la manifestation modérée du paradoxe de calcium. Ceci est important pour la chirurgie cardiaque pour laquelle des solutions cardioplégiques exemptes de calcium sont utilisées. Les bloqueurs de l'entrée de calcium peuvent diminuer le hasard potentiel de l'utilisation de ces solutions.

Resumen

La reperfusión de corazones aislados con una solución de concentración normal de calcio, después de un breve período de perfusión sin calcio, produce un perjuicio irremediable de la célula (paradoja del calcio). Este fenómeno se caracteriza por una penetración excesiva de calcio en las células, una aparición rápida de una contractura miocárdica, un agotamiento de los fosfatos de alta energía en el tejido, una liberación masiva de componentes celulares y un notable perjuicio ultra-estructural. La paradoja del calcio puede ser considerada como la forma más severa de necrosis miocárdica que puede producirse experimentalmente.

Bajo las condiciones experimentales descritas en este estudio, los inhibidores de la penetración intracelular de calcio verapamilo, nifedipino, diltiazem y lidoflazina no lograron disminuir el masivo escape de enzimas que ocurre en la forma severa de la paradoja del calcio. Estos inhibidores, sin embargo, pueden moderar los acontecimientos que ocurren durante el desarrollo de la paradoja del calcio y pueden tener un efecto protector en forma ligera contra la paradoja del calcio.

Esto es de interés para la cirugía cardíaca en la cual se usan frecuentemente soluciones cardioplégicas sin calcio. Los inhibidores de la penetración intracelular pueden disminuir los riesgos potenciales del uso de estas soluciones.

Zusammenfassung

Werden isolierte Herzen nach einer kurzen Periode kalziumfreier Perfusion von einer kalziumhaltigen Lösung durchströmt, so entstehen irreversible Zellschäden. Bei diesem Phänomen sind ein übermässiger Kalziumeinstrom in die Zellen, ein schnelles Einsetzen der Myokardkontraktion, eine Erschöpfung der energiereichen Gewebephosphate, ein massives Freiwerden von Zellbestandteilen, und umfangreiche ultrastrukturelle Schäden zu beobachten. Das Kalziumparadoxon kann als die schwerste Form experimentell hervorgerufener Myokardnekrose betrachtet werden.

Bei den hier beschriebenen experimentellen Umständen waren die Kalziumeintritthemmer Verapamil, Nifedipin, Diltiazem und Lidoflazin nicht imstande, die bei einer schweren Form des Kalziumparadoxon hervorgerufene massive Freisetzung von Enzymen zu vermindern. Sie können jedoch den Zeitverlauf der Ereignisse, die bei der Entwicklung des Kalziumparadoxon auftreten, beeinflussen.

Kalziumeintritthemmer können bei einer leichten Form des Kalziumparadoxon eine schützende Wirkung haben. Dies ist bei Herzchirurgie von Bedeutung, wo kalziumfreie Lösungen vielfach zur Kardioplegie gebraucht werden. Kalziumeintritthemmer können das mögliche Risiko einer Anwendung dieser Lösungen herabsetzen.

Introduction

Coronary perfusion with a calcium-free solution results in the development of an electromechanical dissociation (Mines, 1913), but may in addition lead to an increase of the sarcolemmal permeability to calcium (Frank *et al.*, 1977). As a consequence, reperfusion of the heart with calcium-containing solution results in a massive influx of calcium into the cells, followed by exhaustion of tissue high-energy phosphates, the rapid onset of myocardial contracture, massive release of cell constituents, and extensive ultrastructural damage (Zimmerman *et al.*, 1967; Boink *et al.*, 1976; Hearse *et al.*, 1978). This phenomenon was first described by Zimmerman and Hülsmann (1966) and termed the calcium paradox.

In an attempt to reduce the damaging effect of sequential perfusion with calcium-free and calcium-containing medium, calcium entry blockers (verapamil, nifedipine, diltiazem or lidoflazine) were added to the perfusion fluids. Cell damage was quantitated in terms of enzyme leakage, depletion of high-energy phosphates, and ultrastructural damage.

Materials and methods

Perfusion Technique

Male Wistar rats of 200-250 g were anesthetized with diethyl ether. The rats were heparinized and the hearts quickly removed and subsequently perfused at 37°C by the Langendorff technique (1895) at a constant pressure of 10.0 kPa (75 mm Hg). The standard perfusate had the following composition (mmol $.l^{-1}$): NaCl, 124; KCl, 4.7; $CaCl_2$, 1.3; $MgCl_2$, 1.0; $NaHCO_3$, 24.0; Na_2HPO_4, 0.5; glucose, 11.0. During calcium-free perfusion, calcium was omitted from the standard medium; no correction was made for the small change of osmolarity. After equilibration of the perfusion fluids with 95% O_2 - 5% CO_2, the pH was 7.40 ± 0.05.

After a 15 minute stabilization period, during which the hearts were perfused with calcium-containing standard medium, the perfusion was changed to the calcium-free solution. After 4 or 10 minutes of calcium-free perfusion, the hearts were reperfused with the calcium-containing solution. The concentration of the calcium entry blockers verapamil, nifedipine, diltiazem and lidoflazine in the perfusion fluids amounted to 1 mg $.l^{-1}$.

Analytical Procedures

Samples of the effluent medium were collected and analyzed for creatine kinase (CK) activity. CK activity was assayed with the use of a Vitatron Automatic Kinetic Enzyme System (AKES) at 25°C. Enzyme activity was expressed in IU released $.15$ $min^{-1}.g^{-1}$ dry heart tissue (± SD).

127

The perfusion of hearts on which creatine phosphate (CP) and adenosine triphosphate (ATP) determinations were to be made, was terminated by freezing the hearts between large aluminium tongs, precooled in liquid nitrogen. The frozen tissue was assayed for CP and ATP as previously described (Boink et al., 1976). Myocardial CP and ATP content was expressed in μmol .g^{-1} dry weight ($\pm$ SD).

The Student t test was used in Table 1 and Figure 1, taking P = 0.05 as the limit of significance.

Electron Microscopy

Control hearts were perfused for 15 minutes with standard medium and then perfusion-fixed with 4% glutaraldehyde prepared in 0.2 mol . l^{-1} sodium cacodylate buffer (pH 7.3). Other hearts were perfused with calcium-free solution for 4 minutes, reperfused with calcium-containing solution for either 30 seconds or 30 minutes, with or without verapamil, and subsequently perfusion-fixed. After 10 minutes of glutaraldehyde perfusion, the hearts were removed from the Langendorff apparatus, and biopsy specimens of the left ventricle free wall were excised and cut into 1 mm^3 cubes. These were immersion-fixed in the glutaraldehyde solution for 2 hours, then postfixed for 2 hours in 1% OsO_4. Samples were then stained en bloc with uranyl acetate, dehydrated and embedded in epoxy resin. Sections were examined in a Philips 301 electron microscope. Morphometric analysis of the micrographs was carried out as previously described (Ruigrok et al., 1980).

Results

Effect of calcium entry blockers on the release of CK during reperfusion

During the stabilization period and the subsequent 10 minute period of perfusion with calcium-free solution, the hearts released negligible amounts of CK into the coronary effluent. Reintroduction of calcium in the perfusion fluid resulted in massive release of CK (Table 1).

Table 1: Effect of verapamil, nifedipine, diltiazem, and lidoflazine (1 mg .l^{-1}) on the calcium paradox in isolated rat hearts.

Experiment	CK release (IU . 15 min^{-1} . g^{-1} dry wt) during reperfusion
Untreated	2065 $\pm$ 250
Verapamil	2135 $\pm$ 185 NS
Nifedipine	2255 $\pm$ 195 NS
Diltiazem	2270 $\pm$ 160 NS
Lidoflazine	2265 $\pm$ 70 NS

The hearts were perfused for 15 minutes at 37°C with calcium-containing solution, followed by 10 minutes of calcium-free perfusion and 15 minutes of reperfusion with calcium-containing solution. In the treated hearts, the drug was present throughout the entire perfusion. Results are expressed as mean $\pm$ SD (n = 6). NS: not significantly different from the untreated hearts.

The presence of verapamil, nifedipine, diltiazem or lidoflazine (1 mg .l⁻¹) throughout the entire experiment had no significant effect on the calcium-induced release of CK. Enzyme activity was measured in the coronary effluent collected during the first 15 minutes of reperfusion with calcium-containing solution.

In a previous investigation (Ruigrok *et al.*, 1980) the effect of 1 mg .l⁻¹ verapamil, which was present during 4 minutes of calcium-free perfusion and the reperfusion phase, was studied. CK release was measured in samples of the coronary effluent collected during 30 seconds or 1 minute at timed intervals. The enzyme release pattern in the verapamil-treated hearts was not significantly different from that in the untreated hearts. In another study (Boink *et al.*, 1980) it was shown that 4 minutes of calcium-free perfusion at 37°C was sufficient to obtain maximal CK release upon reperfusion with calcium-containing solution.

Effect of verapamil on the depletion of tissue CP and ATP stores during reperfusion

At the end of the stabilization period myocardial CP and ATP stores amounted to 29.6 ± 2.1 and 18.8 ± 0.8 μmol. g⁻¹ dry weight, respectively (Figure 1).

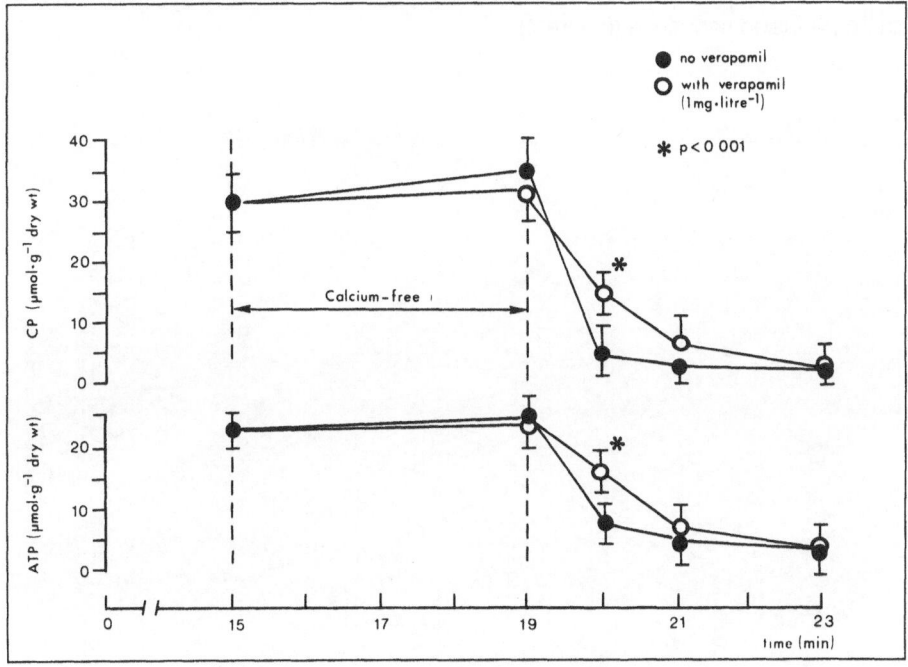

Figure 1: Effect of verapamil (1 mg . l⁻¹) on the depletion of myocardial CP and ATP stores, induced by reperfusion with calcium after a calcium-free period of 4 minutes. When verapamil was present, it was added to the calcium-free medium and the reperfusion medium. Values are given as mean ± SD (n = 4). Tests of significance relate to the significance of the difference between CP and ATP levels in hearts perfused in the presence and absence of verapamil. In certain cases, for the purpose of clarity, only one SD bar has been given. Reprinted with permission from The American Journal of Pathology **98**, 769-790 (1980).

Subsequent calcium-free perfusion for 4 minutes resulted in a slight increase in the endogenous stores of CP and ATP, irrespective of whether verapamil was present. During the first minute of reperfusion with calcium, myocardial CP fell from 35.6 ± 2.9 to 4.6 ± 3.2 μmol. g^{-1} dry weight in the absence of verapamil, and from 33.1 ± 2.6 to 15.0 ± 2.2 μmol . g^{-1} dry weight in the presence of verapamil (P < 0.001). In the same period myocardial ATP fell from 20.8 ± 1.4 to 6.3 ± 2.7 μmol . g^{-1} dry weight in the absence of verapamil, and from 20.6 ± 1.5 to 13.2 ± 1.2 μmol . g^{-1} dry weight in the presence of verapamil (P < 0.001). Figure 1 shows that although the rate of consumption of the tissue stores of ATP and CP during reperfusion was slower in the verapamil-treated than in the untreated hearts, after 4 minutes of reperfusion there was no difference between the ATP and CP content of treated and untreated hearts.

Effect of verapamil on the ultrastructure during reperfusion

At the end of the 15 minute stabilization period of perfusion with standard medium, the ultrastructure of the hearts was normal (Figure 2). Morphometric analysis showed that the mean sarcomere length amounted to 2.18 μ. After a subsequent calcium-free period of 4 minutes, followed by 30 seconds of reperfusion with calcium-containing solution, most cells showed contracted myofibrils and contraction bands (Figure 3). Many cells of the verapamil-treated hearts, however, contained relaxed myofibrils after the same perfusion sequence (Figure 4).

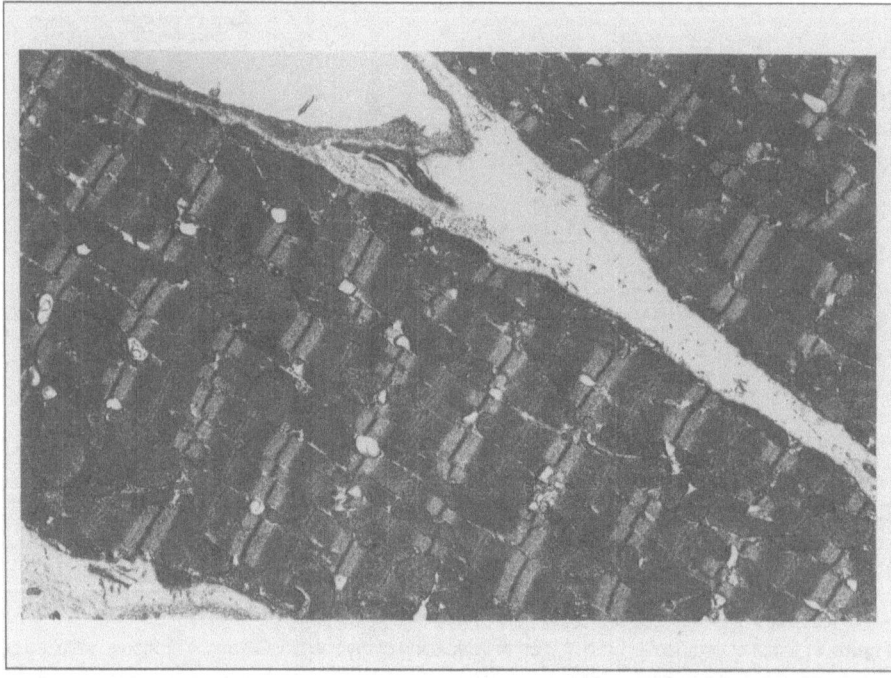

Figure 2: Control heart perfused for 15 minutes with standard medium. The heart has the appearance of normal myocardium. Myofibrils are in register and mitochondria have an electron-opaque matrix (x 7500).

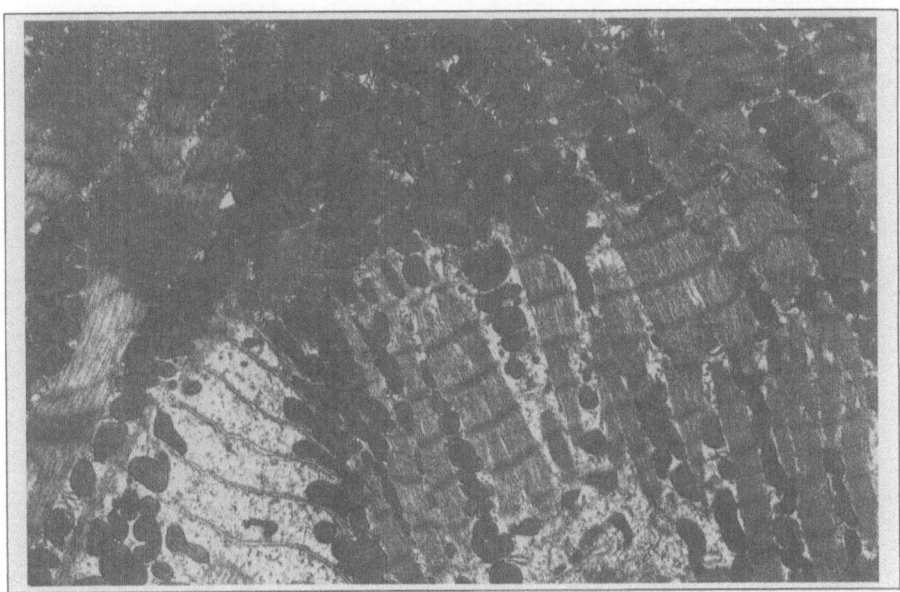

Figure 3: Heart perfused for 15 minutes with standard medium, followed by 4 minutes of calcium-free perfusion and 30 seconds of reperfusion with calcium-containing medium. This figure shows contracted myofibrils and contraction bands. The mitochondria have an electron-opaque matrix (x 7500).

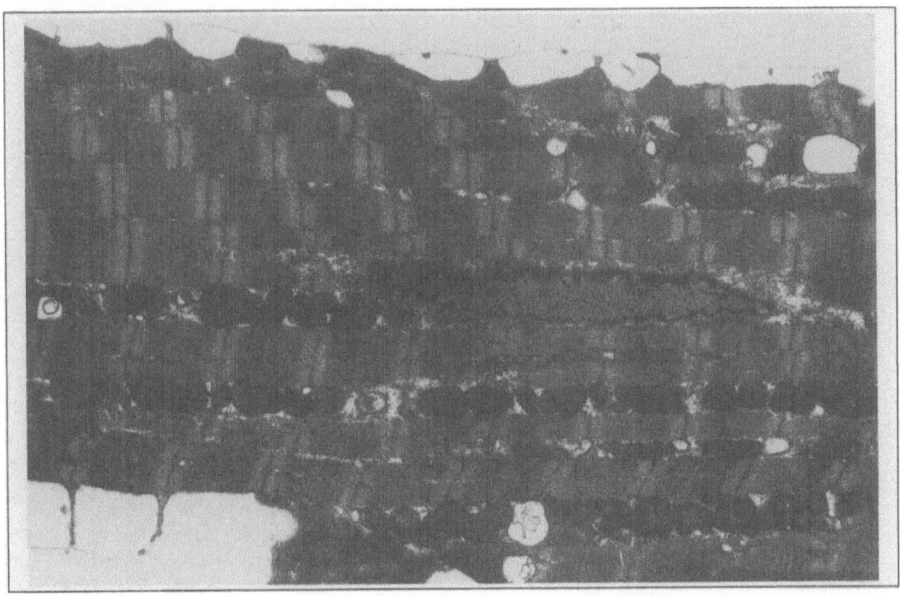

Figure 4: Heart perfused for 15 minutes with standard medium, followed by 4 minutes of calcium-free perfusion and 30 seconds of reperfusion with calcium-containing medium. The calcium-free medium and the reperfusion medium contained 1 mg . l⁻¹ verapamil. Myofibrils are relaxed and mitochondria have an electron-opaque matrix. This micrograph shows a separation of the basement membrane and formation of blebs (x 7500).

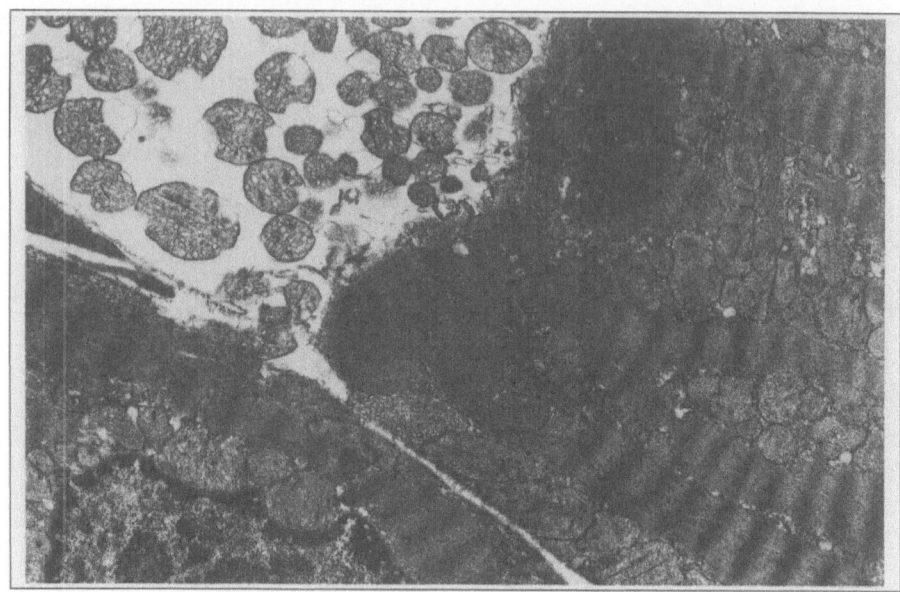

Figure 5: Heart perfused for 15 minutes with standard medium, followed by 4 minutes of calcium-free perfusion and 30 minutes of reperfusion with calcium-containing medium. Myofibrils are heavily contracted; mitochondria are swollen and contain electron-dense deposits (x 7500).

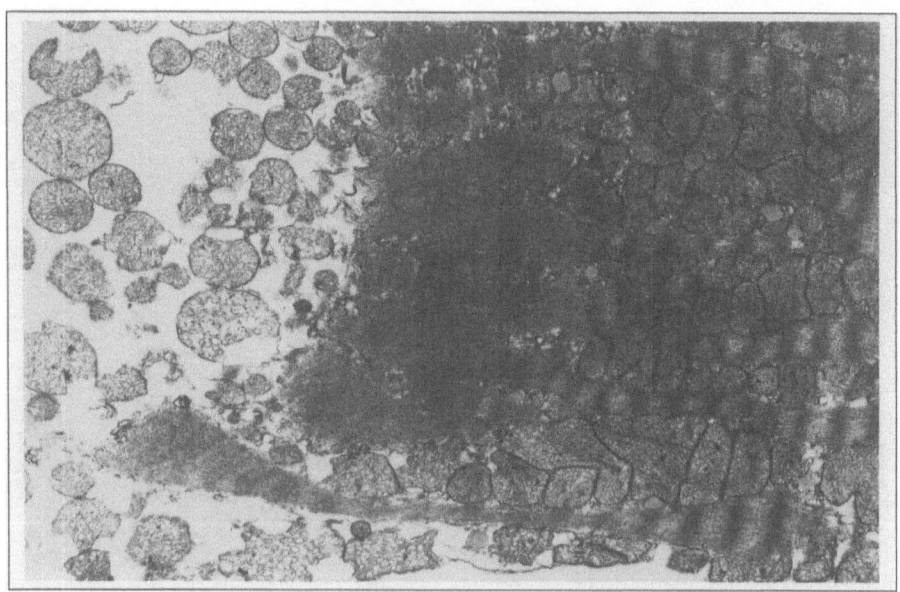

Figure 6: Heart perfused for 15 minutes with standard medium, followed by 4 minutes of calcium-free perfusion and 30 minutes of reperfusion with calcium-containing medium. The calcium-free medium and the reperfusion medium contained 1 mg . l⁻¹ verapamil. This cell shows severe contracture of the myofibrils. The mitochondria are swollen and contain electron-dense material (x 7500).

The untreated series appeared to have a mean sarcomere length of 1.08 μ, whereas the verapamil-treated series had a mean sarcomere length of 1.33 μ. This difference was significant (P < 0.001). After 30 minutes of reperfusion with calcium-containing solution the hearts all showed evidence of extensive damage, irrespective of whether verapamil had been added (Figure 5 and 6). Every field showed gross tissue damage and severe contracture, and no quantitative analysis was undertaken.

Discussion

During calcium-free perfusion the myocardial cell membrane is altered in such a way that reperfusion with calcium-containing solution leads to a net gain in tissue calcium. The possible routes of calcium entry that occurs during the phase of calcium repletion have recently been reviewed (Grinwald and Nayler, 1981). These routes included the glycocalyx, the slow channels, the Na^+-Ca^{2+} and K^+-Ca^{2+} exchange mechanisms, passive diffusion, and abnormal sites of calcium entry (e.g. damaged areas of the inter-calated discs, and distorted ion selective channels). The present results (Table 1) show that under our experimental conditions the calcium entry blockers verapamil, nifedi-pine, diltiazem and lidoflazine did not reduce the massive enzyme release, which is one of the characteristics of the calcium paradox. Moreover, Alto and Dhalla (1979) and Nayler and Grinwald (1981) demonstrated that verapamil and D600 did not pre-vent the massive gain in calcium that occurs during the calcium paradox.

Our enzyme release data contrast with the results of Hearse and co-workers (Hearse, Baker and Humphrey, 1980; Hearse and Baker, 1981; Baker and Hearse, 1981), who reported that the calcium entry blockers nifedipine, verapamil, D600, diltiazem, terodi-line and fendiline were able to reduce protein leakage by up to one third. There is growing evidence that calcium entry blockers may be protective in a submaximal or mild form of the calcium paradox. Van Belle et al. (1982) demonstrated that lidoflazine had a protective effect in a submaximal calcium paradox, which was induced by successive perfusion with 15 μmol .l[-1] calcium for 5 minutes, and reperfusion with 1.25 mmol .l[-1] calcium. Ohhara, Kanaide and Nakamura (1982) investigated the effect of verapamil on severe and mild forms of the calcium paradox. Verapamil did not in-fluence the severe calcium paradox, but had a marked protective effect on the mild calcium paradox. The mild paradox was produced by reducing the coronary flow rate during the calcium-free period. These findings may be of interest for cardiac surgery where cold calcium-free cardioplegic solutions are widely used to induce cardiac ar-rest. It has been claimed (Tyers, 1975; Jynge, Hearse and Braimbridge, 1977) that the use of these solutions may adversely affect membrane permeability and integrity, and may predispose the heart to some form of the calcium paradox. It is worth noting that Ashraf et al. (1982) found a complete inhibition of the calcium paradox injury by a com-bination of diltiazem treatment and hypothermia.

Although our results show that calcium entry blockers do not protect rat hearts against the severe form of the calcium paradox, the time course of the events that occur during the development of the paradox may be altered. Verapamil had an energy-sparing effect (Figure 1) and reduced the decrease of the mean sarcomere length (Figures 3 and 4) during the first few minutes of reperfusion. A reduction of the rate of calcium entry during the early phase of calcium repletion may be responsible for these effects.

Acknowledgment

The authors are grateful to Dr. C. Borst for his constructive criticism.

References

Alto, L.E. and Dhalla, N.S. Myocardial cation contents during induction of calcium paradox. *Am. J. Physiol.*, **237**, H713 (1979).

Ashraf, M., Onda, M., Benedict, J.B. and Millard, R.W. Prevention of calcium paradox-related myocardial cell injury with diltiazem, a calcium channel blocking agent. *Am. J. Cardiol.*, **49**, 1675 (1982).

Baker, J.E. and Hearse, D.J. A comparison of the ability of slow channel calcium blockers to reduce tissue damage during the calcium paradox in the rat heart. *J. Mol. Cell. Cardiol.*, **13** (Suppl. 1), 6 (1981).

Boink, A.B.T.J., Ruigrok, T.J.C., Maas, A.H.J. and Zimmerman, A.N.E. Changes in high-energy phosphate compounds of isolated rat hearts during Ca^{2+}-free perfusion and reperfusion with Ca^{2+}. *J. Mol. Cell. Cardiol.*, **8**, 973 (1976).

Boink, A.B.T.J., Ruigrok, T.J.C., De Moes, D., Maas, A.H.J. and Zimmerman, A.N.E. The effect of hypothermia on the occurrence of the calcium paradox. *Pfluegers Arch.*, **385**, 105 (1980).

Frank, J.S., Langer, G.A., Nudd, L.M. and Seraydarian, K. The myocardial cell surface, its histochemistry, and the effect of sialic acid and calcium removal on its structure and cellular ionic exchange. *Circ. Res.*, **41**, 702 (1977).

Grinwald, P.M. and Nayler, W.G. Calcium entry in the calcium paradox. *J. Mol. Cell. Cardiol.*, **13**, 867 (1981).

Hearse, D.J. and Baker, J.E. Verapamil and the calcium paradox: a reaffirmation. *J. Mol. Cell. Cardiol.*, **13**, 1087 (1981).

Hearse, D.J., Baker, J.E. and Humphrey, S.M. Verapamil and the calcium paradox. *J. Mol. Cell. Cardiol.*, **12**, 733 (1980).

Hearse, D.J., Humphrey, S.M., Boink, A.B.T.J. and Ruigrok, T.J.C. The calcium paradox: metabolic, electrophysiological, contractile and ultrastructural characteristics in four species. *Eur. J. Cardiol.*, **7**, 241 (1978).

Jynge, P., Hearse, D.J. and Braimbridge, M.V. Myocardial protection during ischemic cardiac arrest; a possible hazard with calcium-free cardioplegic infusates. *J. Thorac. Cardiovasc. Surg.*, **73**, 846 (1977).

Langendorff, O. Untersuchungen am überlebenden Säugetierherzen. *Pfluegers Arch.*, **61**, 291 (1895).

Mines, G.R. On functional analysis by the action of electrolytes. *J. Physiol.* (London), **46**, 188 (1913).

Nayler, W.G. and Grinwald, P.M. The effect of verapamil on calcium accumulation during the calcium paradox. *J. Mol. Cell. Cardiol.*, **13**, 435 (1981).

Ohhara, H., Kanaide, H. and Nakamura, M. A protective effect of verapamil on the calcium paradox in the isolated perfused rat heart. *J. Mol. Cell. Cardiol.*, **14**, 13 (1982).

Ruigrok, T.J.C., Boink, A.B.T.J., Slade, A., Zimmerman, A.N.E., Meijler, F.L. and Nayler, W.G. The effect of verapamil on the calcium paradox. *Am. J. Pathol.*, **98**, 769 (1980).

Tyers, G.F.O. Metabolic arrest of the heart. *Ann. Thorac. Surg.*, **20**, 91 (1975).

Van Belle, H., Xhonneux, R., Borgers, M. and Flameng, W. Cardioprotective effect of adenosine, lidoflazine and R 51 469. International Symposium on Adenosine, Charlottesville (USA) (1982).

Zimmerman, A.N.E. and Hülsmann, W.C. Paradoxical influence of calcium ions on the permeability of the cell membranes of the isolated rat heart. *Nature* (London), **211**, 646 (1966).

Zimmerman, A.N.E., Daems, W., Hülsmann, W.C., Snijder, J., Wisse, E. and Durrer, D. Morphological changes of heart muscle caused by successive perfusion with calcium-free and calcium-containing solutions (calcium paradox). *Cardiovasc. Res.*, **1**, 201 (1967).

Myocardial oxygen deprivation and calcium deprivation: ultrastructural characteristics and clinical significance

G.R. Bullock, D.J. Hearse

Summary

This contribution defines the ultrastructural characteristics of two very different conditions which can both lead to very extensive, and in some ways rather similar, myocardial injury. The two conditions are oxygen depletion and repletion and calcium depletion and repletion. Both conditions are of clinical relevance and both have been studied extensively in the laboratory, revealing in the process a great deal of valuable information about cellular injury and its prevention.

Résumé

Cette contribution définit les caractéristiques ultrastructurales de deux situations très différentes qui toutes deux peuvent conduire à des lésions du myocarde très étendues et d'une certaine manière, assez semblables. Ces deux situations sont l'épuisement et la réplétion d'oxygène et l'épuisement et la réplétion de calcium. Ces deux situations sont intéressantes sur le plan clinique et toutes deux ont été étudiées longuement en laboratoire, processus au cours duquel elles ont révélé bon nombre d'informations précieuses au sujet de la lésion cellulaire et de la prévention de celle-ci.

Resumen

Esta contribución define los característicos ultraestructurales de dos condiciones muy distintas que pueden conducir ambas a una lesión miocardíaca muy importante y, en algunos casos, bastante similar. Las dos condiciones son agotamiento y saturación de oxígeno y agotamiento y saturación de calcio. Ambas condiciones son de valor clínico y han sido objeto de estudios exhaustivos en el laboratorio, revelando en el proceso gran cantidad de información valiosa en cuanto a lesiones celulares y su prevención.

Zusammenfassung

Dieser Beitrag definiert die ultrastrukturellen Charakteristika zweier äusserst verschiedener Zustände, die beide zu umfangreichen, und in bestimmter Hinsicht ähnlichen Myokardschäden führen können. Diese zwei Zustände sind Sauerstoffmangel bzw. -übersättigung und Kalziummangel bzw. -übersättigung. Beide sind klinisch wichtig, und ihre ausführliche Untersuchung im Labor hat eine Fülle wertvoller Informationen über Zellschäden und deren Vorbeugung erbracht.

1. Clinical significance

(i) Oxygen Deprivation

Myocardial oxygen deprivation can arise as a consequence of an impairment or a cessation of coronary flow (ischaemia) or a reduction in the PO_2 of the coronary blood (hypoxia). Regional or localised ischaemia may arise as a consequence of a variety of circumstances such as severe coronary artery narrowing or occlusion with a thrombus. In both instances a complex sequence of progressively more severe cellular events is initiated (Hearse and De Leiris, 1979) which unless rapidly treated will result in cell death and tissue necrosis — the whole process being myocardial infarction. Global or whole heart ischaemia occurs during cardiac surgery when the coronary blood supply may be halted for several hours (Hearse *et al.*, 1981) — again unless appropriate preventative steps are taken, cell death may result. It is important to appreciate that with both regional and global ischaemia the reduction of coronary flow not only limits oxygen and substrate supply to the myocardium, but also reduces the removal of toxic metabolic products such as carbon dioxide and lactate.

This contrasts with hypoxia where coronary flow and hence substrate delivery and metabolite removal may remain normal or may even be elevated. It therefore follows that the metabolic characteristics and cellular consequences of hypoxia and ischaemia are different. Although less frequently encountered clinically, myocardial hypoxia may occur under a variety of circumstances, for example at high altitude, during respiratory arrest or with pulmonary embolism. Both hypoxia and ischaemia can be mimicked in a variety of *in vivo, ex vivo* and *in vitro* experimental models (Hearse *et al.*, 1981).

(ii) Calcium depletion

Reduction of extracellular calcium can be achieved through the addition of various specific chelating agents to the blood. However, the clinical situation of most interest relates to the use of calcium-free aqueous cardioplegic solutions during cardiac surgery. At the present time myocardial injury during cardiac surgery, arising as a consequence of the necessary induction of global ischaemia, is minimised by the intermittent coronary infusion of cold (4°C-20°C) cardioplegic solutions. These solutions are designed to cool and protect the heart and also maintain a state of diastolic arrest (Hearse *et al.*, 1981). A number of solutions in clinical use (Bretschneider *et al.*, 1975) are devoid of calcium and their use has been strongly criticised (Hearse *et al.*, 1981; Jynge *et al.*, 1977) because of the possibility of the induction of a calcium paradox (Zimmerman and Hulsmann, 1966; Zimmerman *et al.*, 1967; Hearse *et al.*, 1978).

(iii) Oxygen repletion

Reperfusion after ischaemia occurs under a number of pathological and clinical circumstances such as after the relief of coronary spasm, during reperfusion after cardiac surgery and following thrombolysis and coronary artery surgery. Reoxygenation after hypoxia may be seen after the treatment of respiratory arrest or during hyperbaric or oxygen therapy. Interest in reperfusion and reoxygenation has arisen as a result of many experimental studies, demonstrating that under certain circumstances these apparently desirable events may cause an apparent exacerbation of injury induced by the preceding period of ischaemia or hypoxia (Hearse *et al.*, 1978; Hearse, 1977).

(iv) Calcium repletion

This may occur clinically during reperfusion following cardioplegia with calcium-free solutions. Numerous experimental studies have shown that brief periods of complete calcium depletion (as little as 3 minutes) followed by calcium repletion, can result in massive myocardial injury — the so-called calcium paradox (Zimmerman and Hulsmann, 1966, Zimmerman *et al.*, 1967, Hearse *et al.*, 1978). Injury of this nature may have been responsible for deaths during cardiac surgery where "stone heart" conditions were observed (Cooley *et al.*, 1972; Katz and Tada, 1972; Hearse *et al.*, 1977).

2. Oxygen and calcium depletion and repletion — a common link?

Although very different in their origins, tissue injury associated with the "oxygen paradox" (Hearse *et al.*, 1978) is in many ways similar to that seen with the calcium paradox, and certain common processes have been implicated (Hearse *et al.*, 1978) in the development of injury. Intracellular calcium overload is thought to be of primary importance in the overall injury process. In the following section some of the ultrastructural characteristics of these processes will be compared and contrasted.

3. Ultrastructural changes

(i) Hypoxia and ischaemia

The first phase of ischaemia is associated with intracellular oedema and loss of glycogen, the subendocardial region being most affected. The response is heterogeneous

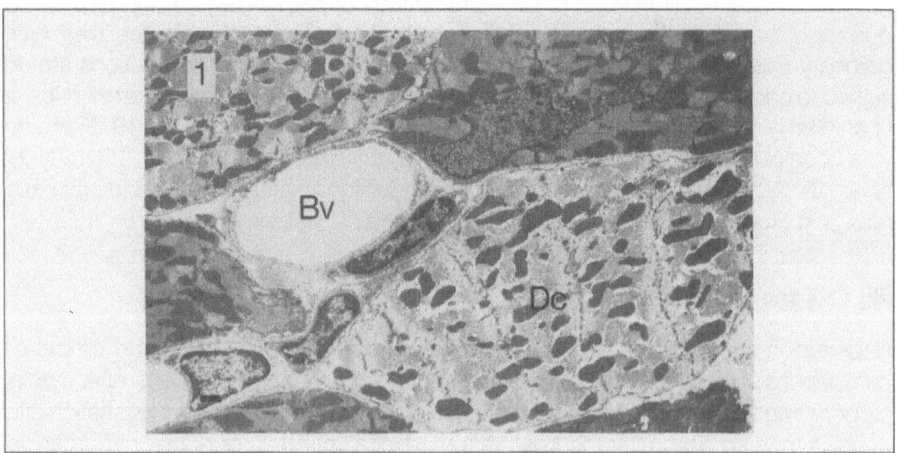

Figure 1: Micrograph illustrating the heteregeneous nature of the response to hypoxia. DC = damaged cell. BV = blood vessel./Bar = 1 μm (micron) unless otherwise stated.

138

(see Fig. 1) with some cells affected much earlier than others, the relatively undamaged cells being those which can still be salvaged. After 1 hour, protein coagulation occurs, seen as thickening of the striations or Z bands, and contraction of the muscle cells also takes place. A feature of interest is the integrity of the intercalated discs which remain patent until gross tissue damage has taken place (Fig. 2).

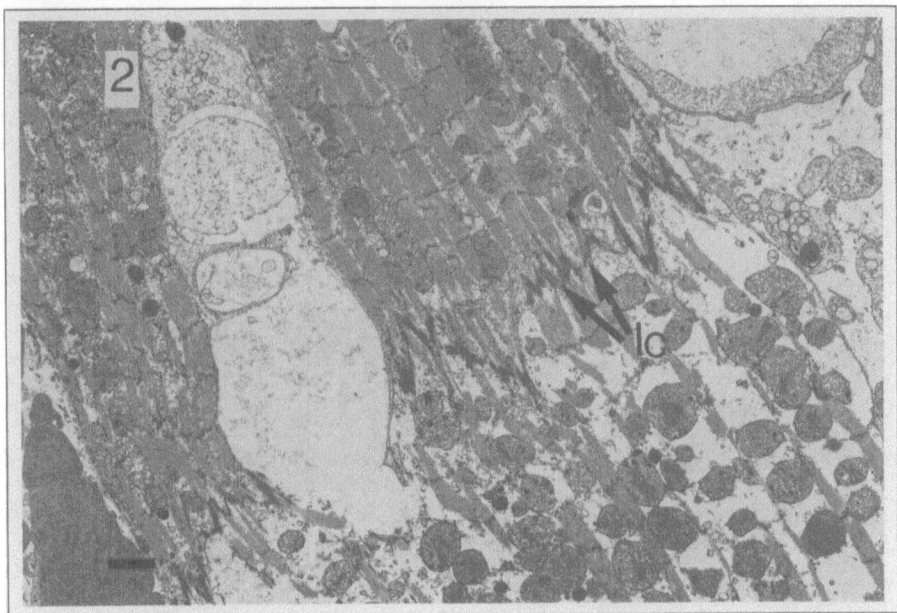

Figure 2: A badly damaged cell adjacent to a partially damaged cell. The intercalated disc (IC) is clearly intact.

The mitochondria swell at first losing their normal granules and after 2-3 hours, so-called "ischaemic granules" can be seen within them (Fig. 3). The muscle cell membrane (sarcolemma) stays visibly intact for a long period, but eventually breaks can be seen, again associated with marked tissue damage. In human material separation of the outer layers of the membrane from the inner layers has been described (Flameng *et al.*, 1982), suggesting changes in permeability of these cells which could be associated with loss of metabolic integrity.

(ii) Calcium depletion

Tissue response to calcium depletion induced by "zero" calcium perfusion is very rapid ((3-5 minutes). However, the changes are very specific with the bulk of the myocardial cell appearing to be unaffected and relaxed. The heterogeneous response seen during hypoxia is only found when hypothermic protection (29-32°C) is introduced (Baker *et al.*, 1983).

One very significant change is that seen in the intercalated discs. Here the junction between two cells which provides both electrical and ionic contact becomes loosened by the loss of calcium and cell shrinkage giving vesiculation and loss of electron opacity

139

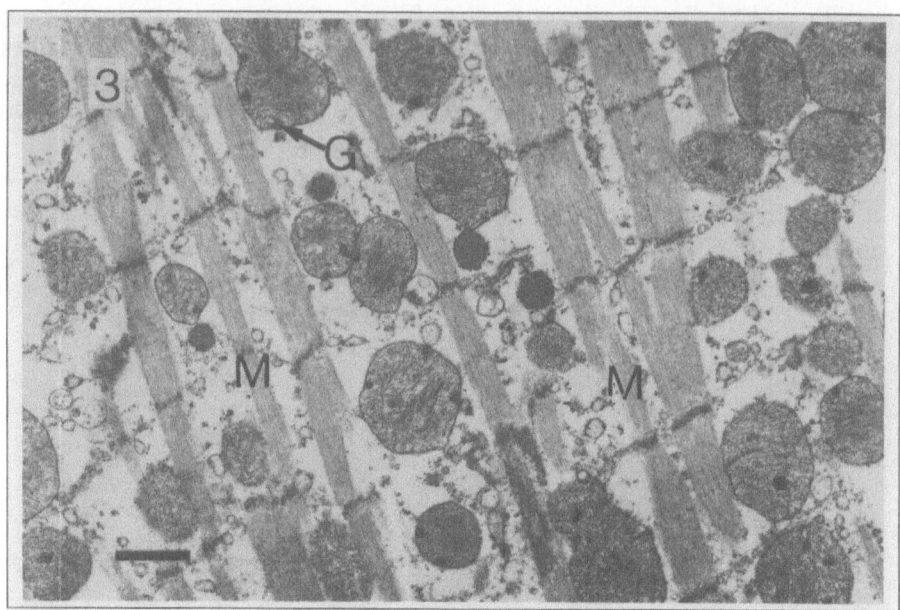

Figure 3: A badly damaged cell containing swollen mitochondria with ischaemic granules (G). Most of the cytoplasm is lost and the myofibrils (M) show evidence of thinning.

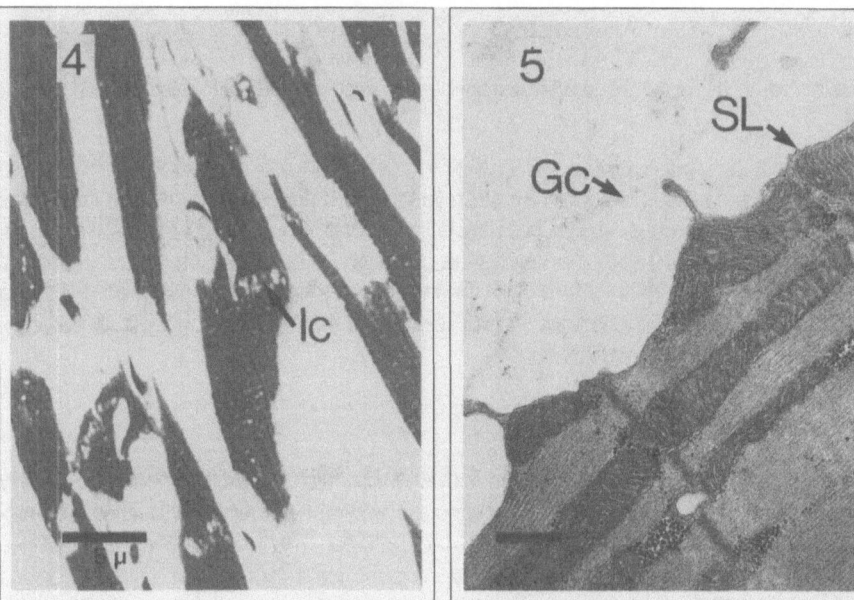

Figure 4: Light micrograph showing vesiculation and partial separation of the intercalated discs (IC). Cells somewhat shrunken with intercellular oedema.

Figure 5: Electron micrograph of a calcium depleted cell showing separation of the outer layers of the glycocalyx (GC) from the inner layers and sarcolemma (SL).

140

(Fig. 4). The second change is seen in the sarcolemma where separation of the outer layers of the glycocalyx from the inner layers and true membrane is a consistent feature (Fig. 5).

(iii) Reoxygenation and reperfusion

With restoration of oxygen and flow to heart cells, the ultrastructural changes are dependent on the length of the ischaemic or hypoxic period. The earlier phases of mitochondrial swelling and intracellular oedema are largely reversible emphasising the necessity of restoring oxygen as rapidly as possible following ischaemia. However, once a critical point has been passed, the damage becomes irreversible and widespread with contracted, leaking cells containing swollen mitochondria and mitochondrial ischaemic granules. The myofibrillar organisation breaks down and is beyond recovery.

It has been shown by using both ultrastructural and histochemical techniques that reperfusion is beneficial for reversibly injured tissue but it accelerates the decay of irreversibly-injured tissue. (Schaper and Schaper, 1983)

(iv) Calcium repletion

At the end of a period of calcium deprivation at 37°C, restoration of calcium (2.4 mM) causes a very marked change in cardiac ultrastructure. This is seen as massive contracture of the cells accompanied by total disruption of the intercalated discs and extrusion of the mitochondria (Fig. 6).

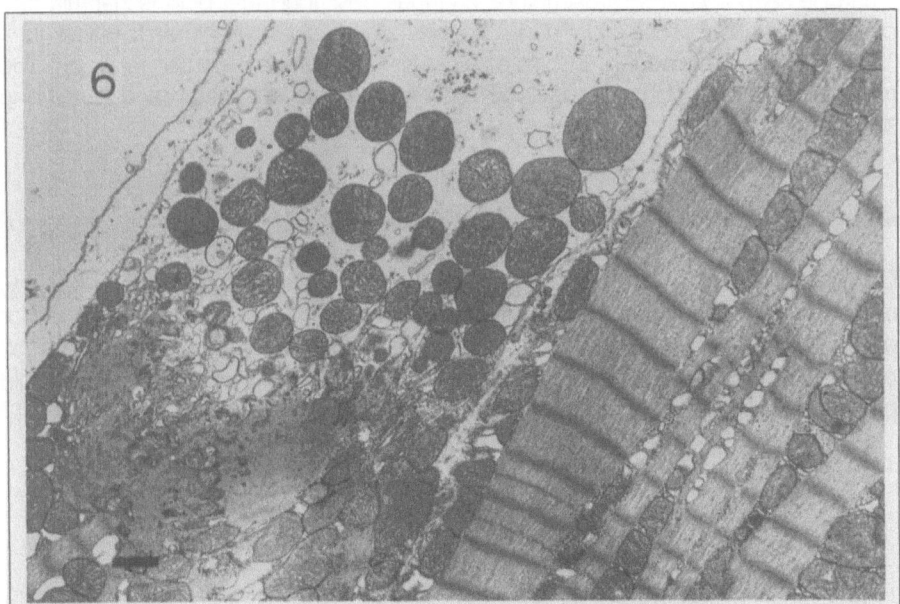

Figure 6: End of a cardiac cell in contracture showing extrusion of mitochondria and some cytoplasmic contents.

141

An interesting feature of the prevention of damage by hypothermia is that it is an all or none effect in that a cell will either go into contracture and lose cell contents or remain structurally apparently normal (Fig. 7).

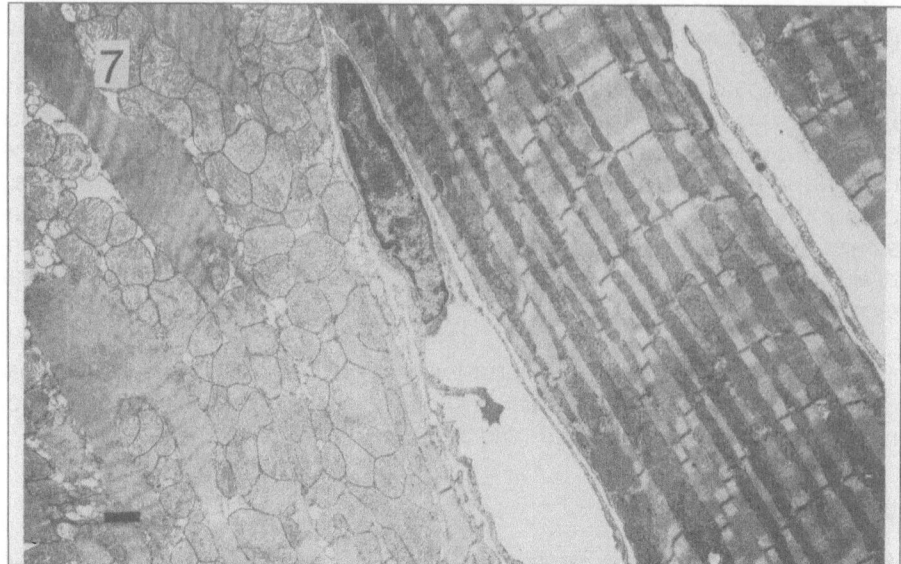

Figure 7: Heterogeneous response to calcium repletion seen when the temperature of the calcium-free period is reduced to 29°C. A "normal" cell lies adjacent to a damaged cell.

It can be seen from the ultrastructural changes described that both ischaemia and calcium depletion cause significant changes during these treatments which then "allow" the development of the damage seen during reperfusion or repletion. The mechanisms may not be identical, but the effect on the cell membrane has strong similarities.

4. Concluding comments

Despite a growing body of knowledge concerning various types of cellular injury, much remains to be learnt, particularly in relation to the development of methods for preventing or slowing the development of injury. In the cases of the oxygen paradox and the calcium paradox, the possible clinical relevance of these conditions should provide great stimulus for further investigation.

References

Baker, J.E., Bullock, G.R. and Hearse, D.J. The temperature dependence of the calcium paradox: enzymatic, functional and morphological correlates of cellular injury. *J. Molecular & Cellular Cardiology* (In press) (1983).

Bretschneider, H.J., Hubner, G., Knoll, D., Lohr, B., Nordbeck, H. and Spieckermann, P.G. Myocardial resistance and tolerance to ischemia: physiological and biochemical basis. *J. Cardiovascular Surg.*, **16**, 241-260 (1975).

Cooley, D.A., Reul, G.J. and Wukasch, D.C. Ischemic contracture of the heart: "Stone heart". *Am. J. Cardiol.*, **29**, 575-577 (1972).

Flameng, W., Xhonneux, R. and Borgers, M. Myocardial protection in open-heart surgery. In: Protection of tissues against hypoxia, pp. 403-416. Eds. Wauquier, A., Borgers, M. and Amery, W.K., Elsevier Biomedical Press, Amsterdam, New York, Oxford (1982).

Hearse, D.J., Braimbridge, M.V. and Jynge, P. Protection of the ischemic myocardium: cardioplegia. Raven Press, New York (1981).

Hearse, D.J., Garlick, P.B. and Humphrey, S.M. Ischemic contracture of the myocardium: mechanisms and prevention. *Am. J. Cardiol.*, **39**, 986-993 (1977).

Hearse, D.J., Humphrey, S.M. and Bullock, G.R. The oxygen paradox and the calcium paradox: two facets of the same problem? *J. Molecular & Cellular Cardiology*, **10**, 641-668 (1978).

Hearse, D.J. Editorial. Reperfusion of the ischemic myocardium. *J. Molecular & Cellular Cardiology*, **9**, 605-616 (1977).

Hearse, D.J. and De Leiris, J. Enzymes in Cardiology: Diagnosis and Research. John Wiley, Chichester (1979).

Jynge, P., Hearse, D.J., Braimbridge, M.V. Myocardial protection during ischemic cardiac arrest. A possible hazard with calcium-free cardioplegic infusates. *J. Thorac. Cardiovasc. Surg.*, **73**, 846-855 (1977).

Katz, A. and Tada, M. The "Stone Heart". A challlenge to the biochemist. *Am. J. Cardiol.*, **29**, 578-580 (1972).

Schaper, J. and Schaper, W. Reperfusion of ischemic myocardium: ultrastructural and histochemical aspects. *J. Am. Coll. Cardiol.*, **1**, 1037-1046 (1983).

Zimmerman, A.N.E., Dalms, W., Hulsmann, W.C., Snyder, J., Wisse, E. and Durrer, D. Morphological changes of heart muscle caused by successive perfusion with calcium-free and calcium-containing solutions (calcium paradox). *Cardiovascular Research*, **1**, 201-209 (1967).

Zimmerman, A.N.E. and Hulsmann, W.C. Paradoxical influence of calcium ions on the permeability of the cell membranes of the isolated rat heart. *Nature*, **211**, 646 (1966).

Basic and clinical aspects of myocardial protection by calcium entry blockers

M. Borgers, W. Flameng

Summary

Our morphologic and cytochemical observations on myocardial ischemia in man, dog and rabbit strongly suggest that lidoflazine alleviates myocardial injury by preserving the cell surface structure. Whether this effect is achieved indirectly through energy preservation, lowering of oxygen consumption or through a direct interaction with membrane components, such as phospholipids, is not known at present. In view of the lack of obvious morphologic protective effects to mitochondria during the ischemic episode whilst marked preservation of the sarcolemma-glycocalyx is prominent, we favor the hypothesis of direct interaction between the drug and the sarcolemma-glycocalyx.

Résumé

Nos observations morphologiques et cytochimiques sur l'ischémie myocardique chez l'homme, le chien et le lapin suggèrent résolument que la lidoflazine soulage la lésion myocardique en préservant la structure de la surface cellulaire. On ne sait pas encore à l'heure actuelle si cet effet est obtenu indirectement par une préservation d'énergie, une réduction de la consommation d'oxygène ou par une interaction directe avec les composantes membraneuses telles que les phospholipides. En égard au manque d'effets protecteurs morphologiques manifestes sur la mitochondrie pendant l'épisode ischémique alors que la préservation du sarcolemme-glycocalyx est manifeste, nous penchons en faveur de l'hypothèse d'une interaction directe entre la substance et le sarcolemme-glycocalyx.

Resumen

Nuestras observaciones morfológicas y citoquímicas en isquemia miocardíaca en el hombre, el perro y el conejo indican que lidoflazina alivia el daño miocardíaco protegiendo la estructura de la pared celular. No se sabe, en este momento, si este efecto se realice indirectamente por preservación de energía, disminución de la consumición de oxígeno o por una interacción directa con compuestos de membrana, tales como los fosfolípidos. Dado la carencia de obvios efectos protectores morfológicos en mitocondrias, durante el período isquémico, mientras la preservación marcada del sarcolema-glicocalix está destacada, preferimos la hipótesis de la directa interacción de la droga con el sarcolema-glicocalix.

Zusammenfassung

Unsere morphologischen und zytochemischen Beobachtungen über Myokardischämie bei Mensch, Hund und Kaninchen deuten darauf hin, dass Lidoflazin durch Schutz der Zelloberflächenstruktur die Myokardschäden verringert. Ob diese Wirkung auf indirektem Weg durch Energieeinsparung und Erniedrigung des Sauerstoffverbrauches, oder durch eine direkte Wechselwirkung mit Membrankomponenten, wie den Phospholipiden erfolgt, ist zur Zeit noch ungeklärt. In Anbetracht des Fehlens klarer morphologischer Schutzwirkungen gegenüber den Mitochondrien während der Ischämieperiode bei deutlichem Vorhandensein einer Sarkolemm-Glycocalyx-Konservierung, befürworten wir die Hypothese einer direkten Wechselwirkung zwischen dem Arzneimittel und dem Sarkolemm-Glycocalyx.

146

Introduction

The complex biochemical events involved in ischemia and post-ischemic reperfusion of the myocardium have raised widespread interest and form the basis of a vast number of research papers and reviews (Jennings and Ganote, 1976; Hearse and de Leiris, 1979; Kloner and Braunwald, 1980). The regulatory role played by calcium in some key metabolic functions of the cardiac cell is well established (Katz, 1977; Nayler et al., 1979; Racker, 1980). In order to maintain the homeostatic balance of calcium, the cell is equipped with a multiplicity of regulatory devices.

In a cell at rest, the out-in Ca^{2+}-concentration gradient is at least 10^4, whereas in an activated cell the cytosol concentration rises some 10^2 fold. These Ca^{2+} have to be removed from the cytosol in order to regain the rest state. In order for these Ca^{2+}-movements to occur, the cell possesses membrane-associated Ca-pumps, ionic exchange mechanisms, Ca-binding proteins, etc. Disturbances of one or more of these Ca-controlling mechanisms may lead to the loss of Ca-homeostasis, Ca-overload and consequently cellular dysfunction (Nayler et al., 1979; Langer, 1978). Such disturbances are seen following excessive metabolic stimulation, ischemia, hypoxia and physicochemical aggression of the sarcolemma-glycocalyx (SG) complex.

Once a too high amount of Ca^{2+} is allowed to enter the cytosol through a defective SG a number of biochemical processes are initiated which compromise further cell function and survival (Nayler and Grinwald, 1981). The cardioprotective effects of a number of compounds belonging to the heterogenous class of Ca^{2+}-entry blockers in myocardial ischemia have been reported (Nayler and Grinwald, 1981; Clark et al., 1977; Hearse et al., 1978; Kloner and Braunwald, 1980; Flameng et al., 1981; Nayler, 1980). The exact mode by which drugs such as lidoflazine, verapamil, nifedipine, diltiazem exert their cardioprotective effects is not clarified. The obvious reason why a simple explanation is not at hand is first of all the inadequate understanding of the biochemical events that control Ca^{2+}-movements within the cell. This lack of understanding fosters the current confusion around Ca^{2+}-entry blockers.

Secondly, the pharmacological properties of the Ca^{2+}-entry blockers are complex and the Ca^{2+}-antagonistic profile of some is quite at variance from that of the others. Differences in selectivity for tissues (e.g. blood vessels versus heart), in affinity for membrane channels (e.g. voltage- versus receptor-operated) or in selectivity for a physiopathologic change (e.g. normoxia versus hypoxia) have been described for different members of this group (Rahwan et al., 1979; Van Nueten and Vanhoutte, 1981; Godfraind, 1981). Lidoflazine is a good example to illustrate the complexity of the tissue. In contrast to verapamil, nifedipine and diltiazem, this compound has little affinity for the voltage-activated channels (e.g. does not shorten the plateau phase of the action potential and exerts only weak negative inotropism in isolated heart muscle). On the other hand, this drug clearly antagonizes Ca^{2+}-dependent vasoconstrictive responses in a multitude of blood vessels (Van Nueten and Wellens, 1979) and prevents myocardial Ca^{2+}-overload in ischemic and post-ischemic reperfused myocardium (Nayler, 1980; Flameng et al., 1981). In this paper we will focus on the structural protection of the heart during ischemia in animals and in man afforded by acute lidoflazine treatment.

Animal studies

Using a rabbit Langendorff-isolated heart preparation, Nayler (1980) demonstrated the cardioprotective effects of lidoflazine in the ischemic myocardium. Acute as well as chronic pretreatment with this drug suppressed the steep rise in end-diastolic contracture that occurred during the post-ischemic reperfusion phase. The lidoflazine-pretreated hearts showed a good recovery of developed tension. The functions of mitochondria, determined after measurement of oxidative phosphorylation, ATP generation and calcium content, were significantly better preserved in the drug treated hearts.

In dogs subjected to 1 hour normothermic global ischemia followed by reperfusion, lidoflazine exerted a remarkable protective effect of both function and structure of the aggressed myocardium (Flameng et al., 1981). Essentially, none of the untreated dogs could be weaned from the extracorporeal bypass, indicating the severity of the model. Light- and electron-microscopic examination showed that the loss of the structural integrity of the sarcolemma and mitochondria were prominent features at the end of the ischemic arrest period (Fig. 1).

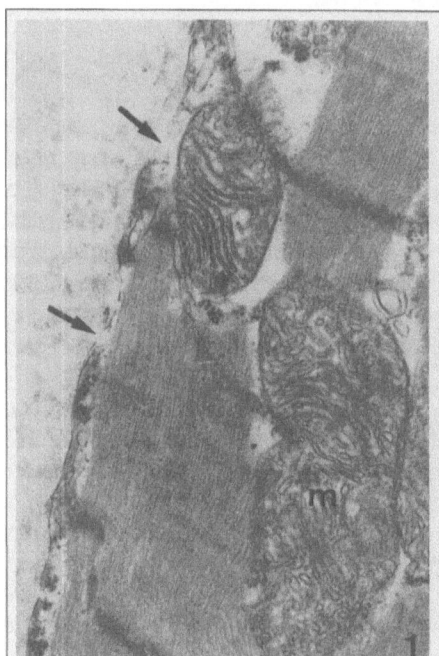 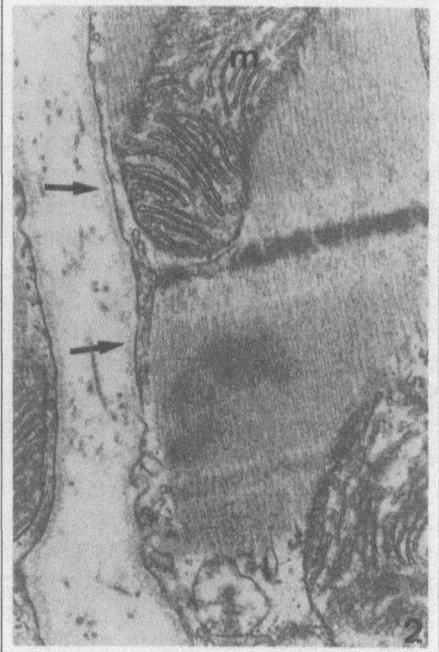

Figures 1 - 4: LV(=left ventricle) biopsies of the dog subendocardial areas.

Figure 1: Untreated dog after 60 min ischemia. Mitochondria (m) are swollen and the sarcolemma-glycocalyx is frequently interrupted (arrows) (x 32,400).

Figure 2: Lidoflazine-treated dog after 60 min ischemia. The SG-complex appears to be intact (arrows) whereas mitochondria (m) are altered to a similar extent as in the untreated dog (x 41,500).

Intracellular edema, contracture of the sarcomeres and further degeneration of the sarcolemma and mitochondria developed during the initial minutes of post-ischemic reperfusion. Such degeneration went along with massive uptake of cytochemically demonstrable calcium in the damaged mitochondria and nuclei (Fig. 3). All lidoflazine-pretreated dogs showed rapid recovery after 1 hour normothermic arrest and could be weaned from the extracorporeal bypass with excellent hemodynamics. The structural injury seen at the end of 1 hour ischemia was largely limited to mitochondrial swelling and cristae disruption, the sarcolemma-glycocalyx remained intact (Fig. 2). The mitochondrial alterations were rapidly reversed upon reperfusion and the amount of calcium confined to their matrices was limited. After 30 min of reperfusion most of the cells completely regained a normal ultrastructure of all subcellular entities (Fig. 4). Similar histologic protection by lidoflazine has been reported by Godfraind et al. (1980) in rats injected with a high dose of isoprenaline that provoked cardionecrosis.

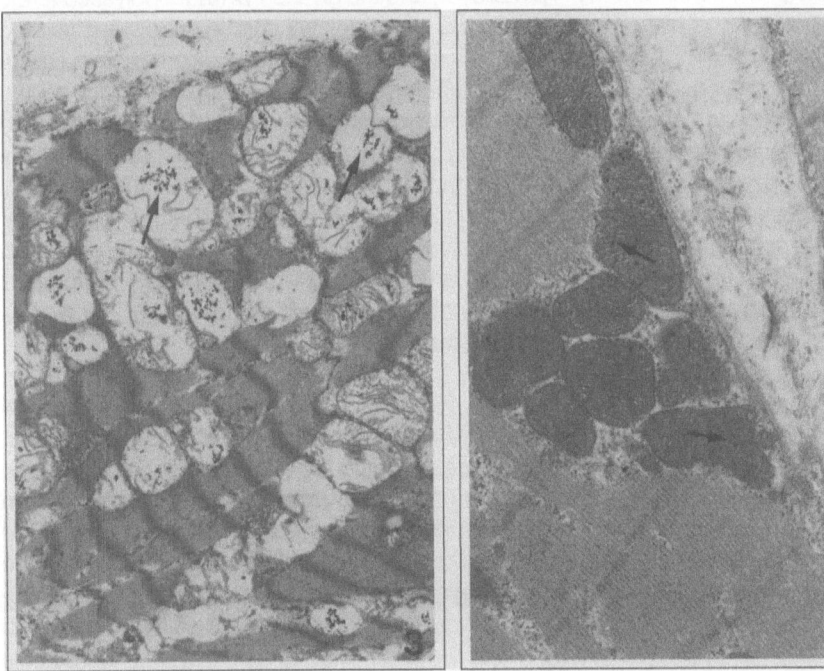

Figure 3: Untreated dog after 60 min ischemia and 30 min post-ischemic reperfusion. Calcium precipitate (arrows) is demonstrated in the hugely swollen and disrupted mitochondria. The SG-complex is very ill-defined (x 8,500).

Figure 4: Lidoflazine-treated dog after 60 min ischemia and 30 min post-ischemic reperfusion. The amount of calcium (arrows) in the mitochondria is limited to few fine granules. Mitochondrial recovery is almost complete and the cell surface retains its normal structure (x 22,700).

Our ultrastructural investigations on ischemic myocardium were recently extended and, in view of the above described effects of lidoflazine in preserving the sarcolemma, particular attention has been paid to the surface structure.

149

Cardioprotection through sarcolemma-glycocalyx (SG) stabilization

Although mitochondrial alterations were prominent to a similar extent in controls and lidoflazine-treated dog hearts subjected to 1 hour normothermic global ischemia (vide supra), disruption of the SG-complex was largely prevented in the treated hearts. We recently confirmed this membrane protective effect in the ischemic rabbit heart (unpublished observations) again without clear preservation of mitochondrial ultrastructure during the ischemic event. A direct link between mitochondrial recovery during the early post-ischemic reperfusion and the maintenance of SG integrity during ischemia is suggested by these observations. In other words, the degree of damage to the SG-complex might be a determinant for the all or none reversibility of cellular function and structure after an ischemic insult. Structurally, the SG-complex is composed of the sarcolemma (plasma membrane or lipid bilayer) and the glycocalyx (mucopolysaccharide coat or basement membrane). This latter 50 nm thick layer can be subdivided into the surface coat, which is an integral part of the sarcolemma, and the external lamina. Both layers of the glycocalyx contain fixed negatively charged sites, mainly due to the abundant presence of sialic acid. The anionic residues of sialic acid bind strongly and preferentially to calcium (Frank et al., 1977; Langer, 1978). Langer et al. (1981) proposed that the control of calcium in-out movements resides in at least two different compartments of the cell surface, one being the glycocalyx, the other the lipid bilayer itself. These authors clearly evidenced that the removal of sialic acid residues produced a marked increase in the membrane Ca^{2+}-permeability. Furthermore, the removal of extracellular calcium and hence surface-bound calcium destabilized the SG-complex with subsequent loss of ionic homeostasis.

Bianchi (1969) forwarded the hypothesis that calcium bound to the external surface has a stabilizing effect on the calcium bound to the internal leaflet of the lipid bilayer. We recently localized ultrastructurally a pool of calcium that was specifically bound to the sarcolemma, including T-tubules and intercalated discs, of the myocardial cells in the dog, rabbit and rat (Borgers et al., submitted). In the normal working heart, the amount of sarcolemma-bound calcium varied according to the contractile state of the cell, the more relaxed the cell, the more deposits settled at the sarcolemma and T-tubules. The questions whether this pool actively participates in the excitation-contraction cycle or merely represents structural calcium is not clarified. Anyway, the fact that different concentrations are seen within the contraction cycle suggests that this pool is an exchangeable one. At the end of prolonged ischemia such sarcolemma calcium was completely lost in subendocardial areas which became irreversibly damaged upon reperfusion. Subepicardial cells of the same biopsy, which usually recover after reperfusion, still presented Ca^{2+}-precipitate at their sarcolemma.

In lidoflazine protected hearts, the preservation of SG-complex integrity in all myocardial areas was accompanied with the retention of the membrane calcium binding capacity. There appears thus to be a direct relation between the presence of membrane calcium of cardiac cells and their ability to recover from an ischemic insult. This peculiar interrelation has recently been confirmed by our observations in "the Ca-paradox" (Zimmerman and Hülsmann, 1966).

When isolated rat hearts were perfused with zero calcium, the SG-complex undergoes characteristic changes and loses its calcium bound to the internal surface of the sarcolemma. This situation predisposed the cells to rapid destruction upon readmittance of external calcium. We showed that interventions which prevented such cellular destruction also preserved the calcium-binding capacity of the sarcolemma (Borgers, unpublished observations).

Cardioprotection with lidoflazine in man

The cardioprotective effects of lidoflazine were tested in patients undergoing multiple aortocoronary bypass grafting (Flameng et al., submitted). Myocardial preservation was compared in 3 groups of 10 patients each: an untreated control group, undergoing intermittent aortic cross clamping at 25 - 28°C (four 11 min period of global ischemia, followed by 7 min reperfusion); and two lidoflazine-treated groups in which the drug was administered intravenously at either 0.5 or 1 mg.kg^{-1}, before going on cardiopulmonary bypass. Intermittent cross-clamping procedures were identical to the control group. Changes in high energy phosphates and glycogen content, ultrastructure of the cardiac cells and the recovery of hemodynamics served as markers of myocardial ischemia. No marked differences in hemodynamic response between the 3 groups were noticed.

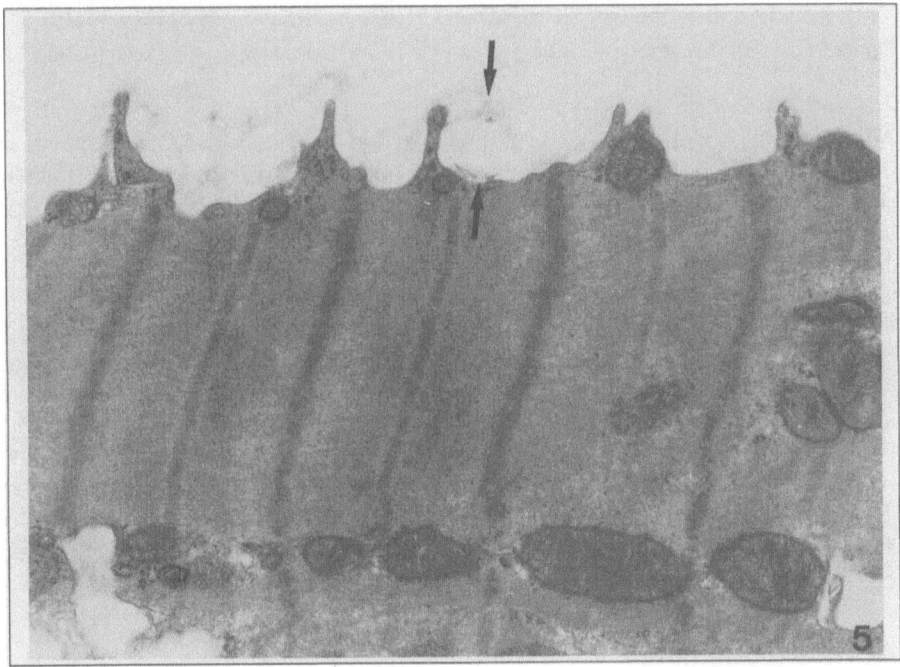

Figures 5-6: LV biopsies of patients undergoing extensive aortocoronary bypass surgery. Postoperative samples of subendocardial areas.

Figure 5: Untreated patient. Edematous blebs are present in between the sarcolemma and the glycocalyx (arrows) (x 28,600).

151

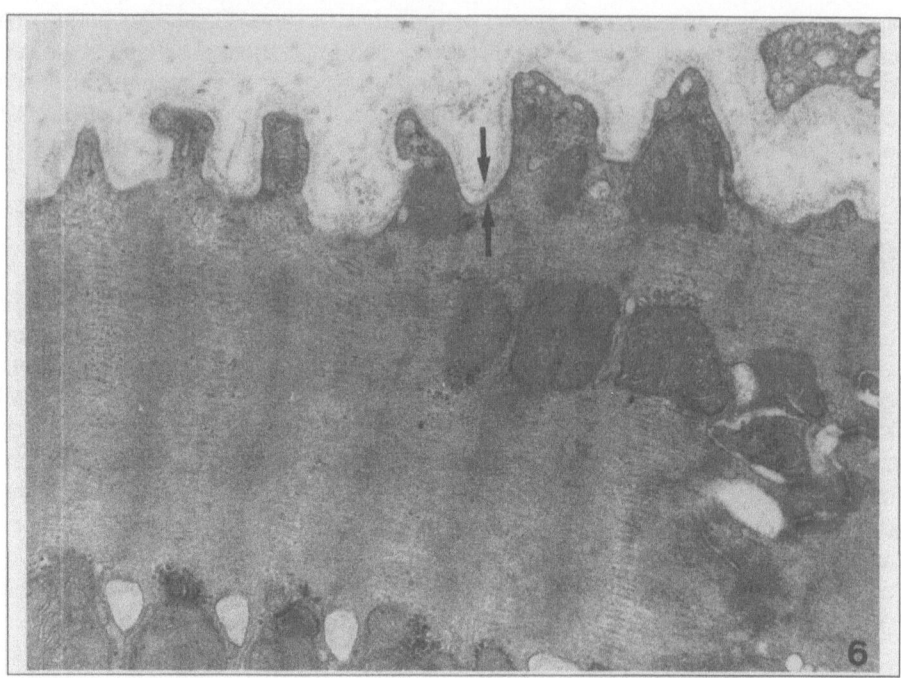

Figure 6: Lidoflazine-treated patient. The glycocalyx is closely apposed to the sarcolemma (arrows) (x 31,900).

Adenosine tri-phosphate, creatine phosphate and glycogen levels, determined in transmural LV biopsies taken at the beginning and at the end of bypass, consistently dropped in the post-ischemic biopsies of the controls, whereas in both treated groups the values were not significantly different between the pre- and post-operative samples. These short periods of hypothermic ischemia did not induce marked changes in ultrastructure. However, one morphologic sign of structural instability was present in the control group: the close apposition of the sarcolemma and glycocalyx was frequently interrupted in a large number of the cells (Fig. 5). Since this phenomenon was already present in the pre-operative sample, we attributed this change, at least in part, to the chronic ischemic situation of the myocardium of these patients. In the lidoflazine-treated group, this membrane instability occurred only in occasional cells in a limited number of samples, most cells showing a fully normal surface structure (Fig. 6). Again this observation indicated that acutely given lidoflazine enables a rapid restoration of the structural stability of the SG-complex, thereby suggesting that this drug primarily exerts its cardioprotective effect at the level of the SG-complex.

Acknowledgement

This work was supported by a grant from I.W.O.N.L.

References

Bianchi, C.P. Pharmacology of excitation-contraction coupling in muscle. Introduction: statement of the problem. *Federation Proc.*, **28**(5), 1624-1628 (1969).

Clark, R.E., Ferguson, T.B., West, P.N., Schuchleib, R.C. and Henri, P.D. Pharmacological preservation of the ischemic heart. *Annals Thor. Surg.*, **24**(4), 307-314 (1977).

Flameng, W., Daenen, W., Borgers, M., Thoné, F., Xhonneux, R., Van de Water, A. and Van Belle, H. Cardioprotective effects of lidoflazine during 1-hour normothermic global ischemia. *Circulation*, **64**, 796-807 (1981).

Frank, J.S., Langer, G.A., Nudd, L.M. and Seraydarian, K. The myocardial cell surface, its histochemistry and the effect of sialic acid and calcium removal on its structure and cellular ionic exchange. *Circ. Res.*, **41**, 702-714 (1977).

Godfraind, T., Khouri, G. and Sturbois, X. The action of flunarizine and lidoflazine on isoprenaline induced cardiac lesions. *Arch. int. Pharmacodyn.*, **244**, 330-332 (1980).

Godfraind, T. Calcium influx and receptor-response coupling. In: "New perspectives on calcium antagonists". Ed. G.B. Weiss, Am. Physiol. Soc., Bethesda, Maryland (1981).

Hearse, D.J., Humphrey, S.M. and Bullock, G.R. The oxygen paradox and the calcium paradox: two facets of the same problem? *J. Mol. Cell. Cardiol.*, **10**, 641-668 (1978).

Hearse, D.J. and de Leiris, J. Enzymes in Cardiology, Publ. John Wiley & Sons, Ltd (1979).

Jennings, R.B. and Ganote, C.E. Mitochondrial structure and function in acute myocardial ischemic injury. *Circ. Res.*, **38**, 81 (1976).

Katz, A.M. Physiology of the heart. Raven Press, New York (1977).

Kloner, R.A. and Braunwald, E. Review: Observations on experimental myocardial ischaemia. *Cardiovasc. Res.(T.M.)*, **14**, 370-395 (1980).

Langer, G.A. The structure and function of the myocardial cell surface. *Amer. J. Physiol.*, **235**, H 461-468 (1978).

Langer, G.A., Frank, J.S. and Philipson, K.D. Correlation of alterations in cation exchange and sarcolemmal ultrastructure produced by neuraminidase and phospholipases in cardiac cell tissue culture. *Circulat. Res.*, **49**, 1289-1299 (1981)

Nayler, W.G. The protective effect of lidoflazine on ischemic and reperfused heart muscle. *R. Soc. Med. Congr. & Symp. Series*, **29**, 79 (1980).

Nayler, W.G. and Grinwald, P. Calcium entry blockers and myocardial function. *Federation Proc.(T.M.)*, **40**, 2855-2861 (1981).

Nayler, W.G., Poole-Wilson, P.A. and Williams, A. Hypoxia and calcium. *J. Mol. Cell Cardiol.*, **11**, 683 (1979).

Racker, E. Fluxes of Ca^{2+} and concepts. *Federation Proc.*, **39**, 2422-2426 (1980).

Rahwan, R.G., Piascik, M.F. and Witiak, D.T. The role of calcium antagonism in the therapeutic action of drugs. *Canad. J. Physiol. & Pharmacol.*, **57**, 443-460 (1979).

Van Nueten, J.M. and Wellens, D. Tissue specificity of calcium-antagonistic properties of lidoflazine. *Arch. int. Pharmacodyn. & Ther.*, **242**, 329-331 (1979).

Van Nueten, J.M. and Vanhoutte, P.M. Calcium entry blockers and vasospasm. In: "Vasodilatation", ed. P.M. Vanhoutte and I. Leusen, Publ. Raven Press, New York (1981).

Zimmerman, A.N.E. and Hülsmann, W.C. Paradoxical influence of calcium ions on the permeability of the cell membrane of the isolated rat heart. *Nature*, **211**, 646-647 (1966).

Effect of calcium entry blockers on impaired left ventricular wall motion

P.F. Cohn

Summary

Left ventricular wall motion abnormalities due to myocardial ischemia can be improved after administration of calcium entry blockers as demonstrated in both animal and human studies. The mechanism of this improvement involves a complex interplay between coronary vasodilatation, systemic vasodilatation and reduced myocardial oxygen requirements.

Résumé

Les anomalies de mouvement de la paroi ventriculaire gauche dues à l'ischémie myocardique peuvent être améliorées après administration de bloqueurs de l'entrée de calcium ainsi qu'on l'a démontré dans des études animales et humaines. Le mécanisme de cette amélioration implique une action réciproque complexe entre la vasodilatation coronaire, la vasodilatation ischémique et la demande réduite d'oxygène myocardique.

Resumen

La mejoría de las anomalías en el movimiento de la pared ventricular izquierda debidas a isquemia miocardíaca puede ser demostrada en estudios, tanto animales como humanos, después de la administración de inhibidores de la penetración intracelular de calcio. El mecanismo de esta mejoría tiene que ver con una interacción compleja entre vasodilatación coronaria, vasodilatación sistémica y reducción de la cantidad requerida de oxígeno miocardíaco.

Zusammenfassung

Bewegungsanomalien der linksventrikulären Wand, die infolge einer Myokardischämie auftreten, können durch Verabreichung von Kalziumeinstromhemmern verbessert werden, wie in Tierversuchen und klinischen Studien gezeigt wurde. Der Mechanismus, der dieser Verbesserung zugrundeliegt, impliziert eine komplizierte Wechselwirkung zwischen Koronarvasodilatation, systemischer Vasodilatation und herabgesetztem Myokardsauerstoffbedarf.

The calcium entry blocking agents are enjoying increasing popularity as antianginal agents because of numerous clinical studies that have been performed in both the United States and Europe. These investigations have documented clinical improvement (relief of anginal symptoms, decrease in nitroglycerin usage) prolongation of exercise time, amelioration of exercise ECG abnormalities, and enhancement of coronary blood flow. The hemodynamic effects have been more variable, especially as they pertain to left ventricular function. These effects have been expressed as alterations in left ventricular systolic and diastolic pressure, mean velocity of circumferential fiber shortening, systolic ejection rate, the end systolic pressure - volume relationship, as well as in segmental shortening and global and regional ejection fraction. In the present communication, we will be particularly interested in the action of these drugs on left ventricular wall motion and ejection phase indices derived from wall motion measurements. The studies to be discussed have been performed during both acute and chronic myocardial ischemia in both animals and humans.

I. Animal studies

The effects of the calcium-entry blockers in animals made ischemic has been studied in a variety of preparations. Smith et al. (1976), using ultrasonic crystals, measured several parameters of myocardial function in both nonischemic and ischemic segments of the left ventricle. The level of ischemia was controlled by graded occlusion of a carotid-to-coronary artery shunt. When perfusion pressure was reduced in the shunt, impaired wall motion (hypokinesia) resulted. After verapamil was administered intravenously, contractility was further reduced in all five dogs studied. There was no similar depression of contractility in the normal myocardium. The authors postulated that the decrease in contractility might be beneficial in reducing the degree of ischemia by reducing local myocardial oxygen requirements.

Different and beneficial effects of this class of drugs were noted by Henry et al. (1979) using nifedipine. In these experiments ultrasonic crystals were again employed to measure myocardial shortening, but instead of a carotid-to-coronary artery shunt the left anterior descending coronary artery was ligated directly. After control measurements were made, nifedipine was infused intravenously. Following coronary artery occlusion in the control state the ischemic segments failed to shorten during early and mid-systole and were also elongated at the end of both systole and diastole. After nifedipine was given, shortening during left ventricular ejection was improved. These investigators also observed that in some ischemic segments paradoxical systolic elongation reverted to normal. Subsequent studies from the same laboratory (Perez et al., 1980) showed that diltiazem also caused improvement in shortening of ischemic segments. In these studies the calcium entry blockers were clearly superior to nitroglycerine and nitroprusside in this regard. Thus, impairment of ventricular wall motion due to acute ischemia in the animal model appears to be alleviated by some of these agents (nifedipine and diltiazem) but not others (verapamil). The reasons for these discrepancies are not clear.

157

II. Studies in humans

The effect of these agents on the left ventricular function in patients with angina of one type or another has been studied by several groups. Ferlinz et al. (1979) administered intravenous verapamil to 20 patients with chronic, stable angina and angiographically documented coronary disease. Mean velocity of circumferential fiber shortening increased from 0.85 ± 0.39 to 0.97 ± 0.46 circ/sec (p < 0.01) and ejection fraction improved from 55 ± 16% to 61 ± 18% (p < 0.01). Contrary to the animal studies cited earlier (Smith et al., 1976), the drug did not worsen the extent of left ventricular wall motion abnormalities in the majority of patients. Similar results were reported by Johnson et al. (1981) using radionuclide ventriculograms of the equilibrium-gated blood pool type. In their studies of patients with Prinzmetal's angina, orally administered verapamil had no deleterious effect on global ejection fraction, nor for that matter did nifedipine, which was also studied in the same protocol. Tan et al. (1982) used a similar radionuclide protocol both at rest and during exercise in 12 patients with chronic stable angina. During exercise on a placebo, the ejection fraction decreased from 40 ± 9% to 35 ± 11% (p < 0.025). Orally administered verapamil abolished this decrease during exercise. The authors also noted that the ejection fraction was significantly higher at identical work loads than on placebo because of a smaller increase in end-systolic volume.

Nifedipine has been an especially popular drug in clinical studies. Again, the protocols have been varied. Lorell et al. (1981) administered 20 mgm of the drug sublingually before an atrial pacing study, and compared the results to a placebo in 17 patients with multivessel coronary disease. Typical angina developed in all patients during pacing tachycardia before nifedipine but in only three patients during pacing after the drug was administered. The increase in left ventricular end-diastolic pressure usually seen with pacing tachycardia was attenuated by the drug. There was no reduction in contractility since neither left ventricular ejection fraction nor dp/dt was altered appreciably. Ludbrook et al. (1982) reported increases in mean velocity of circumferential fiber shortening and ejection fraction (also determined by contrast ventriculogram) in 32 patients with coronary disease. These increases were more prominent in patients with hemodynamic evidence of impaired baseline left ventricular function.

A drawback to the interpretation of the results of these studies has been the paucity of data concerning **regional** wall motion abnormalities. To overcome this difficulty Serruys et al. (1981) used radiopaque markers implanted during coronary revascularization surgery. Both intravenous and intracoronary nifedipine were administered in their study of 21 patients. These patients had recovery normally from bypass surgery for angina pectoris. Regional shortening was determined from the change in position of the markers during pacing tachycardia before and after administration of the drug. With intravenous injections there was no evidence of a negative inotropic effect and regional function increased. With intracoronary injections (via the bypass grafts) a direct negative inotropic effect was observed. Regional contraction was asynchronous due to delayed relaxation. The authors postulated that the negative inotropic effect of the drug is overridden when given intravenously. This is due to reflex increases in heart rate and contractility triggered by the lowering of systemic arterial pressure usually observed with calcium-entry blocking agents. Since these patients had patent bypass grafts it is not clear that the same drug effects would be observed in patients still prone to develop ischemia because of coronary artery stenosis.

Studies of the regional coronary circulation in man (Engel et al., 1981; Malacoff et al., 1982) have demonstrated the ability of these drugs to increase myocardial perfusion. Could the coronary vasodilatory effect of these drugs cause increases in wall motion in regions subserved by stenosed coronary arteries? This improvement in wall motion abnormalities would be in addition to that expected as a result of the peripheral vaso-dilatory "unloading" effect of the drugs. To evaluate this question we used a computer-assisted method to analyze regional wall motion changes on radionuclide ventriculo-grams at rest and during exercise (Maddox et al., 1979). With this technique, regional ejection fraction images are created from gated modified left anterior oblique images of the cardiac blood pool. Left ventricular wall motion is classified as normal, or abnor-mal based on previously defined comparisons with contrast ventriculograms. When we employed this technique in our laboratory to evaluate the effects of the calcium entry blocker lidoflazine, we first measured resting and exercise values in a control (baseline) state. Regional ejection fraction usually decreased with exercise in regions supplied by coronary arteries with 70% or more luminal stenosis. Patients were then given lidoflazine and the studies repeated at 24 hrs, 6 weeks, and 12 weeks. To com-pare values from different regions, regional ejection fraction was normalized (REFn) by dividing the regional ejection fraction by the normal ejection fraction for that region. Regional wall motion was defined as normokinetic (REFn > .70), hypokinetic (REFn .40 - .70) and akinetic (REFn < .40). Results in 30 regions from 10 patients (Nesto et al., 1981) are presented in Table 1 and indicate that the calcium entry blocker improved regional wall motion in areas of jeopardized, hypokinetic myocardium (rather than in normal or akinetic areas) even though the increase in global ejection fraction pre- and post- lidoflazine was minimal in these patients (0.36 to 0.43).

Table 1: Effect of lidoflazine on regional left ventricular wall motion

Regions (30)	REF$_n$ during exercise		
	Pre-lidoflazine		Post-lidoflazine
Normokinetic (10)	.82	NS	.82
Akinetic (7)	.15	NS	.15
Hypokinetic (13)	.52	p < .01	.67

REF$_n$ = normalized regional ejection fraction

III. Conclusions

The calcium entry blockers inhibit the movement of calcium ions from the extracellular to the intracellular space in both cardiac and arterial smooth muscle. Diminished arte-rial tone and diminished myocardial contractility can result from these actions. Left ven-tricular function — and wall motion — can thus be altered by either the resulting coronary and systemic arterial dilation (the latter resulting in afterload reduction) or by myocardial inotropic depression.

Improvement in left ventricular wall motion abnormalities can be demonstrated in both acute and chronic ischemia with calcium-entry blockers, though this effect is not always seen with all of these drugs in each of the various experimental and clinical protocols employed. The more the technique analyzes **regional** changes the more likely will this effect be observed, especially in clinical studies. These effects are due in part to several physiologic actions of the calcium-entry blockers: 1) systemic unloading of the left ventricle, and 2) reduction in myocardial oxygen requirements; but they are also probably largely due to 3) the drugs' beneficial action on myocardial perfusion. Thus when flow is improved to areas of myocardium subserved by stenosed coronary arteries, function in those areas will also improve. For example, the usual decrease in regional wall motion during stress will be abolished or ameliorated. These beneficial effects demonstrate in an objective, quantitative manner the clinical usefulness of this class of drugs. However, the exact role of each of these physiologic factors in this complex interrelationship is still not clearly defined.

References

Chew, C.Y.C. Influence of severity of ventricular dysfunction on hemodynamic responses to intravenously administered verapamil in ischemic heart disease. *Am. J. Cardiol.*, **47**, 917 (1981).

Engel, H-J and Lichtlen, P.R. Beneficial enhancement of coronary blood flow by nifedipine. Comparison with nitroglycerin and beta blocking agents. *Am. J. Med.*, **71**, 658 (1981).

Ferlinz, J., Easthope, J.L. and Aronow, W.S. Effects of verapamil on myocardial performance in coronary disease. *Circulation*, **59**, 313 (1979).

Henry, P.D. et al. Effect of nifedipine on myocardial ischemia: Analysis of collateral flow, pulsatile heat and regional muscle shortening. *Am. J. Cardiol.*, **44**, 817 (1979).

Johnson, S.M. et al. Effects of verapamil and nifedipine on left ventricular function at rest and during exercise in patients with Prinzmetal's variant angina pectoris. *Am. J. Cardiol.*, **47**, 1289 (1981).

Lorell, B.H., Turi, Z. and Grossman, W. Modification of left ventricular response to pacing tachycardia by nifedipine in patients with coronary artery disease. *Am. J. Med.*, **71**, 667 (1981).

Ludbrook, P.A. et al. Acute hemodynamic responses to sublingual nifedipine: dependence on left ventricular function. *Circulation*, **65**, 489 (1982).

Maddox, D.E. et al. The ejection fraction image: A noninvasive index of regional left ventricular wall motion. *Am. J. Cardiol.*, **41**, 1230 (1978).

Malacoff, R.F. et al. Beneficial effects of nifedipine on regional myocardial blood flow in patients with coronary artery disease. *Circulation*, **65** (Suppl. 1), 32 (1982).

Nesto, R. et al. Beneficial effect of lidoflazine on regional wall motion determined by radionuclide ventriculography. *Circulation*, **64** (Suppl. 4), 105 (1981).

Perez, J.E., Sobel, B.E. and Henry, P.D. Improved performance of ischemic canine myocardium in response to nifedipine and diltiazem. *Am. J. Physiol.*, **239**, H658 (1980).

Serruys, P.W. et al. Regional wall motion from radiopaque markers after intravenous and intracoronary injections of nifedipine. *Circulation*, **63**, 584 (1981).

Smith, H.J. et al. Regional contractility. Selective depression of ischemic myocardium by verapamil. *Circulation*, **54**, 629 (1976).

Tan, A.T.H. et al. Verapamil in stable effort angina: effects on left ventricular function evaluated with exercise radionuclide ventriculography. *Am. J. Cardiol.*, **49**, 425 (1982).

The influence of Ca²⁺-entry blockers on hemodynamics and coronary blood flow, and its importance for the treatment of angina pectoris

P.R. Lichtlen, W. Rafflenbeul, I., Amende, R. Simon and G. Reil

Summary

The way calcium-entry blocking agents, especially nifedipine, act in angina pectoris, is a complex one and is still not completely understood. Nifedipine, through its profound relaxing effect on vascular smooth muscle tone and its predilective action for certain vascular regions, e.g. the peripheral systemic arteriolar system as well as the large coronary arteries, is especially suitable for the treatment of angina pectoris. On the one hand, nifedipine leads to a significant decrease in afterload by reducing blood pressure and peripheral resistance; this results in a considerable decrease in myocardial oxygen consumption, although heart rate, cardiac output and contractility, due to the rise in sympathetic tone, increase mildly. On the other hand, the direct dilating effect on the coronary arteriolar system, increasing coronary blood flow and by this oxygen delivery, especially also in the poststenotic, ischemic region, is strong enough to counteract an autoregulatory drop in coronary flow brought about by the decrease in oxygen consumption, yet not large enough to lead to a steal phenomenon. In this regard, nifedipine behaves differently from nitroglycerin and beta-blocking agents whose effect is accompanied with a decrease in coronary flow in the poststenotic zone, provoked by a drop in the rate-pressure-product and, in the case of beta-blockers also in contractility, i.e., by the decrease in oxygen consumption (Engel and Lichtlen, 1981). The additional effect on some of the high-grade coronary obstructions, especially the eccentric ones, observed both in patients with stable and unstable angina pectoris, has to be regarded as a supporting, not yet well-defined action. However, in Prinzmetal's angina, the main action of the calcium blocking agents is to be found solely on the large coronary arteries, releasing the spasm and by this transmural ischemia. This effect, although often observed only after high doses of nifedipine, is so overwhelming that calcium antagonists are regarded as the drugs of choice in this disease, preventing and also interrupting the ischemic attacks. Nevertheless, it should be stressed that due to their different sites of action, nitroglycerin and nifedipine act synergistically in these cases.

Hence, the action of nifedipine in relieving angina pectoris differs considerably from all previous drugs, especially beta-blocking agents, but also nitrates, although the latter also act on vascular smooth muscle tone.

Résumé

La manière dont les agents bloqueurs de l'entrée de calcium, en particulier la nifédipine, agissent sur l'angine de poitrine est complexe et n'est pas encore pleinement comprise. La nifédipine, du fait de son profond effet relâchant sur la tonicité du muscle lisse vasculaire et de sa prédilection pour certaines régions vasculaires telles que le système artériolaire systémique périphérique et les grandes artères coronaires est particulièrement propice pour le traitement de l'angine de poitrine. D'une part, la nifédipine conduit à une diminution significative de la postcharge en réduisant la tension artérielle et la résistance périphérique. Il en résulte une diminution considérable de la consommation d'oxygène myocardique, bien que la fréquence, le débit et la contractilité cardiaque augmentent modérément suite à un accroissement de la tonicité sympathique. D'autre part, l'effet dilatateur direct sur le système artériolaire coronarien, augmentant le débit coronarien et donc l'apport d'oxygène, en particulier dans la région ischémique poststénotique, est suffisamment fort pour contrecarrer une chute autorégulatrice dans le débit coronarien, due à une diminution de la consommation d'oxygène et n'est cependant pas assez puissant pour conduire à un phénomène de détournement. La nifédipine réagit différemment à cet égard, de la nitroglycérine et des agents bêta-bloquants dont l'effet est accompagné d'une diminution du débit coronarien également dans la zone poststénotique, due à une diminution du produit-fréquence-pression et, dans le cas des bêta-bloquants, de la contractilité, c'est-à-dire par la diminution de la consommation d'oxygène (Engel et Lichtlen, 1981). L'effet additionnel observé sur certaines obstructions coronariennes d'un degré élevé, en particulier les obstructions excentriques, se manifestant chez les patients atteints d'angine de poitrine tant stable qu'instable, doit être considéré comme une action de support encore mal définie. Toutefois, pour l'angine de Prinzmetal, l'action principale des agents bloqueurs de calcium ne se situe que sur les grandes artères coronaires, antagonisant le vasospasme et donc l'ischémie transmurale. Cet effet, bien que n'étant souvent observé qu'après de fortes doses de nifédipine est tellement important que les antagonistes de calcium sont considérés comme des substances de choix dans cette maladie, prévenant et coupant les attaques ischémiques.

Néanmoins, il convient de souligner qu'en raison de leurs sites d'action différents, la nitroglycérine et la nifédipine agissent de façon synergiste dans ces cas. Dès lors, l'action de la nifédipine dans le soulagement d'angine de poitrine diffère considérablement de celle de toutes les substances précédentes, ainsi de la nitroglycérine bien que son effet prinicipal est aussi la diminution de la tonicité du muscle vasculaire lisse.

Resumen

La manera como los agentes inhibidores de la penetración intracelular de Ca^{2+} actúan en angina de pecho, especialmente nifedipino, es muy complicada y no se entiende completamente. Nifedipino es específicamente apropiado para el tratamiento de angina de pecho, por su profundo efecto relajador de la tonicidad del músculo liso vascular y su acción selectiva en ciertas regiones vasculares, p.ej. el sistema periférico arteriolar tanto como las arterias coronarias anchas. Por un lado, nifedipino conduce a una significante disminución en la postcarga del corazón, reduciendo la presión arterial y la resistencia periférica; esto resulta en una considerable disminución de la consumición de oxígeno miocardíaco, aunque la frecuencia cardíaca, el volumen-minuto y la contractilidad suben ligeramente, debido al aumento en el tono simpático. Por otro lado, el directo efecto dilatador en el sistema arteriolar coronario, aumentando el flujo sanguíneo coronario y con esto la distribución del oxígeno, especialmente en la región postestenósica isquémica, es suficientemente fuerte para contrarrestar una gota autorreguladora en el flujo coronario, causada por la disminución de la consumición de oxígeno, lo que no es suficientemente importante para conducir a un efecto de hurto. A este respecto, nifedipino difiere de nitroglicerina y de los agentes beta-bloqueadores, los cuales disminuyen el flujo coronario, también en la zona estenocardíaca, por una gota en el producto frecuencia x presión, y además, difiere de los beta-bloqueadores porque estos disminuyen la contractilidad miocardíaca, y como consecuencia, la consumición de oxígeno (Engel y Lichtlen, 1981). El efecto adicional en algunas de las obstrucciones coronarias de alto grado, especialmente las excéntricas, observadas en pacientes con angina de pecho tanto estable como inestable, es considerado como una acción de apoyo, no bien definida todavía. No obstante, en la angina de Prinzmetal, la acción más importante de los inhibidores de la penetración intracelular de Ca^{2+} reside únicamente en las arterias coronarias largas, relajando el espasmo, y por esto, la isquemia transmural.

Este efecto, aunque muchas veces sólo observado después de altas dosis de nifedipino, es tan abrumador que los antagonistas de Ca^{2+} son considerados como las drogas predilectas en esta enfermedad, *porque impiden y también interrumpen los ataques isquémicos. No obstante, se tiene que insistir en que nitroglicerina y nifedipino actúan sinérgicamente en estos casos, debido a sus distintos lugares de acción. Por lo tanto, la acción de nifedipino en angina de pecho aliviada, difiere considerablemente de todos los fármacos anteriores, especialmente de los agentes beta-bloqueadores, pero también de los nitrates, aunque los últimos no son tan diferentes porque poseen la propiedad de guardar los iones cálcicos fuera del aparato contráctil.*

Zusammenfassung

Die Wirkungsweise von Kalziumantagonisten, besonders von Nifedipin, bei Angina pectoris ist kompliziert und noch immer nicht voll aufgeklärt. Aufgrund seiner stark relaxierenden Wirkung an der glatten Gefässmuskulatur und seiner Prädilektionswirkung auf bestimmte Gefässregionen, z.B. das allgemeine periphere Arteriolensystem und die grossen Koronararterien, ist Nifedipin zur Behandlung von Angina pectoris besonders geeignet. Überdies führt Nifedipin zu einer bedeutenden Abnahme der Nachlast, indem es den Blutdruck und den peripheren Widerstand herabsetzt. Dies führt zu einer erheblichen Abnahme des myokardischen Sauerstoffverbrauches, obwohl Herzfrequenz, Herzminutenvolumen und Kontraktilität wegen des Anstieges des Sympathikotonus leicht zunehmen. Andererseits ist die direkte dilatierende Wirkung auf das Koronararteriolensystem genügend stark, um einer autoregulierenden Verminderung des Koronarflusses infolge einer Abnahme des Sauerstoffverbrauches entgegenzuwirken, jedoch nicht stark genug, um ein Steal-Phänomen hervorzurufen. Ersteres ist durch die Zunahme der koronaren Durchblutung und folglich der Sauerstoffzufuhr, besonders in den poststenotischen, ischämischen Gebieten zu erklären. Nifedipin verhält sich in dieser Hinsicht unterschiedlich gegenüber Nitroglyzerin und Betablockern, deren Wirkung mit einer Verminderung der Koronardurchblutung, auch im poststenotischen Gebiet, einhergeht, welche ihrerseits durch ein erniedrigtes Frequenz-Druck-Produkt verursacht wird; im Falle der Betablocker resultiert ebenfalls eine Verminderung der Kontraktilität, und als Folge ein erniedrigter Sauerstoffverbrauch (Engel und Lichtlen, 1981). Die zusätzliche Wirkung auf bestimmte hochgradige — besonders exzentrische — Stenosen, die bei Patienten mit stabiler bzw. unstabiler Angina beobachtet werden, ist als eine unterstützende, noch ungenügend geklärte Wirkung zu betrachten. Bei Prinzmetal-Angina bezieht sich die Hauptwirkung der Kalziumantagonisten jedoch ausschliesslich auf die grossen Koronararterien, indem Spasmen und dadurch transmurale Ischämien behoben werden. Diese Wirkung, die bei Nifedipin erst bei hohen Dosen auftritt, ist so ausgesprochen, dass Kalziumantagonisten für diese Krankheit als Arzneimittel der Wahl zu betrachten sind: Ischämieanfällen wird vorgebeugt oder sie werden sogar unterbrochen.

Jedoch muss betont werden, dass Nitroglyzerin und Nifedipin, aufgrund ihrer verschiedenen Angriffsstellen in diesen Fällen eine synergistische Wirkung zeigen.

Die Wirkung von Nifedipin auf die Angina pectoris unterscheidet sich damit in erheblichem Masse von allen früheren Arzneimitteln, insbesondere von Betablockern, aber auch von Nitraten, obwohl die letzteren ebenfalls über eine Senkung des Vasomotorentonus wirken.

Ca-entry blockers have become an important additional principle in the treatment of ischemic heart disease, differing considerably in their action from nitrates and beta-blocking agents. As demonstrated in Fig. 1, in the cardiovascular field, there are mainly three systems in which Ca-entry blockers exert their effects, i.e. the conduction system, the vascular smooth muscle system and the myocardium. During the last years it was shown that the various calcium blocking agents affect these systems differently, verapamil and diltiazem, for instance both acting on the cardiac conduction as well as vascular smooth muscle cells whereas nifedipine, which will be the main drug analyzed here, acts predominantly on the muscle cells (Fleckenstein, 1981, Triggle, 1981).

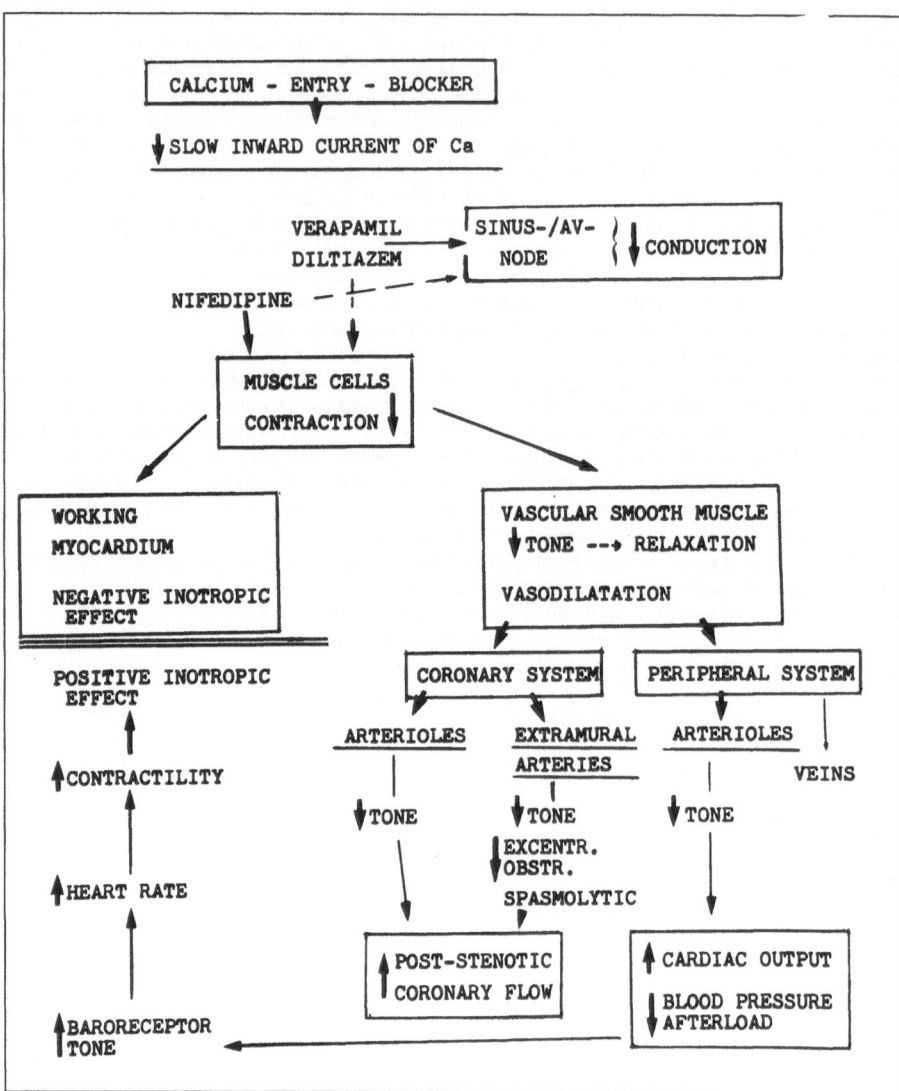

Figure 1 : Schematic diagram of the effect of calcium entry blockers on the conduction system, the peripheral and coronary arteries and the myocardium; for details see text.

All these drugs have in common a marked reduction in contractile function due to partial inhibition of the transmembrane calcium flux across both vascular smooth muscle as well as myocardial cell membranes; this results in relaxation of the vascular tone both of peripheral and coronary arteries and arterioles as well as in a negative inotropic effect on the myocardium. In the following presentation the effects on these various systems will be analyzed more closely.

I. Effect on hemodynamics after sublingual administration of nifedipine

a) Central hemodynamics, systolic function

Hemodynamics were studied in 15 patients using tip-manometers (PC-481, Millar Instruments) to record left ventricular pressures before and during left ventricular angiography taken in a RAO-40°-projection. Left ventricular volumes and wall motion were analyzed by a computerized video system (Grafomed Philips) (for details of the technique, see: Amende et al., 1979). Sublingual administration of 20 mg nifedipine was shown to exert a marked reduction of afterload (Table 1) decreasing systolic blood pressure, especially if elevated, and peripheral resistance and increasing cardiac output, heart rate and dp/dt max.

Table 1: Hemodynamic changes following sublingual nifedipine (20 mg); 7 patients with coronary disease yet normal left ventricles.
Abbreviations: HR = heart rate, CO = cardiac output, Mean AO = mean aortic pressure, PVR = peripheral vascular resistance, Vpm = velocity of fiber shortening, EDVI = end-diastolic volume index, EF = ejection fraction, MNER = mean normalized ejection rate, ET = ejection time, VCF = velocity of circumferencial fiber shortening.

Hemodynamic changes following nifedipine (N = 7)				
	HR (min^{-1})	CO (l/min)	$Mean\ AO$ $(mm\ Hg)$	PVR $(dyn\ sec\ cm^{-5})$	dp/dt_{max} $(mm\ Hg/sec)$
Before	62.6	5.87	87.8	1217	1421
After	75.8	7.33	89.1	1011	1606
Diff.	+13.2	+1.46	+2.3	−206	+185
P <	0.001	0.01	N.S.	0.005	0.05

Isovolumetric and ejection phase parameters before and after nifedipine (N = 7)							
	V_{pm} (ML/sec)	$EDVI$ (ml/m^2)	EF $(\%)$	$MNER$ EF/ET (sec^{-1})	$\overline{V}_{CF}$ $(circ/sec)$	Segmental changes %B	%M	%A
Before	36.0	89.6	58	1.65	0.958	29.8	29.6	33.2
After	35.0	89.6	62	1.83	0.986	30.6	30.4	37.2
Diff.	−1.0	0	+4	+0.18	+0.028	+0.8	+0.8	+4.0
P <	N.S.	N.S.	N.S.	N.S.	N.S.	N.S.	N.S.	N.S.

ML = muscle length; V_{CF} = mean velocity of fiber shortening.

165

The rise in contractility and heart rate is considered to be secondary in nature following the drop in blood pressure and the baroreceptor-mediated increase in sympathetic tone (Lichtlen, 1980).

It is of interest to note that no influence on preload, i.e., on venous return was observed as long as end-diastolic volume was within normal limits; similarly, also no increase in ejection fraction or improvement in wall motion was seen under non-ischemic conditions. It should be stressed, however, that in patients with elevated end-diastolic volumes (> 120 ml/m^2), a decrease in end-diastolic volume as well as an increase in wall motion was demonstrated (Ludbrook, 1980; Paulus, 1981). Furthermore, if measurements of central hemodynamics are performed at a time when blood pressure had dropped significantly, an improvement of wall motion as well as a decrease in end-diastolic pressure and volume might be observed (Rutsch, 1980). These changes in preload, however, have to be regarded as secondary to the increased cardiac output and venous return, rather than as a direct effect on the venous system.

This apparent lack of a direct action of nifedipine on the venous system could be a specific one and explains the increase in cardiac output; hence, this situation is completey different from the one observed under nitroglycerin, always associated with a decrease in preload (Amende, 1979).

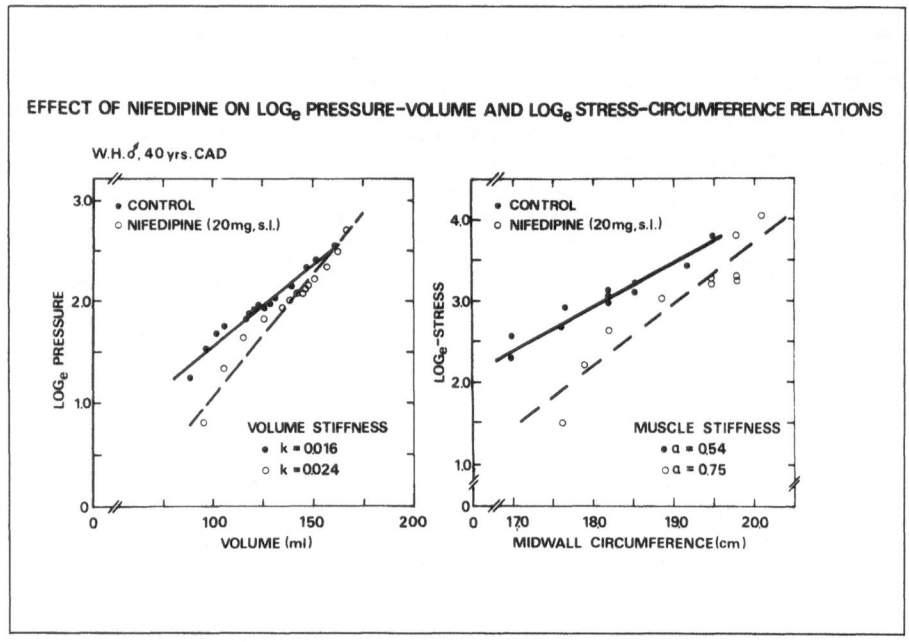

Figure 2: Typical example of the effect of nifedipine on the diastolic pressure-volume (on the left) and stress-circumference relations (on the right). Dots: control values; circles: values after 20 mg nifedipine sublingually; measurements were performed from the lowest diastolic pressure and volume, i.e., midwall circumference up to the beginning of the a-wave. Note that after drug-administration the relation between log-pressure and volume, i.e., circumference becomes steeper indicating an increase in volume stiffness and muscle stiffness.

b) Central hemodynamics, diastolic function

Pressure volume and stress circumference relations were studied in 6 coronary patients with normal left ventricular function, seven minutes after drug administration when coronary flow was already augmented but no significant peripheral effects had occurred (for details of the technique, see: Amende et al., 1979). Volumes and pressures were assessed frame by frame throughout diastole, starting at the lowest diastolic pressure value up to the beginning of the a-wave; LV-pressures and LV-angiograms were again obtained by the aid of tip-manometers (PC-481, Millar Instruments), pressures were immediately digitized and stored on the same frame; the final analysis of the pressure volume relation was performed by a computerized video system (Grafomed Philips).

After administration of 20 mg nifedipine sublingually the **logarithmic pressure volume curve** became steeper, indicating a slight increase in so called volume stiffness; however, these changes were mild, as the end-diastolic pressure and volume were practically unchanged; a typical example is shown on Fig. 2. Similarly, **diastolic stress circumference relation** showed no marked displacement, although the steeper slope reflects a mild increase in so-called muscle stiffness. Similar observations were made during pacing induced ischemia by Lorell et al. (1981).

II. Direct effect on the myocardium observed after intra-coronary administration of nifedipine

If calcium-entry blockers are injected directly into a coronary artery, a depressive effect on the myocardium is to be expected, as the increase in baroreceptor tone due to afterload reduction does not take place. In addition, an immediate effect on the coronary circulation will be observed.

Methods

0.1 mg Nifedipine were injected into bypass grafts in 8 patients and into the left main coronary artery in one patient. Left ventricular pressures (LVSP, LVEDP) and pressure-derived parameters (positive dp/dt max and negative dp/dt min) were assessed over 10 minutes by tip-manometers; coronary blood flow was recorded from the coronary sinus by the aid of the thermodilution technique. Velocity of fiber shortening was recorded from movements of intramyocardial Tantalum-markers placed in the mid-myocardium, three in the anterior and three in the inferior wall, one in the apex, allowing the analysis of percent end-systolic shortening, using cinefilms with 150 frames/sec in RAO-30°-projection (Amende, 1981).

Results

Several important factors were observed (Figs. 3a - 3c): first, the effect on left ventricular pressures and contractility lasted only for approx. 3 minutes, in contrast to the effect on coronary blood flow which was increased for up to 10 minutes; this indicates a different mode of action on the myocardium and on the vascular smooth muscle cell.

167

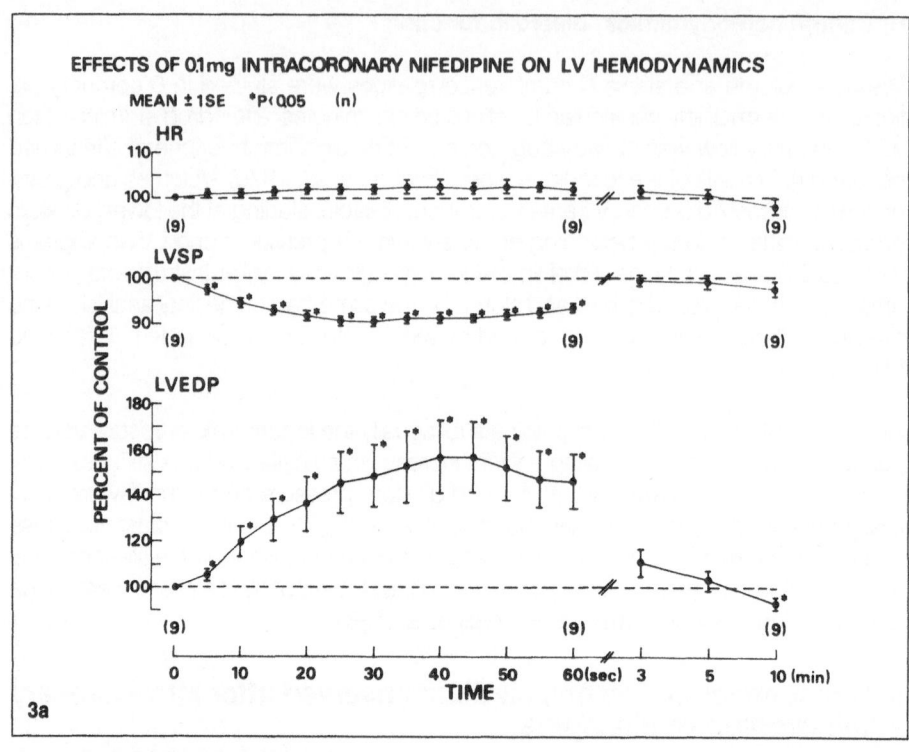

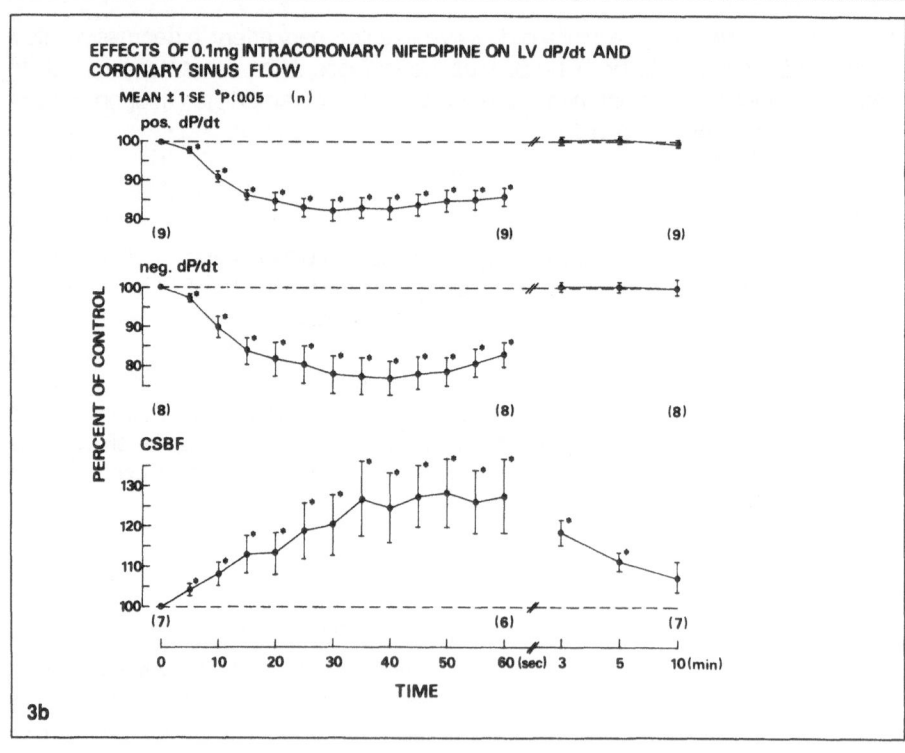

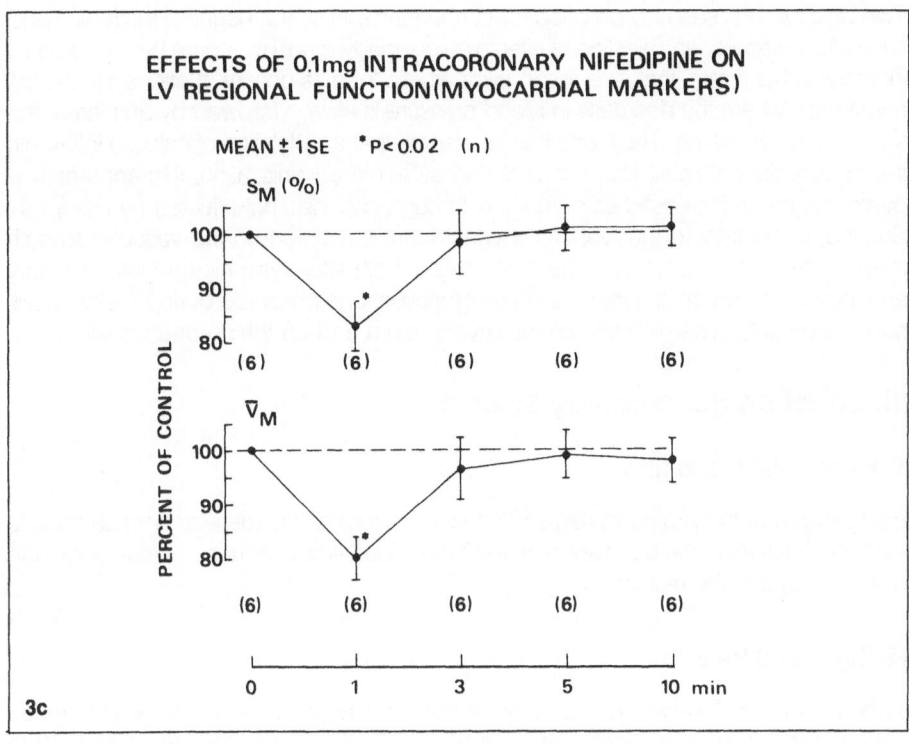

Figure 3a, 3b, 3c: Effects of intracoronary administration of 0.1 mg nifedipine on left ventricular hemody-namics.

3a: Percent changes of heart rate (HR), left ventricular systolic (LVSP) and end-diastolic pressure (LVEDP) over 10 min. Note that after 3 min all changes were normalized.

3b: Percent changes of positive and negative dp/dt and coronary sinus blood flow (CSBF); note the pro-longed effect on CSBF in contrast to positive and negative dp/dt.

3c: Percent changes of LV regional function, measured by the distance of myocardial markers. Note that velocity of shortening is depressed for approximately 2 minutes only and normalized after 3 to 5 minutes; for details see text.

Second, as was to be expected, left ventricular systolic pressure decreased by approx. 10%, positive and negative dp/dt max by approx. 20%, and velocity of fiber shorten-ing by approx. 20%, while ventricular end-diastolic pressure increased by 50% (p < 0.01) (Fig. 3a, 3b). Finally, percent systolic shortening in the midwall circumference (S_M%) as well as velocity of shortening (V_M) decreased significantly by approx. 20%, reaching the maximum after the first minute (p < 0.02) (Fig. 3c). Hence, the partial in-hibition of calcium influx into the myocardium led to a short-lasting, but profound nega-tive inotropic effect and by this to a reduction in oxygen demand which was combined with a marked increase in coronary blood flow by approx. 30% (Amende, 1981). No adverse reactions were observed during these short changes.

Two observations seem to be of special importance. First, the negative inotropic effect seen after intracoronary injection of nifedipine obviously is not overcome by a secondary increase in heart rate, that is, a rise in sympathetic tone as observed after systemic administration where the decrease in blood pressure is always followed by an increase in sympathetic discharge. Thus, one has to assume that an inhibition of calcium influx into the myocardial cell must also occur during systemic administration; this apparently is overcome by an increased calcium influx through channels not affected by nifedipine. Second, in contrast to the working myocardium, the action on the vascular smooth muscle tone of the coronary system is identical both after systemic and intracoronary administration. Hence, the increase in sympathetic tone observed during systemic administration acts synergistically on the myocardium and on the coronary system.

III. Effect on the coronary system

1. Myocardial blood flow

Being aware of the profound relaxing effect of nifedipine on vascular smooth muscle tone, the analysis of the behavior of myocardial blood flow in ischemic areas under the drug was of special interest.

Methods and Patients

Myocardial blood flow was recorded by the use of the regional precordial Xenon residue detection technique (for details, see: Lichtlen, 1979; Engel and Lichtlen, 1981). 10 to 20 mCi 133 Xenon were injected selectively into the main left coronary artery and washout of the isotope was registered by a Pho-gamma-III-camera placed over the precordium in a LAO-projection of 40°, approximately 400 to 600 matrix points covering the heart. The exact position was checked by fluoroscopy and the anatomical distribution of the coronary arteries was verified by coronary angiograms performed in exactly the same projection. A CDC 1700 computer system was used for flow calculation, which followed a monoexponential washout pattern for the first 30 seconds, according to Kety and Schmidt (1945). Flow values were presented both in a digital and analog way, that is, in ml/min/100 g myocardium and as flow image, respectively. Myocardial blood flow was registered in 11 patients both at rest as well as during right atrial pacing increasing heart rate until typical signs of ischemia were present (angina pectoris and/or ST-depression > 0.1 mV); after the injection of Xenon, pacing was continued for another two minutes until washout was completed. After return to control values, 20 mg nifedipine were administered sublingually and, after an interval of 10 minutes, atrial pacing was repeated at the same heart rate and over the same period of time. For this study, only patients with single vessel disease and obstructions > 75% (objectivated by morphometrical measurements) were included, the poststenotic area being perfused by the left anterior descending branch (7 times), by the left circumflex branch (twice) or by the RCA (twice). Normal flow values were obtained from the contralateral artery i.e., from the left circumflex or left anterior descending region of the same patient. Hence, each patient not only served as his own control, but also allowed to compare coronary flow from normal and abnormal regions. The anatomical regionalization of the areas in question was obtained in the same LAO 40° projection.

170

Results

The results are presented in Table 2 and Fig. 4a, b, showing changes of regional myocardial blood flow (RMBF) (precordial Xenon-Clearance) in pacing induced angina after 20 mg sublingual nifedipine. At rest, myocardial blood flow was with 57.1 ± 10.4 ml/min/100 g significantly lower in the poststenotic than in the normal area (70.7 ± 12.8 ml/min/100 g) ($p < 0.0025$). During control pacing, all patients developed ischemic ST-depressions > 0.1 mV and most of them also angina pectoris.

Myocardial blood flow on the average increased significantly in both the normal and the post-stenotic area reaching 91.2 ± 18.5 and 77.6 ± 20.7 ml/min/100 g myocardium respectively; hence, coronary flow remained significantly lower in the ischemic area than in the normal region, where it corresponded to the oxygen demand ($p < 0.005$). As the 133 Xenon technique records transmural flow only, no information can be obtained on myocardial blood flow in the endocardial area where flow — at least in some patients — must have decreased during control pacing (Lichtlen, 1982); this is also suggested from the decrease in poststenotic transmural flow during control pacing below flow levels at rest, observed in one of the patients of this group, who was suffering from severe angina and ST-depressions > 0.2 mV (Fig. 4a).

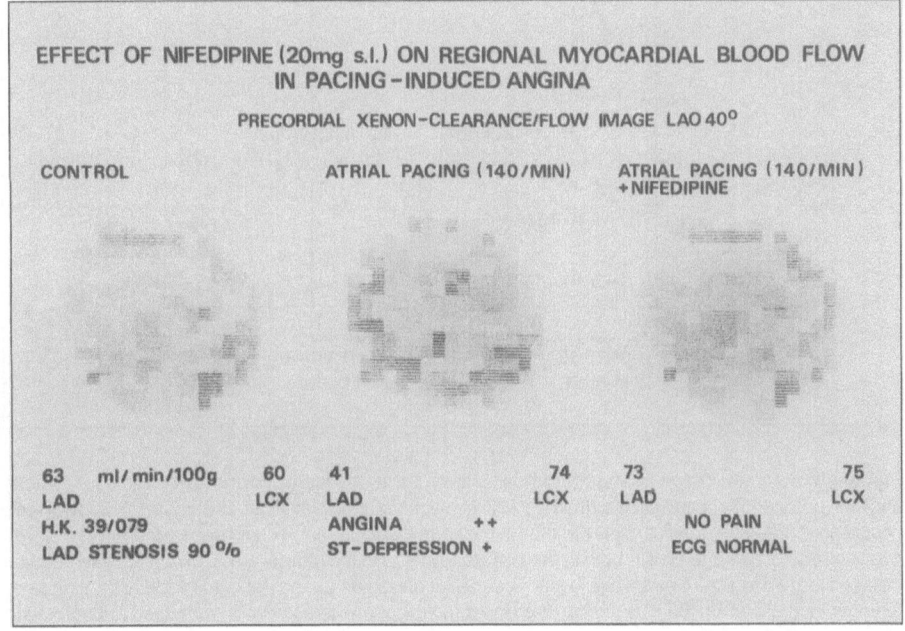

Figure 4a: Typical example: At rest RMBF in the normal and poststenotic area was equal; during control pacing flow decreased in the poststenotic zone and increased in the normal area; this was associated with severe angina and ST-depressions; after drug-administration flow was increased in the poststenotic area and was equal in the normal and poststenotic zone.

- Sublingual nifedipine completely suppressed angina pectoris and ischemia in 7 of 11 patients and reduced angina considerably in the other four patients with ST-depressions < 0.05 mV.

Myocardial blood flow in the previously ischemic area showed a further although not significant increase to 82.3 ± 14.8 ml/min/100 g myocardium whereas in the normal area it remained unchanged with 86.8 ± 14.8 ml/min/100 g myocardium, the difference between the two areas now being insignificant (Fig. 4b).

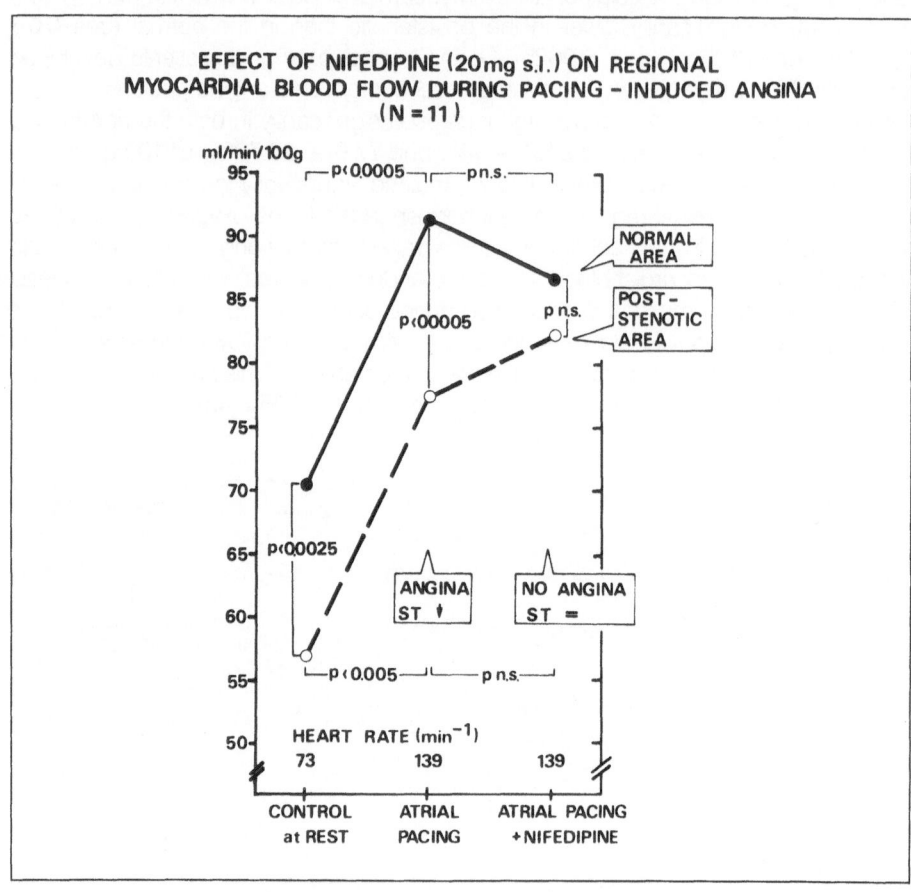

Figure 4b: Summary of flow changes in 11 patients; ordinate: myocardial blood flow in the normal (dots) and the poststenotic area (circles) (ml/min/100 g myocardium). Note that already at rest flow in the poststenotic area was significantly lower than in the normal area; during control pacing there was a significant increase of average RMBF both in the poststenotic and in the normal area, however, the difference between the two regions was still highly significant; after nifedipine during pacing with identical heart rates a further increase of RMBF was seen in the poststenotic zone whereas RMBF remained unchanged in the normal area.

Hence, one must assume that after administration of nifedipine, further arteriolar dilatation occurred in the poststenotic area leading to an increase in flow and oxygen supply, whereas oxygen demand decreased significantly as suggested by the drop in mean aortic pressure from 107.9 to 94.9 mm Hg ($p < 0.005$) (Table 2).

The observation of a further increase of poststenotic flow after nifedipine is difficult to explain, assuming that in the ischemic area coronary reserve is always exhausted, arteriolar dilatation reaching its maximum. One has, therefore, to assume that the additional arteriolar dilatation mainly took place in adjacent areas, i.e., in the mid- and epicardial layers, areas which to a certain extent were probably also underperfused during control pacing. In addition, diastolic volume and muscle stiffness increased mildly as shown in chapter 1.

Table 2: Hemodynamic changes during atrial pacing before and after sublingual administration of nifedipine in 11 patients undergoing recordings of regional myocardial blood flow.

	HEART RATE (BEATS/min)	AORTIC PRESSURE SYSTOLIC (mm Hg)	AORTIC PRESSURE MEAN (mm Hg)	RATE - PRESSURE PRODUCT (mm Hg $\cdot$ min^{-1} $\cdot$ 10^{-2})
REST	72.8	132.5	101.2	96.9
CONTROL RAP	139.5[***]	131.5	107.9	181.7[***]
PACING + NIF	139.5	114.5[***]	94.9[***]	158.6[***]

[***]$P < 0.0005$

2. Effect on coronary obstructions

Postmortem studies have revealed that approximately half of the high-grade obstructions of large epicardial arteries are eccentric in location (Freudenberg, 1981) and a considerable portion of the wall in the area of an obstruction is still normal at histology (Fig. 5); these obstructions are still capable to change their contractile status. It is, therefore, not surprising that after administration of nitrates as well as calcium antagonists such as nifedipine, dilatations of the smallest diameter of an obstruction in the range of more than 20% can be observed in approximately half of the stenoses. The importance of this observation is underlined by the fact that clinically symptomatic obstructions usually have diameters below 1.5 mm, i.e., are in a range where the relation between flow and diameter is an exponential one (Rafflenbeul, 1982); this indicates that small changes in diameter can affect flow quite considerably.

Methods

Coronary obstructions were measured by means of a vernier caliper with an accuracy of 0.05 mm from 35 mm cinefilms projected onto a Tage-Arno reviewer, the tip of the catheter, whose diameter amounts to approx. 1.8 mm both for the SONES as well as for the JUDKINS catheter, serving as reference.

The smallest diameter of an obstruction (D_{sten}) was assessed from multiple projections (2 to 7, average 4) taken within an angle of more than 90°. As intraobserver variability was found to amount to approx. 10%, only changes of D_{sten} by more than 12% were regarded as biologically valid (for details, see: Rafflenbeul, 1979).

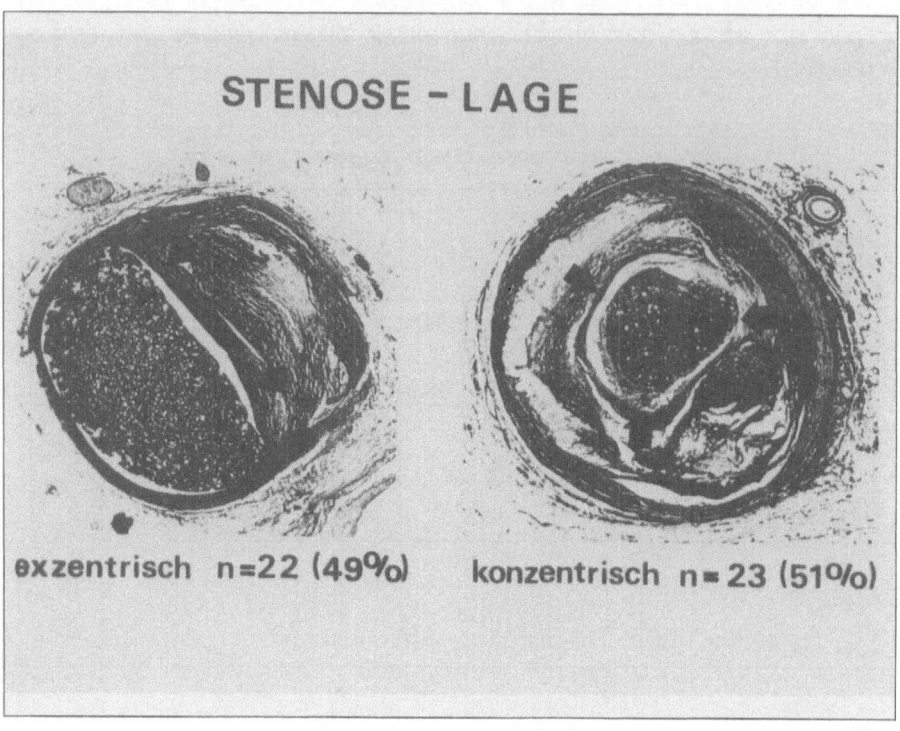

Figure 5: Typical examples of eccentric and concentric obstructions; the eccentric obstruction still shows a large normal wall segment; the rest lumen is filled with contrast medium from postmortem angiography; in 55 consecutive histologic cross-sections an equal distribution between concentric and eccentric obstructions was observed.

Results

The study includes 148 measurements on obstructions, 54 after 0.1 mg sublingual nitroglycerin, 42 after 20 mg sublingual nifedipine and 50 after combined administration of nitroglycerin and nifedipine. As Fig. 6a, b, shows, approx. half of the obstructions analyzed increased their smallest diameter; under nifedipine, 20 of the 42 obstructions by an average of 31%, after nitroglycerin, 25 of the 54 obstructions by an average of 28%, and after combined treatment, 31 of 50 obstructions by an average of 49% (Fig. 6a); hence, the combined effect of nitroglycerin and nifedipine was clearly superior to the isolated administration of the two drugs. This is explained by the different site of action of the two drugs; while nifedipine inhibits the influx of calcium into the cell by blocking approx. 30% of the calcium channels, nitroglycerin seems to act inside the smooth muscle cell by stimulating cGMP and by this smooth muscle relaxation.

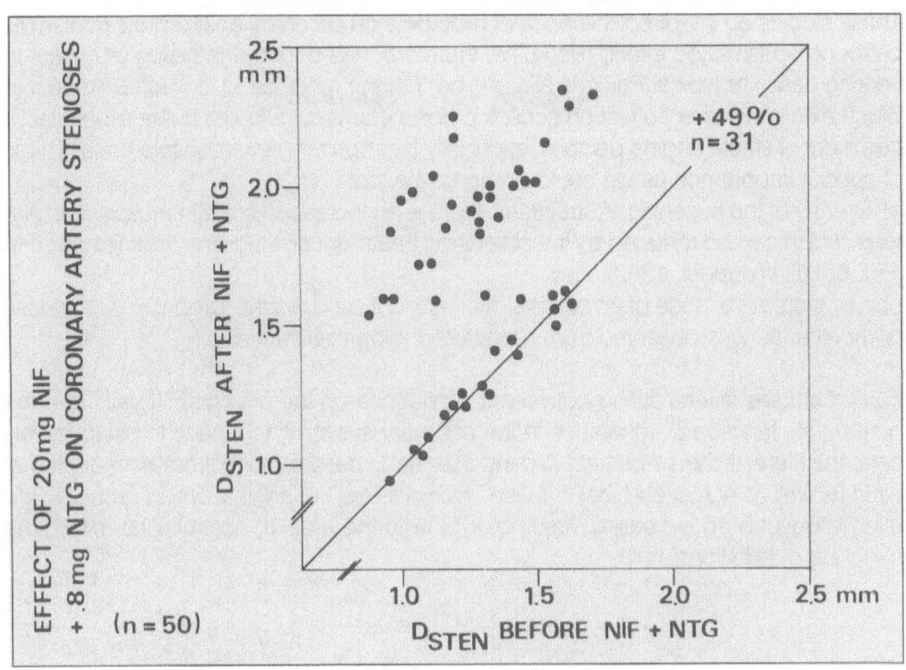

Figure 6a: Combined effect of nifedipine (20 mg s.l.) and nitroglycerin (0.8 mg s.l.) on coronary obstructions: smallest diameter of obstructions before (abscissa) and after drug-administration (ordinate). Note that in 31 of 50 obstructions a significant increase of the smallest diameter was observed, i.e. > 10%, averaging + 49%.

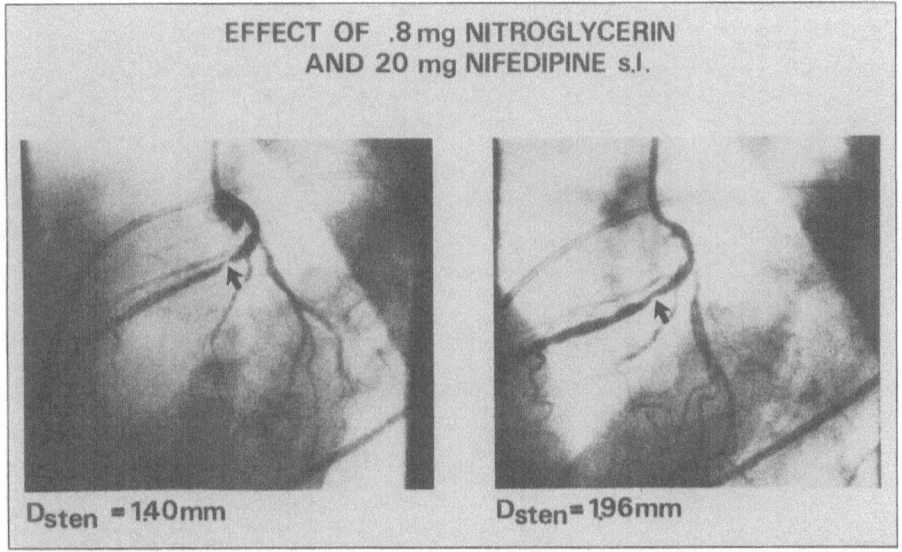

Figure 6b: Typical example of the increase in the smallest diameter of a high-grade obstruction of the left anterior descending branch (arrow) after combined administration of nitroglycerin and nifedipine (left halfaxial projection). Note also the increase in the entire vessel diameter.

175

These studies on the direct influence of nifedipine on coronary obstructions confirm its profound spasmolytic effect; nifedipine, therefore, has become the drug of choice in treating cases of typical Prinzmetal's angina. On the other hand, it is still unknown to which extent this direct effect on eccentric obstructions contributes to the prophylactic treatment of stable angina pectoris, especially by improving exercise tolerance. This is of special importance as we could demonstrate that

a) in many of the eccentric obstructions, there is an increased smooth muscle vascular tone, which can be reduced by the combined treatment of nifedipine and nitroglycerin (Fig. 6b) (Rafflenbeul, 1982), and

b) this "increased" tone often persists over a long period of time, probably over weeks or months, as was observed from repeated angiographic studies.

Further studies differentiating between the influence on the proximal, "fixed" and the peripheral "functional" resistance in the coronary system finally have to establish this concept. Here, it should be kept in mind that many patients suffer from both angina at effort as well as at rest and that in these "mixed forms" of angina, which probably are often based on an increased vasomotor tone in the area of obstructions, nifedipine might be of additional help.

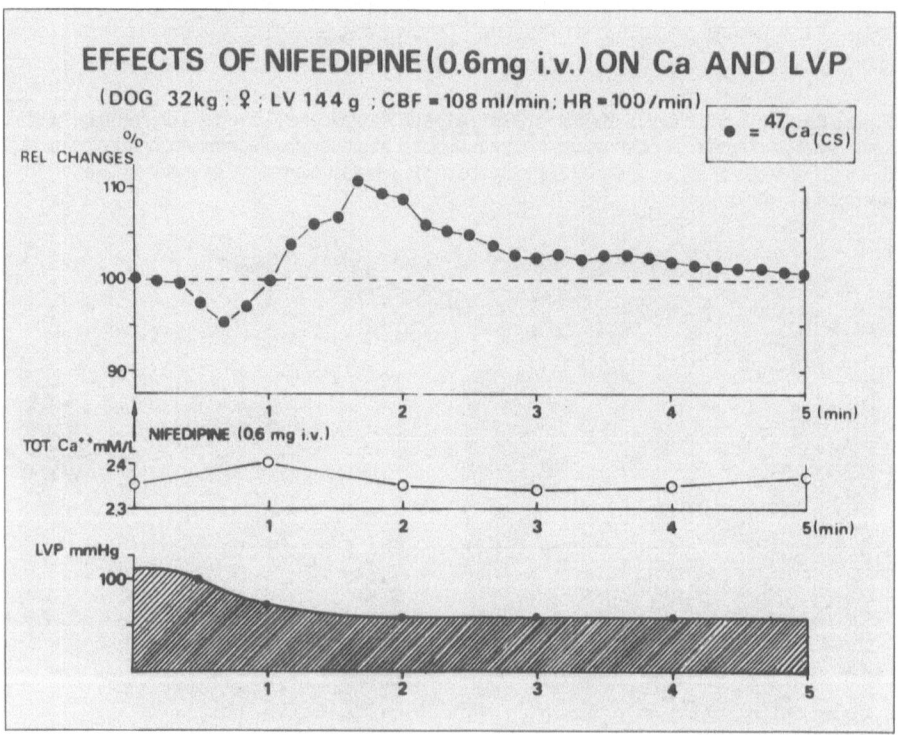

Figure 7: Effects of intracoronary nifedipine on ⁴⁷Ca-activity in coronary sinus blood and on left ventricular pressure in an open-chest dog heart preparation. Before nifedipine was administered a steady state of ⁴⁷Ca-activity was reached (100% value on the ordinate); after intracoronary administration there was a rapid increase of ⁴⁷Ca-activity in the coronary sinus blood to a maximum of 12%, lasting for approximately 5 minutes; at the same time systolic pressure showed a marked decrease.

IV. The influence of calcium-entry blockings agents on [47]calcium influx in the dog heart in situ

In order to quantify calcium fluxes *in vivo*, we performed experiments with the dog heart *in situ* using an open chest preparation (for details, see: Reil, 1981).

Methods

After exposure of the heart, a Gregg-cannula was inserted into the left main coronary artery and the left coronary system was perfused with a constant flow with the aid of a roller pump. After sinus node crash, hearts were paced from the right ventricle at a constant rate of approx. 90 beats/min. A catheter was introduced into the coronary sinus, allowing blood sampling at a constant rate. Pressure measurements were performed from the left ventricle by a cannula introduced through the apex of the heart. During the experimental period, [47]calcium was added to the inflow at a constant rate and sampled from the coronary sinus at 6-second intervals using an automatic sampling; [47]calcium activity was then analyzed in a well counter. In addition, intravascular space was constantly monitored from the coronary sinus using indocyanine green, extravascular space was calculated from dilution curves of ascorbic acid, added to the perfusate and sampled from the coronary sinus. After a steady state had been reached, alterations of calcium flux were induced either by increasing the inotropic state through a rise in heart rate or decreasing it by drugs, especially the intracoronary administration of calcium antagonists (Fig. 7).

Results

Both nifedipine and verapamil reduced [47]calcium uptake by approx. 15 to 18% (Table 3); approx. 2 min after drug administration, a new steady state had been reached, [47]Ca-uptake returning back to baseline, although the negative inotropic effect on the myocardium was still present. This inhibition of calcium flux was observed to be independent of the administered dose of nifedipine and verapamil, suggesting a specific action of the drug on selected calcium channels. It should be mentioned that the model used does not allow a separation of the action on the myocardium from the one on the vascular smooth muscle cells. Nevertheless, from these experiments on the dog heart *in situ*, it seems that the amount of calcium blocked from the entry into the myocardial cell is perhaps smaller than the one found in vascular smooth muscle cell preparations or in isolated hearts.

Table 3: Results of the decrease in [47]Ca-uptake into the myocardium and coronary system after intracoronary administration of nifedipine and verapamil in 4 cases. The absolute values were calculated from wash-in-curves both of [47]Ca and cardiac green as well as ascorbic acid serving as extra-vascular and intra-vascular markers (for details see text).

Exp.	Control $[\mu M\ Ca_{tot}]$	Nifedip. $[\mu m\ Ca_{tot}]$	Differ. $[\mu M\ Ca]$	Differ. [%]
1	1052	865	-187	-18
2	1045	910	-135	-13
3	1388	1178	-210	-14
		Verap.		
4	991	855	-136	-14

References

Amende, I., Simon, R., Hood, W.P., Lichtlen, P.R. The effects of the betablocker Atenolol and Nitroglycerin on left ventricular function and geometry in man *Circulation*, **60**, 836-849 (1979).

Amende, I., Simon, R., Lichtlen, P.R. Early effects of nifedipine on left ventricular diastolic function in man. *Circulation*, **62**, III-259 (1980).

Amende, I., Simon, R., Hood, W.P., Daniel, W., Lichtlen, P.R. Differential effects of intracoronary nitroglycerin and nifedipine on coronary flow and myocardial function in man. *Circulation*, **64**, IV-293 (1981).

Engel, H.J., Lichtlen, P.R. Beneficial enhancement of coronary blood flow by Nifedipine. Comparison with Nitroglycerin and beta blocking agents. *Am. J. Med.*, **71**, 658-666 (1981).

Fleckenstein, A. Fundamental actions of Ca-antagonists on myocardial and cardiac pacemaker cell membranes. In: New perspectives on Ca-antagonists; ed. by G.B. Weiss, Am Physiol. Society, Bethesda, Waverly Press, Baltimore, p. 59-81 (1981).

Freudenberg, H., Lichtlen, P.R. Das normale Wandsegment bei Koronarstenosen, eine postmortale Studie (The normal wall segment in coronary obstructions, a postmortem study). *Z. Kardiol.*, **70**, 863-869 (1981).

Kety, S.S., Schmidt, C.F. The determination of cerebral blood flow in man by the use of nitrous oxide in low concentrations. *Am. J. Physiol.*, **143**, 53-66 (1945).

Lichtlen, P.R., Engel, H.J. Assessment of regional myocardial blood flow using the inert gas washout technique. *Cardiovasc. Radiol.*, **2**, 203-216 (1979).

Lichtlen, P.R., Engel, H.J., Wolf, R., Amende, I. The effect of the Ca-antagonistic drug Nifedipine on coronary and left ventricular dynamics in patients with coronary heart disease. In: Ca-Antagonismus; ed. by A. Fleckenstein and H. Roskamm, Springer-Verlag, Heidelberg, p. 270-81 (1980).

Lichtlen, P.R., Engel, H.J. Relationship between coronary obstructions and regional myocardial blood flow in man during stress provoked by rapid atrial pacing. In: Detection of ischemic myocardium with exercise; ed. by F. Loogen and L. Seipel, Springer-Verlag, Heidelberg, p 98-110 (1982).

Lorell, B.H., Turi, Z., Grossman, W. Modification of left ventricular response to pacing tachycardia by nifedipine in patients with coronary artery disease. *Am. J. Med.*, **71**, 667-675 (1981).

Ludbrook, P.A., Tiefenbronn, A.J., Byrne, J.D., Sobel, B.E. Effects of Nifedipine on left ventricular function: their dependence upon reduced impedance. *Circulation*, **62**, III-259 (1980).

Paulus, W.J., Lorell, B.H., Craig, W E., Wynne, J., Murgo, J.P., Grossman, W. Improved left ventricular diastolic properties in hypertrophic cardiomyopathy treated with nifedipine: altered loading or improved muscle inactivation? *Circulation*, **64**, IV-249 (1981).

Rafflenbeul, W., Smith, L.R., Rogers, W.J., Mantle, J.A., Rackley, C.E., Russell, R.O. Quantitative coronary angiography: coronary anatomy of unstable angina pectoris one year after optimal medical therapy. *Am. J. Cardiol.*, **43**, 699 (1979).

Rafflenbeul, W., Lichtlen, P.R., Kaltenbach, M., Kober, G. Zur dilatierenden Wirkung von Nitroglycerin und Nifedipin auf hochgradige Koronarstenosen. *Z. Kardiol.*, **71**, 166 (1982)

Rafflenbeul, W., Lichtlen, P.R. The concept of dynamic coronary stenosis. *Z. Kardiol.* (im Druck).

Reil, G.H., Frombach, R., Daniel, W., Lichtlen, P.R. Effects of Ca-antagonists on ^{47}Ca-exchange in the dog heart in situ. In: Unstable Angina Pectoris; ed. by W. Rafflenbeul, P.R. Lichtlen, R. Balcon, Thieme, Stuttgart, p. 88-92 (1981).

Rutsch, W., Schartl, M., Krais, T., Schmutzler, W. Der Kalzium antagonistische Effekt auf die zentrale und periphere Hämodynamik, Ventrikelvolumina und die regionale Wandbewegung bei koronarer Herzkrankheit. In: Ca-Antagonismus; ed. by A. Fleckenstein and H Roskamm, Springer-Verlag, Heidelberg, p. 293-299 (1980).

Triggle, D.J. Calcium antagonists: basic chemical and pharmacological aspects. In: New perspectives on Ca-antagonists; ed. by G.B. Weiss, Am. Physiol. Society, Bethesda, Waverly Press, Baltimore, p. 1-18. (1981)

The use of selective calcium antagonism in variant (vasospastic) and classical (effort) angina pectoris

P.H. Kidner

Summary

The calcium-entry blockers as a group are effective in the clinical management of both vasospastic and effort angina. Nifedipine and diltiazem are more effective for the former and diltiazem and verapamil for the latter. Lidoflazine is effective against effort angina. Diltiazem has the lowest incidence of side effects. Verapamil is contra-indicated in the presence of left ventricular dysfunction and high degree of atrio-ventricular block. It should be used with caution with the beta-adrenergic blocking agents. Lidoflazine and nifedipine can be combined with the beta-adrenergic blocking agents and can also be given to patients with left ventricular dysfunction. Lidoflazine must not be given to patients with pre-existing prolongation of the QT interval or with drugs likely to prolong it such as quinidine and disopyramide. The experience with diltiazem is not sufficient to comment usefully on drug combinations nor is it possible to say whether the calcium-entry blockers can be given together with added clinical efficacy or safety.

Résumé

Les bloqueurs de l'entrée de calcium en tant que groupe sont efficaces dans le traitement clinique de l'angor vasospastique et de l'angor d'effort. La nifédipine et le diltiazem sont plus efficaces pour le premier et le diltiazem et le vérapamil le sont davantage pour le second. La lidoflazine est efficace contre l'angor d'effort. Le diltiazem comporte le moins d'effets secondaires. Le vérapamil est contre-indiqué dans le cas d'un dysfonctionnement ventriculaire gauche et d'un bloc auriculo-ventriculaire d'un degré élevé. Il faut être très prudent quand on associe le vérapamil avec agents bloquants bêta-adrénergiques. Quant à la lidoflazine et la nifédipine, elles peuvent être combinées avec des bloquants bêta-adrénergiques et elles peuvent être administrées à des patients présentant un dysfonctionnement ventriculaire gauche. La lidoflazine ne peut pas être administrée à des patients présentant une prolongation préexistante de l'intervalle QT ou recevant des substances susceptibles de le prolonger, comme la quinidine et le disopyramide. L'expérience menée avec le diltiazem n'est pas suffisante pour que l'on puisse se prononcer valablement sur les combinaisons de substances. Il n'est pas possible de dire si la combinaison de divers bloqueurs d'entrée de calcium peut augmenter leur efficacité clinique ou l'innocuité du traitement.

Resumen

Los inhibidores de la penetración intracelular de Ca^{2+} son generalmente eficaces en el tratamiento clínico de angina tanto vasoespástica como de esfuerzo. Nifedipino y diltiazem son más eficaces en la primera, y diltiazem y verapamilo en la segunda. Lidoflazina es eficaz contra angina de esfuerzo. Diltiazem tiene la incidencia más baja de efectos secundarios. Verapamilo está contraindicado en la presencia de disfunción del ventrículo izquierdo y en altos grados de obstrucción atrioventricular. Se debería emplearlo cuidadosamente con agentes bloqueadores beta-adrenérgicos. Nifedipino y lidoflazina pueden ser combinadas con estos últimos, y también administradas a pacientes con disfunción del ventrículo izquierdo. No se puede administrar lidoflazina a pacientes con prolongación preexistente del intervalo QT o con drogas que tienden a prolongarlo, tales como quinidina y disopiramida. La experiencia con diltiazem no es suficiente para poder dar comentario útil en lo de las combinaciones de fármacos, tampoco es posible decir si inhibidores de la penetración intracelular de Ca^{2+} pueden ser administrados juntos para mejorar la eficacia clínica o la seguridad.

Zusammenfassung

Die Kalziumeinstromhemmer sind zur klinischen Behandlung vasospastischer wie auch klassischer Angina erfolgreich zu verwenden. Nifedipin und Diltiazem ergeben bei der erstgenannten, Diltiazem und Verapamil bei der letztgenannten Form die besten Ergebnisse. Lidoflazin ist mit Erfolg bei klassischer Angina zu verwenden. Diltiazem hat die wenigsten Nebenwirkungen. Verapamil ist bei linksventrikulärer Dysfunktion und bei ausgeprägtem Vorhofkammerblock kontraindiziert. Bei gemeinsamer Verabreichung mit Betablockern ist es mit besonderer Vorsicht zu verwenden. Nifedipin oder Lidoflazin darf zusammen mit Betablockern verabreicht werden und ist zur Behandlung von Patienten mit linksventrikulärer Dysfunktion geeignet. Der letztere Stoff darf nicht an Patienten mit verlängertem QT-Intervall oder zusammen mit Arzneimitteln, die voraussichtlich eine solche Wirkung hervorrufen, wie Chinidin und Disopyramid, verabreicht werden. Für Diltiazem besteht keine ausreichende Information, um über mögliche Arzneimittelkombinationen eine Aussage zu machen. Auch weiss man noch nicht, ob nach gleichzeitiger Verabreichung mehrerer Kalziumeinstromhemmer erhöhte klinische Wirksamkeit und Sicherheit bestehen.

"They who are afflicted with it are seized while they are walking, (more especially if it be uphill, and soon after eating) with a painful and most disagreeable sensation in the breast, which seems as if it would extinguish life, if it were to continue; but the moment they stand still, all this uneasiness vanishes." Thus William Heberden (Heberden, 1802) described angina pectoris.

Prinzmetal et al. (1959) described a variant form of angina pectoris which occurs almost exclusively at rest, is not precipitated by physical or emotional stress, and is associated with ST segment elevation rather than depression. This variant angina may be associated with cardiac arrhythmias including ventricular tachycardia and fibrillation, myocardial infarction and sudden death. Its incidence relative to classic angina pectoris is not known.

Both forms of angina pectoris appear to be associated with reduction of blood flow through the coronary arteries, the one, Heberden's, due to atheroma, the other, Prinzmetal's, due to spasm. The former apparently leads to sub-endocardial ischaemia and ST segment depression on the electrocardiogram and the latter to transmural myocardial ischaemia and ST segment elevation. In that the coronary arteries are actively vasomotile, both mechanisms are probably active at varying times and degrees, in patients with transient cardiac pain (Maseri, 1979). Heberden's or effort angina appears to be due to an increase in the metabolic demand outstripping the metabolic supply to the myocardium. Prinzmetal's or vasospastic angina is apparently due to a sudden falling away of the metabolic supply to the myocardium in the face of an unchanged metabolic demand. When spasm and atheroma co-exist in the epicardial (conductance) arteries then the mechanisms may occur together in varying degrees and the onset of spasm in an area of coronary atheroma might possibly lead to the development of unstable angina pectoris with increasingly severe chest pain on exertion and at rest. It might even lead to myocardial infarction. Indeed spasm and atheroma may co-exist in all cases of effort angina, the atheroma in the conductance vessels leading to myocardial ischaemia on exercise with accumulation of metabolic waste products leading to reflex spasm of the intramyocardial resistance arterioles through disturbance of the platelet thromboxane/vessel prostaglandin vasomotor balance (Helstrom, 1982).

Three basic factors determine the metabolic requirements of the myocardium. The first is the heart rate; the faster is beats the more energy the heart requires. The second is the contractile state of the myocardium which is related to the velocity of contraction of the heart fibres. Rapid contraction requires more energy than slow contraction. The third factor is the tension developed in the wall of the ventricle as it contracts, a factor dependant upon the pressure generated within the cavity and related to the blood pressure, and also upon the size of the heart (La Place's Law). All three of these factors are modified in part by the autonomic nervous system.

Alternatively, three basic factors control the blood flow to the myocardium — a diastolic event, which in turn governs the supply of nutrient. Again heart rate is important as tachycardia encroaches on diastole and shortens the time available for blood and thus nutrient flow.

The second factor is the diastolic blood pressure which provides the driving force for the nutrient flow. The third factor is the size of the coronary lumen which can be restricted by atheroma and spasm. To these may be added a fourth — alteration in the viscosity or "flowability" and oxygen-carrying capacity of the blood which may render critical a previously non-significant but otherwise tight stenosis.

In health, the equation (Fig. 1) of metabolic supply and demand remains in balance under practically all circumstances. An increase in metabolic demand is met by an increase in coronary arterial blood flow which occurs mainly by coronary vasodilation (Berne, 1964). This response is severely limited in the presence of severe coronary obstruction which now becomes the over-riding factor in determining the nutrient supply to the myocardium and thus greatly restricting the ability of the heart to respond to stress.

METABOLIC DEMAND	METABOLIC SUPPLY
Heart Rate (Tachycardia ▲)	Heart Rate (Tachycardia ▼)
Contractility	Diastolic pressure
Wall Tension	Coronary Lumen
Blood Pressure	Physiological Tone
Heart Size	Atheroma and Clot
	Spasm

Figure 1: The principal factors affecting the metabolic supply and demand to the myocardium

As a group, calcium-entry blockers depress the myogenic activity and the responsiveness to vasoconstrictor stimuli of the smooth muscle cells of the pre-capillary sphincters. They can thus reduce the afterload of the heart. Calcium-entry blockers also inhibit the contractile response of the smooth muscle cells of the large arteries and can thus reduce or abolish vasospastic episodes. By inhibiting the constrictor responses of the splanchnic capacitance vessels to the sympathetic nervous outflow, they reduce the pre-load of the heart. However, as individuals, the calcium-entry blockers differ in their ability to affect different cardiovascular variables and in the onset and duration of their effect. They also have different degrees of tissue selectivity (Vanhoutte, 1982). This report is an overview of the way in which the vascular effects of the calcium-entry blockers benefit the disordered equation of metabolic supply and demand in patients with effort and vasospastic angina pectoris.

Figure 2 shows the chemical structure of the four calcium-entry blockers currently available for clinical use. To these may be added prenylamine and perhexiline. The latter two agents have not achieved a wide usage possibly due to the frequency of side effects.

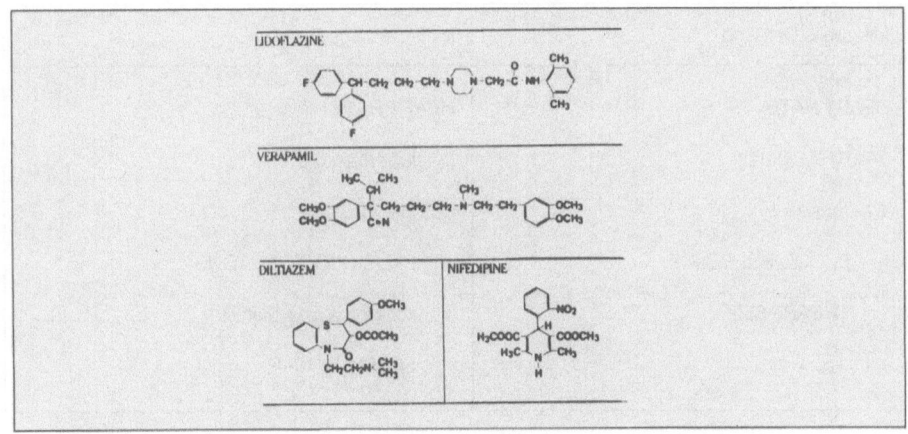

Figure 2: The chemical structure of the four calcium-entry blockers in current clinical use.

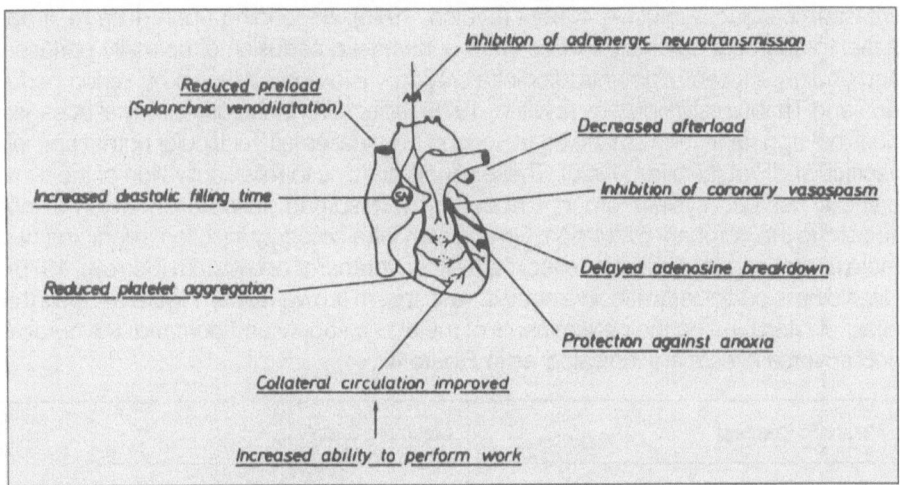

Figure 3: The vascular effects of the calcium-entry blockers (Taken from Vanhoutte, 1982)

Figure 3 summarises the effects of calcium-entry blockers which help to explain their efficacy in the treatment of both forms of angina pectoris. However, not all of the calcium-entry blockers share these effects to the same extent and thus have differing benefits in the treatment of vasospastic and exertional angina. Figure 4 shows the effect of the calcium-entry blockers as a group on the determinants of metabolic supply and demand. The factors which are influenced favourably are in capitals and those influenced unfavourably are italicized.

Nifedipine is a potent vasodilator in general about as potent as nitroglycerine (Henry, 1980). In man it evokes increases in heart rate (± 27%), some decrease in systolic and diastolic pressure, a decrease in peripheral vascular resistance (- 20%) and an in-

185

Metabolic Demand	Metabolic Supply
HEART RATE	HEART RATE
CONTRACTILITY	*Diastolic Pressure*
Wall tension	Coronary Lumen
BLOOD PRESSURE	PHYSIOLOGICAL TONE
? HEART SIZE	Atheroma and Clot
	SPASM

Figure 4: The effect of the calcium antagonists as a group on the determinants of metabolic supply and demand. The factors which are influenced favourably are in capitals and those adversely italicized.

crease in cardiac output (+ 40%) - (Lydten, 1975), depending upon dosage. It appears to augment coronary flow as there is increased perfusion of normally perfused and under-perfused segments after intra-coronary injection as shown by xenon perfusion and Thallium scintigraphy (Lydten, 1975). Nifedipine in the usual clinical dosages does not appear to depress the heart. Indeed it increases left ventricular output and left ventricular dP/dt (Lichtlen, 1980). These effects are due to reflex activation of the sympathetic nervous system brought about by widespread vasodilation which is not specific to the coronary circulation. Given as an intra-coronary injection, nifedipine has more potent negative inotropic effect than either verapamil or diltiazem (Serreys, 1979). Nifedipine is particularly effective against vasospasm (Lown, 1979). Figure 5 shows the effect of nifedipine on the determinants of metabolic supply and demand. Favourable and adverse effects are indicated as in Figure 4.

Metabolic Demand	Metabolic Supply
Heart Rate	*Heart Rate*
? Contractility	*Diastolic Pressure*
Wall Tension	Coronary Lumen
BLOOD PRESSURE	PHYSIOLOGICAL TONE
? HEART SIZE	Atheroma and Clot
	SPASM

Figure 5: The effect of nifedipine on the determinants of myocardial metabolic supply and demand. Favourable effects (capitals) and adverse effects (italics) are indicated as in Fig. 4.

The favourable and unfavourable actions appear to be finely balanced. It is possible the scheme over-simplifies the variables that should be considered or that the favourable and unfavourable actions are not in fact balanced. The effect on coronary arterial tone and/or spasm may outweigh other deleterious effects. Certainly nifedipine does improve myocardial blood flow indeed into regions distal to significant coronary artery obstruction (Lydten, 1975; Malacoff, 1982) which might explain its efficacy in effort angina.

Metabolic Demand	Metabolic Supply
? HEART RATE	? HEART RATE
CONTRACTILITY	*? Diastolic Pressure*
Wall Tension	Coronary Lumen
? BLOOD PRESSURE	PHYSIOLOGICAL TONE
? HEART SIZE	Atheroma and Clot
	SPASM

Figure 6: The effects of verapamil on the determinants of myocardial metabolic supply and demand. Favourable effects (capitals) and adverse effects (italics) are indicated as in Fig. 4.

Verapamil is also a potent vasodilator but somewhat less so than nifedipine and nitroglycerine (Mikkelsen, 1979). In healthy man, intravenous verapamil significantly increases heart rate (+ 14%) and cardiac index (+ 24%) and significantly decreases peripheral resistance (- 33%) and to some extent decreases mean aortic pressure (- 15%) - (Vincenzi, 1976). Given orally to patients with cardiac disease, there is a short-lived decrease in mean arterial pressure, first derivative of left ventricular pressure, systemic resistance and a rise in the left ventricular end-diastolic pressure, but with little change in cardiac output and heart rate (Singh, 1978). Resting heart rate is reduced but peak exercise heart rate is unchanged (Bala Subraminian, 1980). Compared with nifedipine, verapamil has a greater likelihood of depressing myocardial function (Vanhoutte, 1982) especially in patients with cardiac dysfunction (Flaim, 1981). Figure 6 illustrates the effects of verapamil on the determinants of metabolic supply and demand. Favourable and adverse effects are indicated as in Figure 4. This shows that verapamil in theory at least, is likely to be very effective in the treatment of angina pectoris and this appears to be borne out in fact (Bala Subraminian, 1980 and 1982).

Diltiazem is a vasodilator but in contrast to verapamil and nifedipine, it is more selective to the coronary and cerebral circulations (Zelis, 1980). Given orally to patients with coronary artery disease, diltiazem produces small decreases in heart rate (- 6.2%), systolic aortic pressure (- 9.1%), cardiac index (- 5.2%) and peripheral resistance (- 4.1%) - (Kusukawa, 1977). Although a vasodilator, diltiazem produces no tachycardia or minimal sinus bradycardia (Henry, 1980). In comparison with verapamil, in dogs, diltiazem appears to have less effect on contractility and is less negatively inotropic (Walsh, 1979) but in man diltiazem appears to have little or no effect on the contractility indices (Bing, 1979). Figure 7 shows the effects of diltiazem on the determinants of metabolic supply and demand. Favourable and adverse effects are indicated as in Figure 4. Once again, diltiazem would appear to be an effective anti-anginal agent with, in view of its specific vasodilatory properties in the coronary circuit, especial efficacy in vasospastic angina.

Metabolic Demand	Metabolic Supply
HEART RATE	HEART RATE
? CONTRACTILITY	*Diastolic Pressure*
Wall Tension	Coronary Lumen
BLOOD PRESSURE	PHYSIOLOGICAL TONE
? HEART SIZE	Atheroma and Clot
	SPASM

Figure 7: The effects of diltiazem on the determinants of metabolic supply and demand. Favourable effects (capitals) and adverse effects (italics) are indicated as in Fig. 4.

Lidoflazine is a vasodilator and its effect appears to be prolonged (Vanhoutte, 1980). It has little effect on the resting heart rate in normals (De Cock, 1973; Detry, 1976) but appears to reduce it in patients with angina pectoris (Gobel, 1975). It does not reduce the heart rate at maximal exercise (Jenkins, 1981; Shapiro, 1982). In angina sufferers, the stroke volume is improved at rest and upon exercise but the cardiac output only increases on exercise (Gobel, 1975). The mean arterial pressure and systemic vascular resistance fall both at rest and upon maximal exercise. The heart rate — mean arterial pressure product is improved at rest after prolonged oral dosage of lidoflazine but remains unchanged at peak exercise. Lidoflazine is associated with a significant increase in myocardial blood flow (Gobel, 1980) and studies with thallium scintigraphy would suggest this is to regions supplied by significantly obstructed coronary arteries (Shapiro, 1982). Lidoflazine has negligible effects on cardiac contractility in animals (Vanhoutte, 1980) but this may not be so in man (Gobel, 1975). The drug also appears to reduce platelet aggregation significantly and may thus improve blood viscosity leading to improved myocardial perfusion at existing coronary pressures (Vanhoutte, 1980). It also amplifies and prolongs reactive hyperaemia of the myocardium, a function probably associated with its ability to inhibit the uptake into the myocardial cells of adenosine, a potent endogenous vasodilator (Vanhoutte, 1980). Finally, lidoflazine inhibits the influx of calcium into the myocardial cell during the reperfusion phase of prolonged normothermic myocardial ischaemia in dogs. This significantly protects the cell from the deleterious effect of calcium overload with preservation of structural integrity (Flameng, 1980). Figure 8 shows the effects of lidoflazine on the determinants of metabolic supply and demand of the myocardium with favourable and adverse effects indicated as previously.

Metabolic Demand	Metabolic Supply
? HEART RATE	? HEART RATE
Contractility	*Diastolic Pressure*
Wall Tension	Coronary Lumen
BLOOD PRESSURE	PHYSIOLOGICAL TONE
? HEART SIZE	Atheroma and Clot
	SPASM

Figure 8: The effects of lidoflazine on the determinants of myocardial metabolic supply and demand. Favourable effects (capitals) and adverse effects (italics) are indicated as in Fig. 4.

From the foregoing it would appear likely that all four calcium-entry blockers would be effective against both vasospastic and effort angina. Evidence is lacking for the efficacy of lidoflazine in the former but apart from this there is now overwhelming experience attesting to the clinical efficacy of these preparations (Singh, 1978; Bala Subraminian, 1982; Jenkins, 1981; Shapiro, 1982; Parisi, 1982). The mechanism of their action in vasospastic angina appears clear; the calcium-entry blockers relieve the underlying coronary artery spasm. However, the mechanism of their action in effort angina is by no means clear. None of the drugs improves the rate-pressure product at peak exercise and thus an increase in myocardial blood supply to ischaemic areas appears unlikely despite measured increases in total myocardial blood flow. On the other hand, a drug-induced decrease in myocardial oxygen demand seems an unlikely mechanism in view of the apparently small effects of these drugs on the classical determinants of metabolic demand. Diltiazem, verapamil and lidoflazine do lower the resting heart rate and also the heart rate at sub-maximal levels of exercise. This may be one factor explaining their efficacy. However, they do not reduce the heart rate at peak exercise. Redistribution of blood to the ischaemic subendocardium is a possibility as in fibrillating arterially perfused canine hearts, verapamil and nifedipine were reported to relax only small resistive arteries and arterials rather than large (conductance) coronary arteries (Takeda, 1977). However, as mentioned previously, it is very likely that the metabolic demand/supply equation as herein defined grossly over-simplifies the in vivo situation or that advantages conferred by these drugs are underestimated or unknown. Certainly the equation does not explain the prolonged onset of action of lidoflazine nor yet its continued improvement of clinical efficacy over 4-6 months of continued clinical usage (Jenkins, 1981). Perhaps the observation that lidoflazine inhibits calcium overload of the ischaemic cell and thus protects against the effects of ischaemia (Flameng, 1980) provides a clue to at least part of the mechanism of action of calcium-entry blockade in effort angina. At present it is unknown.

Evidence is now available of the relative potencies of the agents in the treatment of angina pectoris. Table I shows the effect of calcium-entry blockers on vasospastic angina from 11 Japanese centres (Kishida, 1975). Verapamil was much less successful than nifedipine and diltiazem in eliminating chest pain (11 %, 77 % and 80 % of cases respectively) though significant improvement was noted in around 90 % of patients with all three drugs. The beneficial effects of the calcium-entry blockers on vasospastic angina pectoris have been amply confirmed elsewhere (Henry, 1980; Lown, 1979; Singh, 1978). Table II shows the comparison of the anti-anginal efficacy of three calcium antagonists with propranolol and placebo (Bala Subraminian, 1982). Although the authors give no subjective data i.e. it is not possible to say from their data whether the patients were any better, the objective exercise data does suggest that the calcium-entry blockers were effective anti-anginal agents, that at submaximal levels of exercise at least, the mechanism of action was one of decrease in metabolic demand, and that verapamil appeared to be the most effective agent followed closely by diltiazem both of whom appeared more effective than nifedipine and propranolol which appeared equipotent in the treatment of angina pectoris.

TABLE I: The effect of the calcium antagonists on vasospastic angina (From Kishida, 1975).

	Total cases (N)	Complete elimination of attacks	Decrease of attacks of less than 50%	% of Effective cases
Nifedipine	149	115	25	94
Diltiazem	87	70	9	91
Verapamil	28	3	21	86

TABLE II: The effect of the calcium-entry blockers on exercise compared with propranolol in patients with effort angina (From Bala Subraminian, 1982).

	P	D	N	V
No. of patients	24	20	28	28
Dosage	240 mg.	360 mg.	60 mg.	360 mg.
Ex. Time	+ 42	+ 67	+ 39	+ 75
Resting HR	- 26	- 20	+ 4	- 8
Max. HR	- 23	- 3	+ 4	- 1
Δ HR	- 43	- 41	- 25	- 37
MST ▼ (CM5)	- 29	- 6	- 3	- 3
IMM Time	+ 73	+ 75	+ 49	+ 82

P = propranolol;
D = Diltiazem;
N = Nifedipine;
V = Verapamil;
HR = Heart Rate;
ΔHR = heart rate increase per minute of exercise;
Ex. Time = The time required to reach angina;
MST ▼ = Peak ST depression;
(All values are expressed as percentage changes compared with placebo).

Table III: Adverse effects attributed to calcium-entry blocking agents.

Nifedipine:	Ankle oedema, headache, dizziness, tinnitus, fatigue, nasal congestion, flushing, hypotension.
Verapamil:	Constipation, headache, dizziness, nausea, sleepiness, palpitation, increases PR interval (higher degress of A-V block after I.V. injection or with beta blockers).
Diltiazem:	Headaches, flushing, dizziness, nervousness, sleeplessness.
Lidoflazine:	Dizziness, headache, tired/painful legs, tinnitus, blurred vision, ventricular arrhythmias.

The oral daily dose of verapamil is 240-480 mg., of diltiazem 180-270 mg., of nifedipine 30-80 mg. and of lidoflazine 180-360 mg. The dose of the latter should be built up over three weeks. Table III gives the adverse effects attributable to the calcium-entry blocking agents. The incidence of side effects with nifedipine is high (17% of patients). It is lower with verapamil (9%) and lowest with diltiazem (4%) - (Flaim, 1981). The overall incidence of side effects with lidoflazine is not known from the literature. However, lidoflazine prolongs the QT interval on the electrocardiogram and a few instances of ventricular tachycardia with syncope have been reported in patients receiving the drug. This matter is currently under review.

References

Bala Subraminian, V., Bowles, M.J., Khurmi, N.S., Davies, A.B. and Raftery, E.B. Comparison of the anti-anginal efficacy of four calcium ion antagonists with propranolol. *Am. J. Cardiol.*, **49** (Abstr.), 929 (1982).

Bala Subraminian, V., Paramisavan, R., Lahii, A. and Raftery, E.B. Verapamil in chronic stable angina. *Lancet*, **1**, 841 (1980).

Berne, R.M. Regulation of coronary blood flow. *Physiological reviews*, **44**, 1 (1964).

Bing, R.J. New drug therapy with a calcium antagonist. Princeton, Excerpta Medica 3-257 (1979).

De Cock, W , Schuermans, V., Jagenau, A., De Cree, J. and Brugmans, J. Heart rate and S.T.I. in normal men after lidoflazine *Arzneim. Forsch.*, **23**, 1450 (1973).

Detry, J.M., Rosseau, M.F., Filleul, R., Frans, A., Clerbeaux, T. and Brasseur, L.A. Haemodynamic effects of lidoflazine in normal subjects. *European J. Cardiol.*, **4**, 165 (1976).

Flaim, S. and Zelis, R. Clinical use of calcium-entry blockers. *Fed. Proc.*, **40**, 2877 (1981).

Flameng, W., Daenen, W., Xhonneux, R., Van de Water, A., Thone, F. and Borgers, M. Lidoflazine protection against normothermic myocardial ischaemia in the dog. In: Myocardial protection and exercise tolerance: the role of lidoflazine, a new anti-anginal agent. Royal Soc. Med., Int. Cong. Symp. Series, **29**, 89-95 (1980)

Gobel, F.L., Nordstrom, L.A., Nelson, R.R. and Ketola, E. The effect of lidoflazine on myocardial performance and blood flow in patients with angina pectoris. In: Proceeding of 2nd international lidoflazine symposium, Perimed Verlag, p. 139 (1975).

Gobel, F.L. The effect of lidoflazine on myocardial blood flow during exercise in patients with angina pectoris. In: Myocardial protection and exercise tolerance: the role of lidoflazine, a new anti-anginal agent. Royal Soc. Med., Int. Cong. Symp. Series, **29**, 43-49 (1980).

Heberden, W. Commentary on the history and cure of diseases. London (1802).

Helstrom, R.H. The injury-spasm (ischaemia-induced haemostatic vasoconstrictive) and vascular auto regulatory hypothesis of ischaemic disease. *Am. J. Cardiol.*, **49**, 802 (1982).

Henry, P.D. Comparative pharmacology of calcium antagonists: nifedipine, verapamil and diltiazem. *Am. J. Cardiol.*, **46**, 1047 (1980).

Jenkins, M.D., Swallow, E.A., Hadi, O.A. and Kidner, P.H. Angina pectoris: effects of lidoflazine on exercise tolerance and chest pain. *Am. J. Cardiol.*, **48**, 140 (1981).

Kishida, H. Application of calcium antagonists in patients with Prinzmetal angina pectoris. In: Lochner, W., Braasch, W., Kroneberg, G. Editors. 2nd international Adalat symposium. New Therapy of ischaemic heart disease. Berlin: Excerpta Medica, p. 246 (1975).

Kusukawa, R., Kinoshita, M., Shimono, Y., Tomonaga, G. and Hosino, T. Haemodynamic effects of a new anti-anginal drug, diltiazem hydrochloride. *Arzneim. Forsch.*, **27**, 878 (1977).

Lichtlen, H., Engel, J., Wolf, R. and Amende, I. The effect of the calcium antagonistic drug nifedipine on coronary and left ventricular haemodynamics in patients with coronary heart disease. In: Fleckenstein, A., Roskamm, H., editors. Calcium-antagonismus, Heidelberg, Springer Verlag, p. 270 (1980).

Lown, B. Symposium on nifedipine and calcium flux inhibition in the treatment of coronary artery spasm and myocardial ischaemia. *Am. J. Cardiol.*, **44**, 779 (1979).

Lydten, H., Lohmoller, G., Lohmoller, R., Schmitz, H. and Walter, I. Haemodynamic studies on Adalat in healthy volunteers and in patients. In: Lochner, W., Braasch, W., Kroneberg, G. Editors. 2nd international Adalat symposium. New Therapy of ischaemic heart disease. Berlin: Excerpta Medica, p. 112 (1975).

Malacoff, R.F., Beverly, L.H., Mudge, G.H., Holman, L.B., Idoine, J., Bifolck, L. and Cohn, P.F. Beneficial effects of nifedipine on regional myocardial blood flow in patients with coronary artery disease. *Circulation*, **65** (Suppl. 1), 32 (1982).

Maseri, A., L'Abbate, A., Cherchia, S., Parodi, O., Sever, S., Biagini, A., Distante, A., Marzelli, M. and Ballestra, A.M. Significance of spasm in the pathogenesis of ischaemic heart disease. *Am. J. Cardiol.*, **44**, 788 (1979).

Mikkelsen, E., Andersson, K.E. and Lederballe Pederson, O. Verapamil and nifedipine inhibition of contractions induced by potassium and noradrenaline in human mesenteric arteries and veins. *Acta Pharmacol. Toxicol.* (Copenh.), **44**, 110 (1979).

Parisi, A.F., Strauss, W.E., McIntyre, K.M. and Sasahara, K.M. Considerations in evaluating new anti-anginal drugs. *Circulation*, **65** (Suppl. 1), 38 (1982).

Prinzmetal, M., Kennamer, R., Merliss, R., Wada, T. and Bor, N. A variant form of angina pectoris. *Am. J. Med.*, **27**, 375 (1959).

Serreys, P.W. and van den Brand, M. Effects of nifedipine on left ventricular isovolumic contraction following intravenous or intracoronary administration. *Circulation*, **60** (Suppl. 2), 82 (1979).

Shapiro, W., Narahara, K.A. and Park, J. The effects of lidoflazine on exercise performance and thallium stress scintigraphy in patients with stable angina pectoris. *Circulation*, **65** (Suppl. 1), 43 (1982).

Singh, B.N., Ellrodt, G. and Peter, C.T. Verapamil: a review of its pharmacological properties and therapeutic use. *Drugs*, **15**, 169 (1978).

Takeda, K., Nakagawa, Y., Katano, Y. and Imai, S. Effects of coronary vasodilators on large and small coronary arteries in dogs. *Jap. Heart J.*, **18**, 92 (1977).

Vanhoutte, P.M. and Van Nueten, J.M. The pharmacology of lidoflazine. In: Myocardial protection and exercise tolerance: the role of lidoflazine, a new anti-anginal agent. Royal Soc. Med., Int. Cong. Symp. Series, **29**. p. 61-77 (1980).

Vanhoutte, P.M. Calcium-entry blockers and vascular smooth muscle. *Circulation*, **65** (Suppl. 1), 11 (1982).

Vincenzi, M., Allegri, P., Gabaldo, S., Maiolino, P. and Ometto, R. Haemodynamic effects caused by intravenous administration of verapamil in healthy subjects. *Arzneim. Forsch.*, **26**, 1221 (1976).

Walsh, R., Badke, F. and O'Rourke, R. Differential effects of diltiazem and verapamil on left ventricular performance in conscious dogs. *Circulation*, **60** (Suppl. 2), 15 (1979).

Zelis, R. and Schroder, J.S. Calcium, calcium antagonists and cardiovascular disease. *Chest*, **78**, 121 (1980).

Calcium entry blockers in cardiovascular therapy.
Influence of diltiazem on hemodynamics and coronary blood flow

M.G. Bourassa

Summary

Diltiazem possesses the usual properties of calcium entry blockers but, because the drug has the distinct advantage of being a negative chronotropic agent, it has the potential of leading to a greater reduction in myocardial oxygen consumption in some clinical situations. Other advantages include a longer duration of action and the causation of minimal side effects, even at relatively high calcium entry blocking doses.

Diltiazem can be considered as one of the drugs of choice in the treatment of patients with documented variant angina. The drug can also be useful in the management of stable and unstable angina, particularly in patients who do not respond adequately to nitrates and beta-adrenergic blocking agents or who experience side effects to these drugs. Diltiazem can be used as a first choice medication in patients with supraventricular tachyarrhythmias or as an alternative to verapamil. Finally, the efficacy of diltiazem in reducing infarct size and in improving the overall prognosis of patients with recent myocardial infarction remains to be determined.

193

Résumé

Le diltiazem possède les mêmes propriétés que les bloqueurs d'entrée de calcium mais, cette substance présentant l'avantage particulier d'être un agent chronotrope négatif, elle est en mesure de conduire à une plus forte réduction de la consommation d'oxygène myocardique dans certaines situations cliniques. Elle compte d'autres avantages parmi lesquels une durée d'action accrue et une diminution des effets secondaires, même à des doses relativement élevées de blocage d'entrée de calcium.

Le diltiazem peut être considéré comme une substance de choix dans le traitement de patients présentant un angor variant documenté. Le substance peut également être utile dans le traitement d'un angor stable ou instable, en particulier chez des patients ne répondant pas de façon appropriée avec nitrates et aux agents bloquants bêta-adrénergiques ou qui sont sujets à des effets secondaires de la part de ces substances. Le diltiazem peut être utilisé comme médication de premier choix chez des patients présentant des tachyarythmies supraventriculaires ou en tant qu'alternative au vérapamil. Enfin, l'efficacité du diltiazem quant à réduire l'étendue de l'infarctus et à améliorer le pronostic général de patients ayant eu un infarctus du myocarde dans un passé récent doit encore être déterminée.

Resumen

Diltiazem posee las propiedades corrientes de los inhibidores de la penetración intracelular de Ca^{2+}, pero, puesto que la droga tiene la clara ventaja de ser un agente cronotrópico negativo, puede conducir a una mayor reducción de la consumición de oxígeno miocardíaco en algunas situaciones clínicas. Otras ventajas se deben al hecho de que la duración de su acción es más larga, y sus efectos secundarios ligeros, incluso con dosis inhibidoras de la penetración intracelular de Ca^{2+} relativamente altas. Diltiazem puede ser considerado como una de las drogas predilectas en el tratamiento de pacientes con angina de Prinzmetal probada. La droga puede también ser útil en el tratamiento de angina estable e inestable, particularmente para pacientes que no responden adecuadamente en nitratos y agentes bloqueadores beta-adrenérgicos o para los que experimentan efectos secundarios con estas drogas. Diltiazem puede emplearse como una medicación predilecta en pacientes con taquiarritmias supraventriculares o como una alternativa de verapamilo. Finalmente, la eficacia de diltiazem queda por determinar en cuanto a la reducción de la extensión del infarto y al mejoramiento del prognóstico global de pacientes con reciente infarto miocardíaco.

Zusammenfassung

Diltiazem hat die üblichen Eigenschaften von Kalziumeinstromhemmern, kann aber weiterhin aufgrund seiner negativ chronotropen Wirkung in bestimmten klinischen Situationen eine grössere Abnahme des myokardialen Sauerstoffverbrauches herbeiführen. Andere Vorteile sind seine lange Wirkungsdauer und, sogar bei verhältnismäßig hohen Dosen, ein Minimum an Nebenwirkungen.

Diltiazem ist als eines der bevorzugten Arzneimittel bei der Behandlung von Patienten mit Prinzmetal-Angina in der Anamnese zu betrachten. Das Arzneimittel kann sowohl bei stabiler als auch bei instabiler Angina verwendet werden, insbesondere bei Patienten, die auf Nitrate und Betablocker nicht ansprechen bzw. unter solcher Medikation mit Nebenwirkungen reagieren. Diltiazem ist bei Patienten mit supraventrikulärer Tachyarrhythmie als Mittel der Wahl oder als Alternative für Verapamil anzuwenden.
Die Wirkung von Diltiazem beim Verringern des Infarktherdes und beim Verbessern der allgemeinen Prognose bei Patienten mit rezentem Myokardinfarkt ist noch zu untersuchen.

Diltiazem shares the different basic properties of calcium entry blockers, a new class of cardiovascular drugs which has assumed great clinical importance recently. Like other calcium channel blockers, diltiazem also possesses several specific hemodynamic, pharmacologic and electrophysiologic characteristics which set it apart as an anti-anginal and anti-arrhythmic agent.

Mechanisms of action of calcium channel blockers calcium ions and excitation-contraction in smooth muscle and cardiac muscle

Calcium ions play major roles in many tissues, but they are particularly critical to the function of cardiac tissue and vascular smooth muscle (Fleckenstein, 1977; Braunwald, 1982). Myocardial cell depolarization (transmembrane action potential) is composed by an initial sharp spike followed by a prolonged plateau. The former is caused by the movement of sodium ions into the cell, whereas the latter results largely from the inward movement of calcium into the cell as well as release of calcium from storage sites in the sarcoplasmic reticulum. The intracellular accumulation of free calcium leads to the formation of a calcium-troponin complex which, by inhibition of tropomyosin, leads to the formation of actomyosin and to mechanical contraction.

The energy required for the formation of actomyosin is supplied by the hydrolysis of ATP by myofibrillar ATPase which is also under the control of calcium. Thus, calcium plays an essential role coupling myocardial and smooth muscle cell excitation to contraction.

Calcium entry can be blocked by a variety of drugs. These substances vary markedly in their chemical structures and in their hemodynamic, pharmacologic and electrophysiologic properties. Their site of action appears limited to the cell membrane. They produce structural changes in cell membranes and bring about profound alterations in cardiovascular function.

Consequences of selective calcium influx inhibition through the cell membrane

Calcium entry blockers exert a selective action on the cardiovascular system: the vascular smooth muscle where they antagonize vasoconstriction, and the myocardium where they exert negative inotropic, chronotropic and dromotropic effects (Antman, 1980; Stone, 1980; Henry, 1980; Low, 1982; Mitchell, 1982).

In coronary and systemic arteries, calcium entry blockers have potent, dose related antivasoconstrictor effects both in vitro and in vivo. Many calcium entry blockers also have major, dose dependent cardiac depressant effects in vitro. However, in anesthetized and conscious animals and in man, these effects are variable, being opposed by reflex sympathetic stimulation. Reduced afterload and reflex baroreceptor activation exert strong positive inotropic and chronotropic effects which antagonize the direct negative cardiac action of these drugs.

Afterload reduction induced by systemic vasodilatation, and decreased arterial pressure and peripheral vascular resistance, tends to increase heart rate and cardiac contractility. These effects are roughly proportional to the drop in systemic blood pressure.

In the coronary circulation, calcium entry blockers increase coronary blood flow in large capacitance vessels and in small vessels including collaterals, and they relieve coronary vasospasm.

Influence of diltiazem on hemodynamics and coronary blood flow

The precise mechanisms by which diltiazem exerts its anti-anginal effects have not been fully determined, but it is believed to be brought about largely by its role as a vascular smooth muscle relaxant and, to a lesser extent, as a negative chronotropic agent (Bourassa, 1980; Théroux, 1980).

Under resting conditions, diltiazem produces a dose dependent, but usually moderate drop in blood pressure and a slight reduction in heart rate. These hemodynamic changes result in a moderate reduction in myocardial oxygen requirements. Studies to date, particularly in patients with good ventricular function, show that cardiac output, ejection fraction and left ventricular end diastolic pressure are not affected.

The effects on heart rate, systemic blood pressure and myocardial oxygen consumption are accentuated during submaximal and maximal exercise, without adverse consequences on left ventricular function (Wagniart, 1982b; Hossack, 1982a; Subramanian, 1983).

Diltiazem dilates both large and small coronary arteries, relieves coronary spasm and increases coronary blood flow. Myocardial oxygen delivery is increased directly in patients with variant angina. There is indirect evidence suggesting that diltiazem also increases myocardial oxygen supply during exercise in patients with chronic effort-related angina (Wagniart, 1982b; Hossack, 1982a; Subramanian, 1983).

Finally, diltiazem produces a moderate prolongation of AH conduction time and of AV node functional and effective refractory periods (Rowland, 1983).

Effects of diltiazem in variant angina

Calcium channel blockers now represent the first line of drugs for the treatment of patients with variant angina. Diltiazem has been found very effective in relieving coronary spasm both in controlled and uncontrolled clinical studies (Kimura, 1981; Waters, 1981a; Waters, 1981b; Rosenthal, 1980; Pepine, 1981; Feldman, 1982; Rosenthal, 1983).

Mechanism of coronary spasm

The cause of coronary spasm in patients with variant angina is still unclear. Vascular, neurohumoral and platelet factors appear to play a role in its pathogenesis (Yasue, 1983). Stimulation of alpha-adrenergic receptors with epinephrine after beta-blockade with propranolol can cause coronary spasm in susceptible patients. Metacholine, a parasympathetic agent, treadmill exercise and the cold pressor test frequently induce coronary spasm in patients with variant angina, presumably through sympathetic reflexes. Several alpha-adrenergic blocking agents are capable of suppressing coronary spasm in these patients.

Contraction and tone of vascular smooth muscle depend on an increase of free intracellular calcium available to the contracting proteins. Alpha-adrenergic stimulation increases intracellular calcium ions and causes contraction of vascular smooth muscle cells.

Coronary spasm can be regarded as an abnormal contraction of smooth muscle of the coronary artery induced by an increase in intracellular calcium ions, and neurohumoral factors that influence intracellular calcium ions may play an important role in the production of coronary spasm. Administration of diltiazem and other calcium entry blockers which dilate coronary arteries by blocking the entry of calcium ions into coronary vascular smooth muscle cells, prevents coronary spasm and increases myocardial oxygen delivery in patients with variant angina.

Comparison of the effectiveness of diltiazem and other calcium channel blockers

A large Japanese collaborative study (Kimura, 1981), involving 11 clinical centers and a total of 279 patients, recently showed that both diltiazem and nifedipine suppressed attacks of variant angina in 75-80% of patients. They reduced the rate of attacks to less than half in 10-15% of patients and were not effective in 6-9% of patients. Verapamil was less effective, suppressing the attacks in only 11% of patients and having no effects in 14%. The association of diltiazem and nifedipine was almost invariably effective.

In a recent study (Waters, 1981b), 27 patients were successively given, in a random order, diltiazem, nifedipine and verapamil. The overall results of the ergonovine test during treatment with diltiazem and nifedipine were similar and slightly better than with verapamil. For the patients taking a calcium blocker that had converted their ergonovine test to negative, the follow-up was angina-free in 93%, compared to only 33 percent of those taking a drug that had been associated with a persistently positive test.

The long term prognosis of variant angina also appears equally good following chronic therapy with diltiazem, nifedipine and verapamil (Waters, 1981a).

Effects of diltiazem in chronic stable angina

In patients with chronic stable angina and fixed coronary obstructions, diltiazem has been shown to significantly reduce the frequency of anginal attacks and/or nitroglycerin consumption, and to increase the duration of treadmill exercise in several controlled studies (Subramanian, 1983; Strauss, 1982; Hossack, 1982b; Pool, 1982).

Improvement in exerise tolerance is observed at dose levels varying between 120 and 360 mg per day, but the best reduction of anginal attacks and nitroglycerin consumption, enhancement of exercise capacity and improvement of objective ischemic variables are observed at dose levels of 240 mg per day or greater.

Mechanisms of action

The hemodynamic disturbances in effort related angina are complex. The action of diltiazem appears to be related primarily to a reduction of myocardial oxygen demand, although there is indirect evidence that myocardial oxygen delivery is also increased in these patients (Wagniart, 1982b; Hossack, 1982a).
Reduction in myocardial oxygen consumption is probably caused by a decrease in blood pressure brought about by the reduction of peripheral resistance and by a decrease in heart rate.

These effects are small at rest, but become important during exercise resulting in increased exercise duration and increased time to onset of angina and/or ischemic ST depression during maximal exercise. During submaximal exercise, heart rate, blood pressure and pressure-rate product are lower after diltiazem, indicating a lower myocardial oxygen requirement at fixed submaximal workload.

The extent of ST segment depression is decreased during maximal exercise, and ejection fraction is frequently improved, suggesting decreased myocardial ischemia and improved coronary blood flow. This increased myocardial oxygen delivery is probably related to dilatation of large and small coronary vessels, and to redistribution of coronary flow to the subendocardial ischemic areas.

Experimental data

In dogs (Clozel, 1983), myocardial blood flow to the ischemic zones is significantly increased after diltiazem as compared to placebo 4 hours after left circumflex occlusion. Increased regional blood flow is observed in hypokinetic ventricular segments, but not in dyskinetic segments, and is compatible with increased retrograde flow through coronary collaterals. The endocardial/epicardial coronary flow ratio is also improved after diltiazem, suggesting redistribution of flow to subendocardial areas. Thus diltiazem appears to increase myocardial oxygen delivery to ischemic areas, through dilatation of the large capacitance vessels with increased antegrade coronary flow whenever possible, through dilatation of small vessels and increased retrograde flow through collaterals, and through redistribution of coronary flow from the epicardial to the subendocardial ischemic areas.

Clinical data

Intravenous diltiazem, 30 μg/kg/min or approximately 2 mg/min, was infused for 10 min in 10 patients with chronic angina and fixed coronary obstructions demonstrated at coronary angiography (Bourassa, 1980). Mean arterial pressure decreased by 15 percent and systemic vascular resistance decreased by 20 percent. Heart rate, cardiac index and left ventricular end diastolic pressure remained unchanged. Coronary sinus blood flow increased by 20 percent and coronary vascular resistance decreased by 24 percent. Thus at these intravenous doses, diltiazem produced mild to moderate systemic and coronary vasodilatation at rest.

The hemodynamic response and the diltiazem plasma levels were monitored in 6 patients after a single intravenous dose of 20 mg and in 11 patients after a single oral dose of 120 mg (Taeymans, 1982a). After the intravenous bolus the only hemodynamic change observed was a transient fall in systolic blood pressure. Heart rate, cardiac output, pulmonary pressure and systemic vascular resistance remained unchanged for the 10 hour observation period. After oral administration, heart rate fell slightly and systolic blood pressure and systemic vascular resistance fell moderately. Peak effects occurred at 3 hours. The hemodynamic effects of diltiazem correlated well with the plasma level; the vasodilating effects were present at concentrations above 100 ng/ml.

In a recent study of 12 patients with chronic effort angina (Wagniart, 1982b), 3 hours after a single oral dose of 120 mg of diltiazem or placebo, heart rate, systolic and diastolic blood pressure were slightly reduced at rest.

During exercise, heart rate and systolic blood pressure were lower than with placebo at an identical submaximal workload; pressure-rate product was 14 percent lower than with placebo during submaximal exercise. At peak exercise, heart rate, systolic and diastolic blood pressure and pressure-rate product were similar with diltiazem and placebo. However, exercise duration was significantly longer after diltiazem than after placebo and time to 1 mm ST depression or termination of exercise increased 20 percent.

Maximum depth of ST depression in any lead at peak exercise was decreased by 25 percent as compared with placebo, and the sum of ST depression in all 12 leads was decreased by 54 percent after diltiazem.
To assess the duration of action of diltiazem on exercise tolerance and exercise-induced ECG ischemia, we studied 9 men with chronic angina and fixed obstructive lesions using a double-blind randomized protocol (Wagniart, 1982a). The effects of diltiazem were manifest as early as 1 hour, were maximal at 3 hours and persisted for as long as 8 hours.

Comparison of the effects of diltiazem and other calcium channel blockers

The effects of a single dose of 120 mg diltiazem and 20 mg nifedipine were compared to placebo using a randomized double-blind protocol in 12 patients with coronary stenoses $\geq$ 70 percent and exercise-induced ST segment depression $\geq$ 0.01 mv (Wagniart, 1983).

Compared to placebo, nifedipine increased peak work capacity at 1 and 3 hours and diltiazem at 3 and 8 hours. The magnitude of improved exercise tolerance was similar (25 percent versus 29 percent, respectively) at 3 hours. During submaximal exercise, diltiazem reduced the chronotropic response and reduced the pressure-rate product by 10 percent, whereas nifedipine increased the heart rate response and did not change the pressure-rate product. Thus, although both drugs improved exercise tolerance to a similar degree at 3 hours, diltiazem has the advantages of a much longer duration of action and of a significant negative chronotropic response during submaximal exercise.

Effects of diltiazem in unstable angina

Unstable angina is usually diagnosed when anginal episodes increase in either frequency, severity or duration. The exact pathophysiological mechanism in the majority of patients with unstable angina remains unclear. Increased oxygen demand with fixed severe coronary stenoses, coronary spasm and coronary artery thrombosis have been proposed as possible mechanisms, and they may occur independently or coexist in this obviously heterogeneous population.

The usual treatment of unstable angina includes hospitalization, bed rest, administration of oral and intravenous nitrates and beta-adrenergic blocking agents, and coronary arteriography and coronary bypass surgery, if symptoms persist in spite of intensive medical therapy. Few clinical studies have assessed the therapeutic usefulness of calcium channel blockers in this situation (Taeymans, 1982b; André-Fouet, 1981).

Sixty-four consecutive patients hospitalized in the coronary care unit for unstable angina were randomized within 12 hours of admission to either 240 mg propranolol per day or 360 mg diltiazem per day (Taeymans, 1982b). After 3 days, 74 percent of patients receiving propranolol and 76 percent receiving diltiazem were angina-free. Mean resting heart rate, systolic blood pressure and pressure-rate product were similar for both drugs. After 1 month of follow-up, death or myoardial infarction had occurred in 8 percent of patients treated with propranolol compared with 13 percent treated with diltiazem; angina had recurred in 64 percent of patients treated with propranolol and 50 percent of patients treated with diltiazem. No major side effects were observed with either drug. These data suggest that propranolol and diltiazem produce similar hemodynamic and clinical effects in patients with unstable angina.

Effects of diltiazem in recent myocardial infarction

Recent data suggest that coronary thrombosis is the primary process in acute myocardial infarction and that coronary spasm rarely plays a major role (DeWood, 1980). However, calcium entry blockers could be expected to decrease the determinants of myocardial oxygen consumption and to protect the ischemic myocardium from excessive intracellular calcium accumulation during the acute phase of myocardial infarction (Clark, 1977).

The hemodynamic effects of a single oral dose of calcium entry blockers were studied in 34 stable patients, after an acute myocardial infarction and before withdrawal of Swan-Ganz and intra-arterial catheters (Théroux, 1980). Twelve patients received 120 mg of diltiazem, 12 patients 20 mg of nifedipine and 10 patients 180 mg of verapamil. Serial hemodynamic measurements were obtained at intervals of 15, 30, 60,90, 120, 180 and 240 min after ingestion of the drugs.

Diltiazem 120 mg p.o. produced hemodynamic changes that could be detected 15 - 30 min after ingestion, had a peak between 180 and 240 min and persisted for more than 240 min. Heart rate, systolic and diastolic blood pressure, and the pressure-rate product fell significantly. Systemic vascular resistance decreased moderately, but not significantly and cardiac index was unchanged.

The effects of an oral dose of 20 mg of nifedipine appeared 15 min after ingestion, reached a peak at 30 and 60 min and persisted for 180 min. Heart rate increased as systolic and diastolic blood pressure decreased significantly. Cardiac index increased moderately but not significantly and the pressure-rate product was unchanged.

With verapamil 180 mg p.o. significant hemodynamic effects were present at 30, 60 and 90 min after ingestion and lasted for 180 min. The most striking effect was a reduction in systolic and diastolic blood pressure, with a reduction in the pressure-rate product. Heart rate, cardiac index and pulmonary wedge pressure remained unchanged.

Statistical analysis revealed significant differences between the effects of diltiazem and nifedipine and verapamil on heart rate, and between the effects of diltiazem and the other 2 drugs on pressure-rate product.

Thus diltiazem is the calcium channel blocker with the longest duration of action, the most potent negative chronotropic effect and the most potent reduction of myocardial oxygen consumption. These effects could be of value in some patients with recent myocardial infarction.

Electrophysiologic effects of diltiazem

In man intravenous diltiazem in doses of 20 mg prolongs AH conduction time and AV node functional and effective refractory periods by approximately 20 percent. In patients with sick sinus syndrome, diltiazem significantly prolongs sinus cycle length (up to 50 percent in some cases). Chronic oral administration of diltiazem in doses up to 360 mg per day has resulted in small increases in PR interval.

In dogs, the increased AH interval occurs at plasma concentrations higher than 85 ng/ml, and increased nodal functional refractory period with plasma concentrations higher than 175 ng/ml. These changes are strongly correlated to the plasma concentrations (unpublished data).

In a recent study (Betriu, 1983), we tested the effectiveness and safety of intravenous diltiazem in the management of paroxysmal supraventricular tachyarrhythmias in 39 patients, 21 with organic heart disease and 7 in heart failure. Fifteen patients presented with supraventricular tachycardia, 12 with atrial fibrillation and 12 with atrial flutter. End points were conversion to sinus rhythm or slowing of the ventricular rate to 100 beats/min or less. Diltiazem was given as an intravenous bolus of either 150 or 300 μg/kg over 2 min. A second injection was administered to patients who received the lower dose and failed to reach either end point within 30 min.

The overall success rate was 82 percent (32 of 39 patients). Time to end point was 5 min or less in 20 patients. Conversion to sinus rhythm occurred in 13 of 15 patients (87 percent) with supraventricular tachycardia and in 2 of 12 patients with atrial fibrillation. Treatment side effects included a slow ventricular rate in one patient who had a sick sinus syndrome and hypotension in 2 patients that rapidly responded to fluid administration.

Thus we conclude that intravenous diltiazem is effective and well tolerated and we advocate its use in the management of paroxysmal supraventricular tachyarrhythmias.

Clinical implications

At rest, diltiazem exerts moderate peripheral vasodilator effects, with a moderate reduction of blood pressure and systemic vascular resistance. In contrast to nifedipine and verapamil, diltiazem also reduces resting heart rate and thus usually brings about a greater reduction in myocardial oxygen consumption than these other drugs.

In vivo, diltiazem possesses neither positive nor negative inotropic activity and cardiac output, left ventricular end diastolic pressure and ejection fraction usually remain unchanged at rest in patients with adequately preserved left ventricular function.

Diltiazem leads to a moderate dilatation of large and small coronary arteries and increases resting coronary blood flow. Like nifedipine and verapamil, diltiazem has been shown experimentally to increase retrograde flow through coronary collaterals and to redistribute effective coronary flow towards the more ischemic subendocardial areas. Diltiazem, nifedipine and verapamil appear to be similarly effective in relieving coronary vasospasm.

Diltiazem depresses atrioventricular conduction moderately, and to a lesser extent than verapamil.

Heart rate, blood pressure and pressure-rate product are significantly decreased during submaximal exercise after diltiazem, as compared to a placebo.

Maximal heart rate, blood pressure and pressure-rate product are similar after diltiazem and placebo. However, total duration of exercise and time to onset of angina and/or ST segment depression are markedly increased after diltiazem.

The extent of myocardial ischemia using the 12-lead electrocardiogram is significantly decreased after diltiazem as compared to a placebo, suggesting that diltiazem does not only decrease myocardial oxygen demand but also increases myocardial oxygen delivery in patients with ischemic heart disease and fixed coronary obstructions.

These effects are dose related and diltiazem is most effective at doses of 240 mg per day or greater. At these higher doses, side effects have been minimal.

References

André-Fouet, X., Viallet, M., Gayet, C., Thizy, J.F., Wilner, C. and Pont, M. Diltiazem versus propranolol. A randomized trial in unstable angina. *Circulation*, **64** (Suppl. IV), IV-293 (1981).

Antman, E.M., Stone, P.H., Muller, J.E., and Braunwald, E. Calcium channel blocking agents in the treatment of cardiovascular disorders. Part I: Basic and clinical electrophysiologic effects. *Ann. Intern. Med.*, **93**, 875 (1980).

Betriu, A., Chaitman, B.R., Bourassa, M.G., Brévers, G., Scholl, J.M., Bruneau, P., Gagné, P. and Chabot, M. Beneficial effect of intravenous diltiazem in the acute management of paroxysmal supraventricular tachyarrhythmias. *Circulation*, **67**, 88 (1983).

Bourassa, M.G., Côté, P., Théroux, P., Tubau, J.F., Genain, C. and Waters, D.D. Hemodynamics and coronary flow following diltiazem administration in anesthetized dogs and in humans. *Chest*, **78**, 224 (1980).

Braunwald, E. Mechanism of action of calcium channel blocking agents. *N. Engl. J. Med.*, **307**, 1618 (1982).

Clark, R.E., Ferguson, T.B., West, P.N., Shuchleib, R.C., and Henry, P.D. Pharmacological preservation of the ischemic heart. *Ann. Thorac. Surg.*, **24**, 307 (1977).

Clozel, J.P., Théroux, P. and Bourassa, M.G. Effects of diltiazem on experimental myocardial ischemia and on left ventricular performance. *Circ. Res.*, **52** (Suppl. I), 120 (1983).

DeWood, M.A., Spores, J., Notske, R., Mouser, L.T., Burroughs, R., Golden, M.S. and Lang, H.T. Prevalence of total coronary occlusion during the early hours of transmural myocardial infarction. *N. Engl. J. Med.*, **303**, 897 (1980).

Feldman, R.L., Pepine, C.J., Whittle, J. and Conti, C.R. Short and long term responses to diltiazem in patients with variant angina. *Am. J. Cardiol.*, **42**, 554 (1982).

Fleckenstein, A. Specific pharmacology of calcium in myocardium, cardiac pacemakers, and vascular smooth muscle. *Ann. Rev. Pharmacol. Toxicol.*, **17**, 149 (1977).

Hamm, C.W. and Opie, L.H. Protection of infarcting myocardium by slow channel inhibitors: Comparative effects of verapamil, nifedipine, and diltiazem in the coronary-ligated, isolated working heart. *Circ. Res.*, **52** (Suppl. I), 129. (1983)

Henry, P.D. Comparative pharmacology of calcium antagonists: nifedipine, verapamil and diltiazem. *Am. J. Cardiol.*, **46**, 1047 (1980).

Hossack, K.F., Bruce, R.A., Ritterman, J.B., Kusumi, F. and Trimble, S. Divergent effects of diltiazem in patients with exertional angina. *Am. J. Cardiol.*, **49**, 538 (1982a).

Hossack, K.F., Pool, P.E., Steele, P., Crawford, M.H., DeMaria, A.N., Cohen, L.S. and Ports, T.A. Efficacy of diltiazem in angina of effort: A multicenter trial. *Am. J. Cardiol.*, **49**, 567 (1982b).

Kimura, E. and Kishida, H. Treatment of variant angina with drugs: A survey of 11 Cardiology Institutes in Japan. *Circulation*, **63**, 844 (1981).

Low, R.I., Takeda, P., Mason, D.T. and DeMaria, A.N. The effects of calcium channel blocking agents on cardiovascular function. *Am. J. Cardiol.*, **49**, 547 (1982).

Mitchell, L.B., Schroeder, J.S. and Mason, J.W. Comparative clinical electrophysiologic effects of diltiazem, verapamil and nifedipine: a review. *Am. J. Cardiol.*, **49**, 629 (1982).

Pepine, C.J., Feldman, R.L., Whittle, J., Curry, R.C. and Conti, C.R. Effect of diltiazem in patients with variant angina: A randomized double-blind trial. *Am. Heart J.*, **101**, 719 (1981).

Pool, P.E. and Seagren, S.C. Long-term efficacy of diltiazem in chronic stable angina associated with atherosclerosis: Effect on treadmill exercise. *Am. J. Cardiol.*, **49**, 573 (1982).

Rosenthal, S.J., Ginsburg, R., Lamb, I.H., Baim, D.S. and Schroeder, J.S. Efficacy of diltiazem for control of symptoms of coronary arterial spasm. *Am. J. Cardiol.*, **46**, 1027 (1980).

Rosenthal, S.J., Lamb, I.H., Schroeder, J.S. and Ginsberg, R. Long-term efficacy of diltiazem for control of symptoms of coronary artery spasm. *Circ. Res.*, **52** (Suppl. I), 153 (1983).

Rowland, E., McKenna, W.J., Gulker, H. and Krikler, D.M. The comparative effects of diltiazem and verapamil on atrioventricular conduction and atrioventricular reentry tachycardia. *Circ. Res.*, **52** (Suppl. I), 163 (1983).

Stone, P.H., Antman, E.M., Muller, J.E. and Braunwald, E. Calcium channel blocking agents in the treatment of cardiovascular disorders. Part II: Hemodynamic effects and clinical applications. *Ann. Intern. Med.*, **93**, 886 (1980).

Strauss, W.E., McIntyre, K.M., Parisi, A.F. and Shapiro, W. Safety and efficacy of diltiazem hydrochloride for the treatment of stable angina pectoris: Report of a cooperative clinical trial. *Am. J. Cardiol.*, **49**, 560 (1982).

Subramanian, V.B., Khurmi, N.S., Bowles, M.J., O'Hara, M. and Raftery, E.B. Objective evaluation of three dose levels of diltiazem in patients with chronic stable angina. *J. Am. Coll. Cardiol.*, **1** (4), 1144 (1983).

Taeymans, Y., Clozel, J.P., Caillé, G., Brévers, G. and Théroux, P. Relationship between diltiazem plasma levels and its hemodynamic effects. *Circulation*, **66** (Suppl. II), II-80 (1982a).

Taeymans, Y., Théroux, P., Waters, D.D., Szlachcic, J. and Pelletier, G.B. A prospective randomized study of propranolol versus diltiazem in patients with unstable angina. *Am. J. Cardiol.*, **49**, 896 (1982b).

Théroux, P., Waters, D.D., Debaisieux, J.C.; Szlachcic, J., Mizgala, H.F. and Bourassa, M.G. Hemodynamic effects of calcium ion antagonists after acute myocardial infarction. *Clin. Invest. Med.*, **3**, 81 (1980).

Wagniart, P., Chaitman, B.R., Brévers, G., Ferguson, R.J., Pasternac, A. and Bourassa, M.G. Comparison of nifedipine and diltiazem on exercise tolerance in chronic stable angina pectoris. *J. Am. Coll. Cardiol.*, **1** (2), 625 (abstract) (1983).

Wagniart, P., Chaitman, B.R., Ferguson, R.J., Brévers, G., Scholl, J.M., Clozel, J.P., Pasternac, A. and Bourassa, M.G. Duration of improved exercise performance following oral diltiazem in chronic stable angina. *Am. J. Cardiol.*, **49**, 1000 (abstract) (1982a).

Wagniart, P., Ferguson, R.J., Chaitman, B.R., Achard, F., Benacerraf, A., Delanguenhagen, B., Morin, B., Pasternac, A. and Bourassa, M.G. Increased exercise tolerance and reduced electrocardiographic ischemia with diltiazem in patients with stable angina pectoris. *Circulation*, **66**, 23 (1982b).

Waters, D.D., Szlachcic, J. and Théroux, P. Prognosis of variant angina patients treated with calcium antagonist drugs. *Am. J. Cardiol.*, **47**, 463 (abstract) (1981a).

Waters, D.D., Théroux, P., Szlachcic, J. and Dauwe, F. Provocative testing with ergonovine to assess the efficacy of treatment with nifedipine, diltiazem and verapamil in variant angina. *Am. J. Cardiol.*, **48**, 123 (1981b).

Yasue, H., Omote, S., Takizawa, A. and Nagao, M. Coronary arterial spasm in ischemic heart disease and its pathogenesis: a review. *Circ. Res.*, **52** (Suppl. I), 147 (1983).

Chapter IV:

Calcium entry blockers and cerebral function

Calcium entry blockers and cerebral function: an introduction

B.S. Meldrum

Summary

In many respects calcium plays a key role in the central nervous system. Synaptic release of neuro-transmitters and various post-synaptic potentials, including dendritic spikes, depend on calcium entry. Calcium buffering systems in the neuronal cytosol are described and mechanisms of calcium toxicity are discussed. Selective vulnerability of specific regions in the brain is described and the excessive calcium influx as its underlying mechanism is considered. On this basis calcium entry blockers may serve as protective agents in cerebral hypoxia/ischaemia and may be useful in the treatment of cerebrovascular disorders. Direct actions on cerebrovascular smooth muscle may also be important.

Résumé

A beaucoup d'égards, le calcium joue un rôle-clé dans le système nerveux central. La libération synaptique de neurotransmetteurs ainsi que divers potentiels post-synaptiques, y compris les pointes dendritiques, dépendent de l'entrée de calcium. Les systèmes de tamponnage du calcium dans le cytosol ont été décrits et les mécanismes de la toxicité du calcium ont été discutés. La vulnérabilité sélective de régions spécifiques dans le cerveau a été décrite et on a considéré l'influx excessif de calcium comme son mécanisme sous-jacent. Sur cette base, les agents bloqueurs de l'entrée de calcium peuvent servir en tant qu'agents protecteurs dans les cas d'hypoxie ou d'ischémie cérébrale et peuvent être utiles dans le traitement des troubles cérébrovasculaires. Des actions directes sur le muscle lisse cérébrovasculaire peuvent également être importantes.

Resumen

En muchos respectos el calcio desempeña un papel clave en el sistema nervioso central. Liberación sináptica de neurotransmisores así que varios potenciales postsinápticos, incluso los impulsos de punta neurodendríticos, dependen de la entrada de calcio. Se describen sistemas reguladores de calcio en el citosol neuronal y se discuten los mecanismos de la toxicidad cálcica. Se examinan la vulnerabilidad selectiva de específicas regiones en el cerebro y la excesiva entrada de calcio como su mecanismo subyacente. Sobre esta base, los inhibidores de la penetración intracelular de Ca^{2+} pueden servir como agentes protectores en hipoxia/isquemia cerebral y ser útiles en el tratamiento de trastornos cerebrovasculares. Sus acciones directas en músculos lisos cerebrovasculares también pueden ser importantes.

Zusammenfassung

Kalzium spielt in mancher Hinsicht eine Hauptrolle im Zentralnervensystem. Die Synapsenfreisetzung von Neurotransmittern und die verschiedenen postsynaptischen Potentiale, einschliesslich die der Dendritenden, sind vom Kalziumeinstrom abhängig. Die Kalziumpuffersysteme im neuronalen Zytosol werden beschrieben und die Mechanismen der Kalziumtoxizität diskutiert. Weiter wird die selektive Empfindlichkeit spezifischer Hirnareale beschrieben und ein übermäßiger Kalziumeinstrom als erklärender Mechanismus angedeutet. Davon ausgehend können Kalziumeinstromhemmer als Schutzstoffe für Gehirnhypoxie/Ischämie dienen und zur Behandlung zerebrovaskulärer Störungen benutzt werden. Direkte Wirkungen auf die zerebrovaskulären glatten Muskeln können dabei ebenfalls wichtig sein.

The role of calcium in receptor/response coupling reaches its apotheosis in the central nervous system. In particular, calcium entry into presynaptic terminals is the essential trigger for release of neurotransmitters. Thus blockade of calcium channels in the central nervous system is likely to impair its integrative function. Fortunately, calcium entry blockers show considerable variation in their pharmacokinetic and pharmacodynamic properties.

The cytosolic $[Ca^{2+}]$ is not accurately known for mammalian central neurones, but by analogy from measurements in invertebrate neurones, and by inference from studies using subcellular fractions of mammalian brains it is thought to be in the range 20-170 nM (Alvarez-Leefmans et al., 1981; Baker, 1978; Nicholls & Åckerman, 1982). Extracellular $[Ca^{2+}]$ is approximately 1.3 mM. This concentration difference plus the negative potential across the plasma membrane provides a very powerful electrochemical gradient. Thus calcium enters neurons passively through channels that can be classified as "leak" channels, voltage-dependent channels, and receptor-operated channels. Of these the voltage-dependent channels have been best studied. They are quantitatively sufficient to give rise to regenerating responses (observed when Na^+ channels have been blocked by tetrodotoxin) in the soma of motoneurones (Alvarez-Leefmans & Miledi, 1980) or in the dendrites of cerebellar Purkinje cells (Llinàs & Hess, 1976) or of hippocampal pyramidal neurons (Wong et al., 1979).

The presence of receptor operated Ca^{2+} channels on hippocampal pyramidal neurons is shown by the reduction of extracellular $[Ca^{2+}]$ produced by iontophoretically-applied aspartate, in the presence of tetrodotoxin (Marciani et al., 1982).

Outward pumping of Ca^{2+} from neurons requires energy. This may be utilised directly by a membrane Ca/Mg ATPase, or indirectly by a sodium pump (Na/K ATPase) and a Na^+/Ca^{2+} exchange, which may operate electrogenically, 3 Na^+ moving in for each Ca^{2+} moving out (Baker, 1976). Inward calcium flux during sustained electrical activity exceeds maximal outward calcium transport. Thus intracellular calcium buffering mechanisms are required. These are provided by proteins, by synaptic vesicles, by the endoplasmic reticulum and by the mitochondria.

Cytosolic Ca^{2+} buffering

Two calcium binding proteins are important in neuronal function. One is calmodulin, which is a ubiquitous protein mediating calcium-dependent activation of a very wide range of enzymic processes (Stoclet, 1981). The other calcium binding protein was identified as "vitamin D-dependent calcium binding protein" in the gut, but is found in high concentration in selected cell types in the brain, where it is not vitamin D-dependent (Jande et al., 1981; Baimbridge et al., 1982 a, b). It is particularly prominent in cerebellar Purkinje cells, in hippocampal dentate granule cells and in CA_1 pyramidal cells (but not in CA_3 pyramidal cells).

The endoplasmic reticulum, the synaptic vesicles and the mitochondria provide active sequestration of Ca^{2+}. This has been demonstrated at the fine structural level using oxalate precipitation and complexing with pyroantimonate or X-ray activation analysis

(Henkart *et al.*, 1978; O'Hara *et al.*, 1979; Griffiths *et al.*, 1982, 1984). It is likely that the synaptic vesicles provide a means of extruding Ca^{2+} that compensates for enhanced Ca^{2+} entry during increased activity. Thus during sustained nerve activity in the electric organ of *Torpedo Marmorata* presynaptic mitochondria contain less Ca^{2+} than normal (Schmidt and Zimmerman, 1980) and during sustained seizure activity in the hippocampus there is no increase in $[Ca^{2+}]$ (seen as pyroantimonate deposits) in either vesicles or mitochondria in presynaptic terminals (Griffiths *et al.*, 1982, 1983b).

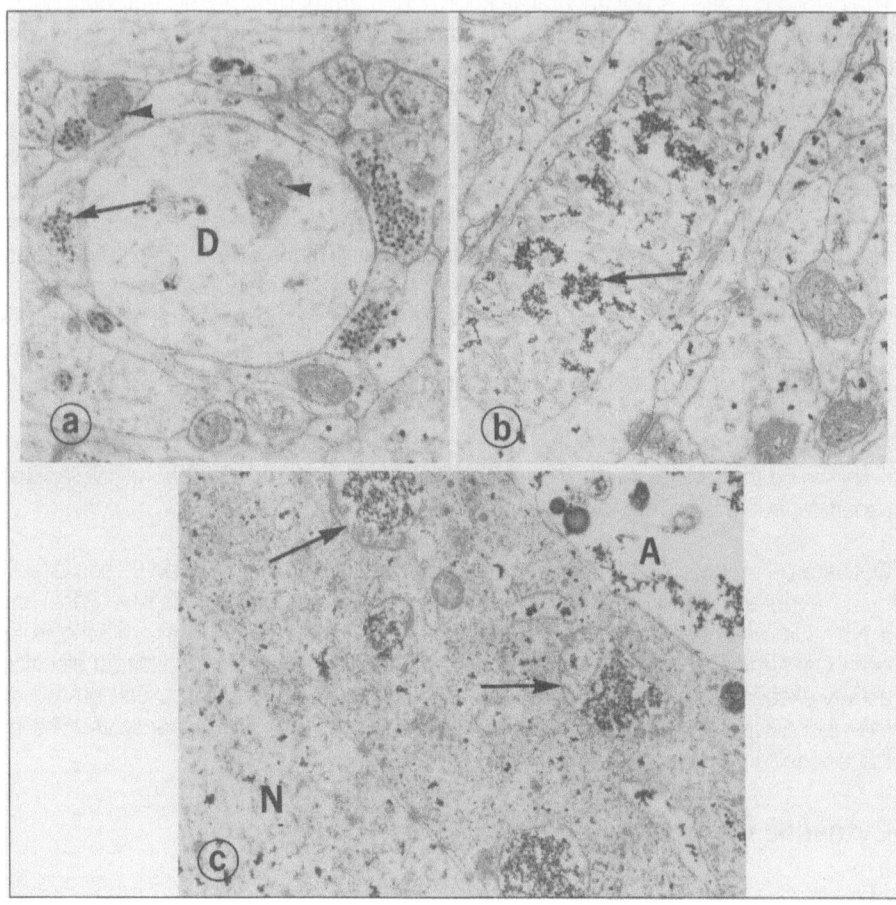

Figure. 1 (a): Transverse section of a pyramidal cell dendrite (D) from a control hippocampus treated with potassium pyroantimonate. Synaptic vesicles each contain a dense spot of calcium pyroantimonate (arrow). A small amount is also found in mitochondria (arrowheads). Mag. x 33,300.

Figure 1 (b): A similar region from an experimental animal (2 h of L-allylglycine induced seizures), shows a dendrite containing a grossly distended mitochondrion. Dense precipitates of calcium pyroantimonate are seen within the mitochondrion (arrow), and also free in the cytoplasm (arrowhead). Mag. x 33,000.

Figure 1 (c): Part of a pyramidal cell soma from the same animal as shown in 1 (b). Its mitochondria are swollen and contain dense precipitates of calcium pyroantimonate (arrows). Precipitate is also present in the nucleus (N), and in an adjacent swollen astrocytic process (A). Mag. x 30,000.

In mitochondria, Ca^{2+} influx and efflux are independently regulated, providing a neutral set point for cytosolic $[Ca^{2+}]$ (Nicholls and Åckerman, 1982). Mitochondrial Ca^{2+} uptake becomes significant with extramitochondrial Ca^{2+} in the range 0.3 - 1 μM, and is half maximal in the range 20-40 μM (Baker, 1976; Nicholls & Åckerman, 1982). This system has an extremely high capacity as the Ca^{2+} can be stored in an inert form as $Ca_3 (PO_4)_2$. It successfully buffers the massive calcium influx into hippocampal pyramidal neurons associated with sustained seizure activity (Griffiths et al., 1982, 1983b) (see Fig. 1). Once cytosolic $[Ca^{2+}]$ is restored to normal by the plasma membrane calcium pump, Ca^{2+} efflux from mitochondria predominates and the Ca^{2+} deposits disappear (Griffiths et al., 1984).

Calcium toxicity

Over the last 10 years substantial evidence has accumulated to show a role for raised cytosolic $[Ca^{2+}]$ in pathological changes occurring in muscles, principally in cardiac or vascular smooth muscle in ischaemia, and in skeletal muscle in various dystrophic disorders (see Table 1). Studies showing the protective action of calcium deficiency, penicillamine and calcium entry blockers (see Wrogemann & Pena, 1976; Borgers, 1981 and Borgers & Flameng in this volume) in experimental syndromes of muscular dystrophy and cardiac ischaemia have provided crucial evidence that the raised cytosolic $[Ca^{2+}]$ is part of a causal sequence leading to pathological change, and not merely secondary to a failure of energy metabolism and hence of calcium regulation. The histological studies demonstrate progressive breakdown of intracellular protein and an increase in fatty acids, consistent with activation of proteases and phospholipases by the raised cytosolic $[Ca^{2+}]$.

Recent experimental studies have shown a toxic effect of excitatory inputs to invertebrate and vertebrate muscle, that is dependent on Ca^{2+} entry (Duce et al., 1983; Leonard & Salpeter, 1982).

In cultured liver cells the cytotoxic action of a wide range of chemical agents has been shown to depend on extracellular $[Ca^{2+}]$ 'Schanne et al., 1979).

In the central nervous system it has not so far proved possible to demonstrate a causal role for raised cytosolic calcium in nerve cell death. Intracellular accumulation of calcium deposits has been observed in association with various stresses leading to nerve cell degeneration (see Table 1). In particular during status epilepticus calcium accumulates post-synaptically in the soma and dendrites of hippocampal pyramidal neurones, with a very strong concentration in swollen mitochondria (Griffiths et al., 1982, 1983b). A similar accumulation of calcium deposits is seen in the cortical neurons of rats exposed to a hypoxic/ischaemic stress (Levine preparation; Van Reempts & Borgers, 1982). Activation of intraneuronal proteases leading to a breakdown of axoplasmic protein structure has been directly demonstrated with high calcium concentration (approx. 1mM) (Rubinson & Baker, 1979). However, activation of various intracellular proteases and phospholipases is observed with much smaller increases in $[Ca^{2+}]$ (in the micromolar range (Baudry et al., 1981). However, these processes appear reversible.

211

Table 1 : Toxicity of raised cytosolic $[Ca^{2+}]$

Tissue	Cause	Pathology	Protection	References
Muscle cardiac vascular skeletal	ischaemia A 23187 Excitotoxins Dystrophy (Duchenne chicks + hamsters)	Mitochondrial swelling + Ca^{2+} accumulation protein breakdown Degeneration Eosinophilia myofibrillar degeneration	Ca^{2+} entry blockers Penicillamine	Flameng et al, 1981 Haack et al, 1975 Nayler et al, 1978 Publicover et al, 1978 Duce et al, 1983 Wrogemann & Pena, 1976 Emery & Burt, 1980
Liver	Various chemical toxins	Cell death		Schanne et al, 1979
Nerve	Electrical stimuli Spinal trauma status epilepticus	Mitochondrial swelling Ca^{2+} accumulation cell loss Axonal degeneration Ca hydroxyapatite Mitochondrial swelling ischaemic cell change		Agnew et al, 1979, 1983 Balantine & Spector, 1977 Griffiths et al, 1982,1984

Selective vulnerability

Brain damage secondariy to focal or generalised ischaemia shows two kinds of selective vulnerability. One concerns the areas of gray matter principally affected, e.g. parietal and occipital cortex, particularly in the depths of sulci, and in arterial boundary zones. The other is the preferential vulnerability of cell types with highest susceptibility shown by certain types of neurons, as for example Purkinje and basket cells in the cerebellum, small pyramidal neurons in lamina III of the neocortex, pyramidal neurons in hippocampal regions CA_1 and CA_{3-4}, small polymorphic neurons in the basal ganglia (see Brierley, 1976). In attempting to define the morphological and functional characteristics of selectively vulnerable neurons, Meldrum (1983) emphasised two types of vulnerable neurons, corresponding to Golgi type I and type II morphology. The Type I neurons have a complex dendritic tree that shows Ca^{2+} spikes and receives powerful excitatory inputs. The vulnerable Golgi type II neurons are the inhibitory GABAergic interneurons. These, e.g. as the aspinous stellate cells of the neocortex, are particularly vulnerable to hypoxia in the infant brain (Sloper et al., 1980) or as the polymorphic neurons in the hippocampal hilar region, are particularly vulnerable during sustained activity induced by kainic acid or electrical stimulation (Sloviter & Damiano, 1981; Sloviter, 1983).

Selective vulnerability is not seen with total ischaemia in the absence of a recovery period (Jenkins et al., 1979). It is seen with moderate durations of total ischaemia (5-30 min) followed by a restitution of circulation, or with periods of oligaemia of variable duration or with a variety of other stresses which include most notably status epilepticus which induces very similar patterns of selective damage. Thus during total ischaemia a latent biochemical lesion is produced that provides the basis for the selective vulnerability during the recovery period. The initial or latent lesion may have two components, one is a sequence of biochemical changes in the selectively vulnerable neuron. The other is a functional impairment in cells that selectively interact with the vulnerable neurons. The latter may be altered properties of endothelial cells or vascular smooth muscle, altered astrocytic function or altered activity in related neurons (e.g. impaired inhibitory activity or abnormal excitatory inputs as with focal bursting activity).

Excessive calcium influx as an explanation for selective vulnerability

The hippocampal neurons that are selectively vulnerable to status epilepticus and to hypoxia/ischaemia either readily show a pathological pattern of burst firing (CA_3 and CA_1 pyramidal neurons) or a physiological pattern of burst firing (hilar, polymorphic inhibitory interneurons, Andersen et al., 1963). Electrophysiological studies show that the burst firing is associated with Ca^{2+} movement into neurons (Schwartzkroin & Wyler, 1979).

These observations were the basis of the hypothesis (Meldrum, 1981, 1983; Meldrum et al., 1982) that selective vulnerability was attributable to membrane properties that gave rise to burst firing and an excessive, sustained entry of calcium. Electron microscope studies with oxalate/pyroantimonate precipitation of Ca^{2+} confirmed that during status epilepticus the selectively vulnerable neurons accumulated Ca^{2+} intracellularly, with the appearance of massive deposits in swollen mitochondria in the dendrites and soma (Griffiths et al., 1982, 1984a). However, these studies have also provided evidence that this massive accumulation of calcium is rapidly reversible (Griffiths et al., 1983a, 1984). Restoration of normal neuronal appearances occurs after massive calcium accumulation.

Similar observations (but without the evidence of selectivity) have been made in the cerebral cortex during ischaemia. Extracellular Ca^{2+} falls rapidly (Harris et al., 1981) and accumulation of calcium in neuronal mitochondria is demonstrable with the oxalate/pyroantimonate method (Van Reempts and Borgers, 1982).

Given the reversibility of the initial Ca^{2+} overload occurring in selectively vulnerable neurons, can a tendency to burst firing and excessive Ca^{2+} entry be retained as the working hypothesis to explain selective neuronal vulnerability? There is ample evidence that ischaemic damage should be considered as a two stage process, with events during the initial ischaemic episode interacting in a complex way with events during the restitution phase to determine the outcome. A plasma membrane permitting a high Ca^{2+} influx during the initial stress (and subsequently) may thus favour pathology. Mechanisms for this are summarised in Table 2. The initial increase in cytosolic Ca^{2+} activates many enzyme systems, including mitochondrial oxidative metabolism. However, phospholipases are activated within a few minutes of onset of ischaemia or seizure activity so that there is an immediate and progressive increase in free fatty acids with a striking percentage increase in the arachidonic acid concentration (Chapman, 1981; Bazan et al., 1971).

Table 2: Calcium entry and neuronal pathology in ischaemia and status epilepticus

Primary events	Secondary events
0-30 min. of ischaemia 0-60 min. of seizure	"restitution" phase

Enhanced Ca^{2+} entry leading to
1. Activation of phospholipases increase in
   free fatty acids, arachidonic acid and
   prostaglandins
	1. Impaired perfusion
	   ? endothelial cell damage
	   ? action of prostaglandins on vessels.
	   ? astrocytic swelling

2. Activation of proteases and peptidases
 	
   exposure of cryptic glutamate receptors
	2. Burst firing due to altered membrane
	   properties or excess excitatory action or
	   impaired inhibition or unequal repolarisation
	   leading to enhanced Ca^{2+} entry

3. Mitochondrial Ca^{2+} overload ? metabolic lesion, failure	3. Enhanced Ca^{2+} entry; raised cytosolic Ca^{2+}

The increase in arachidonic acid concentration will accelerate the formation of prostaglandins and leukotrienes. These may in turn influence tone and permeability in fine vessels. Activation of peptidases and proteases is also a consequence of moderate increases in intracellular $[Ca^{2+}]$ (Baudry et al., 1981; 1983). A possibly highly important effect of this is the exposure of additional membrane glutamate receptors (Baudry et al., 1983). This could be a "latent lesion" making the neurons more susceptible to excitatory inputs and more likely to show burst firing during the restitution periods or any subsequent stresses. Focal seizure activity is a characteristic sign in the first hours of recovery in many animal models of cerebral ischaemia (Naquet, 1966; Levy & Duffy, 1977) and in man after stroke or cardiac arrest (Snyder et al., 1980).

Calcium entry blockers as protective agents in cerebral hypoxia/ ischaemia

The above and other considerations have led to the attempt to protect the brain from hypoxic/ischaemic damage by the administration of calcium entry blockers. In animal models these can of course be given either "prophylactically", prior to the stress (chronically or acutely) or given "therapeutically" during the restitution phase. Studies of this kind have been described by Kazda et al. (1979), Steen et al. (1983), Van Reempts and Borgers (1982, 1983), and Hossmann et al. (1983). They are reviewed here by Dr. Wauquier.

Using objective criteria for evaluating functional or pathological outcome, it should not be difficult in such studies to establish whether there is or is not a protective action of a given calcium entry blocker in a particular model. However, there is not yet agreement on whether verapamil and nimodipine do protect against the pathological consequences of experimental focal or general cerebral ischaemia (Kazda et al., 1979; Steen et al., 1983, Reedy et al., 1983, Harris et al., 1982; White et al., 1982; Hossmann et al., 1983). It is undoubtedly more difficult to evaluate the mechanism of any such protective effect. Table 3 lists some of the systems and responses that are modified by calcium entry blockers and may influence functional or pathological outcome in cerebral hypoxia/ischaemia. It is also difficult to know how appropriate it is to transfer data obtained in an animal model to the clinical situation. The position is simpler if attention is confined to disorders of the cerebral vascular system.

Table 3: Effects of calcium entry blockers relevant to pathological outcome of cerebral ischaemia or status epilepticus

1. Cardiac function
  a) Cardiovascular reflexes activated by hypoxia cerebral ischaemia or status epilepticus.
  b) Late functional changes (including arrhythmias)

2. Vascular function
  a) Peripheral arteriolar tone
  b) Blood viscosity
  c) Cerebral vessels
    (i) physiological responses
    (ii) pathological processes secondary to ischaemia

3. Endocrine effects
  a) Impaired (glucose-induced) insulin release
  b) Altered anterior pituitary responses

4. Altered cerebral activity
  a) depressed synaptic function (lowered metabolic rate)
  b) depression of burst firing or epilepsy (in status epilepticus, and in recovery period after
    ischaemia).

5. Altered blood brain barrier
  a) Raised arterial pressure in status epilepticus
  b) Pathological changes in focal cerebral ischaemia.

Calcium entry blockers and cerebrovascular disorders

Clinical studies of the efficacy of calcium entry blockers in syndromes where cerebral circulation is impaired by a mechanism that includes vasospasm have a strong basis in physiological and pharmacological observations. These are summarised by Van Nueten and Vanhoutte (1980) and by several contributors in part 1 of this volume.

A marked fall in arterial pressure would be disadvantageous in many syndromes of vasospasm. Thus there is a requirement that the calcium entry blocker will be selective either for cerebral vessels (compared with other peripheral vessels) or for vessels undergoing a pathological process leading to spasm. There is substantial evidence that different calcium antagonists act selectively on blood flow to various organs (see for example Hof, 1983).

It has been stated that nimodipine preferentially inhibits contraction of the basilar artery (induced by monoamines, thromboxanes, etc.) compared with similarly induced contractions of the saphenous artery (Towart et al., 1982). Nifedipine in dogs reduces the arterial constriction induced by the subarachnoid injection of blood (Allen et al., 1979). A novel dihydropyridine derivative (PN 200-110) more potently antagonises 5HT induced constriction in basilar than in mesenteric arteries (Müller-Schweinitzer and Neumann, 1983). Such selective actions would be particularly appropriate in the prophylactic or therapeutic management of vasospasm secondary to subarachnoid haemorrhage (due to either aneurysm or neurosurgical intervention) (Towart, 1982; Allen et al., 1983).

The other major neurological disorder involving vasospasm in which calcium entry blockers are theoretically indicated and have shown clinical usefulness in preliminary clinical trials is migraine. A prophylactic action of flunarizine, 10 mg daily has been reported by Amery (1983) and further studies are described here by Dr. Spierings.

References

Agnew, W.F., Yuen, T.G.H., Bullara, L.A., Jacques, D. and Pudenz, R.G. Intracellular calcium deposition in brain following electrical stimulation. *Neurol. Res.*, **1**, 187-202. (1979)

Agnew, W.F., Yuen, T.G.H., and McCreery, D.D. Morphologic changes after prolonged electrical stimulation of the cat's cortex at defined charge densities. *Exp. Neurol.*, **79**, 397-411 (1983)

Allen, G.S. and Bahr, A.L. Cerebral arterial spasm. 10: Reversal of acute and chronic spasm in dogs with orally administered nifedipine. *Neurosurgery*, **4**, 43-46. (1979)

Allen, G.S., Ahn, H.S., Preziosi, T.J., Battye, R., Boone, S.C., Chou, S.N. *et al.* Cerebral arterial spasm — a controlled trial of nimodipine in patients with surarachnoid haemorrhage. *New Engl. J. Med.*, **308**, 619-624. (1983)

Alvarez-Leefmans, F.J. and Miledi, R. Voltage sensitive calcium entry in frog motoneurones. *J. Physiol.*, **308**, 241-257. (1980)

Alvarez-Leefmans, F.J., Rink, T.J. and Tsien, R.Y. Free calcium ions in *Helix aspersa* measured with ion-selective micro-electrodes. *J. Physiol.*, **315**, 531-548. (1981)

Amery, W.K. Flunarizine, a calcium channel blocker: a new prophylactic drug in migraine. *Headache*, **23**, 70-74 (1983)

Andersen, P., Eccles, J.C. and Løyning, Y. Recurrent inhibition in the hippocampus with identification of the inhibitory cell and its synapses. *Nature* (Lond.), **198**, 541-542. (1963)

Baimbridge, K G , Miller, J J and Parkes, C O. Calcium-binding protein distribution in the rat brain. *Brain Res.*, **239**, 519-525. (1982a)

Baimbridge, K.G. and Miller, J J. Immunohistochemical localization of calcium-binding protein in the cerebellum, hippocampal formation and olfactory bulb of the rat. *Brain Res.*,**245**,223-229 (1982b)

Baker, P.F. The regulation of intracellular calcium. In: "Calcium in biological systems", Symposium No 30, Soc. Exp. Biol. Cambridge University Press, Cambridge pp. 67-88. (1976)

Baker, P.F. The regulation of intracellular calcium in giant axons of *Loligo* and *Myxicola*. *Ann. New York, Acad. Sci.* **307**, 250-268. (1978)

Balentine, J.D. and Spector, M. Calcification of axons in experimental spinal cord trauma. *Ann. Neurol.*, **2**, 520-523 (1977)

Baudry, M., Bundman, M.C., Smith, E.K. and Lynch, G.S. Micromolar calcium proteolysis and glutamate binding in rat brain synaptic membranes. *Science*, **212**, 937-938. (1981)

Baudry, M., Siman, R., Smith, E.K. and Lynch, G. Regulation by calcium ions of glutamate receptor binding in hippocampal slices. *Eur. J. Pharmacol.*, **90**, 161-168. (1983)

Bazan, N.G., Bazan, H.E.P., Kennedy, W.G and Joel, C.D. Regional distribution and rate of production of free fatty acids in rat brain. *J. Neurochem.*, **18**, 1387-1393. (1971)

Borgers, M. The role of calcium in the toxicity of the myocardium. *Histochem.J.*, **13**, 839-848. (1981)

Brierley, J.B. Cerebral hypoxia. In Greenfield's Neuropathology edited by W. Blackwood and J.A N. Corsellis, Edward Arnold London pp. 43-85 (1976)

Chapman, A.G. Free fatty acid release and metabolism of adenosine and cyclic nucleotides during prolonged seizures In: Neurotransmitters, Seizures and Epilepsy. Edit. P.L. Morselli, K.G., Lloyd, W. Löscher, B. Meldrum and E.H. Reynolds, Raven Press, New York pp. 165-173. (1981)

Duce, I.R., Donaldson, P.L. and Usherwood, P.N.R. Investigations into the mechanism of excitant amino acid cytotoxicity using a well-characterized glutamatergic system. Brain Res., 263, 77-87. (1983)

Emery, A.E.H., and Burt, D. Intracellular calcium and pathogenesis and antenatal diagnosis of Duchenne muscular dystrophy. Brit. Med. J., 280, 355-357. (1980)

Flameng, W., Daenen, W., Borgers, M., Thone, F., Xhonneux, R., Van de Water, A. and van Belle, H. Cardioprotective effects of lidoflazine during 1-hour normothermic global ischaemia. Circulation, 64, 796-807. (1981)

Griffiths, T., Evans, M.C. and Meldrum, B.S. Intracellular sites of early calcium accumulation in the rat hippocampus during status epilepticus. Neurosci. Lett., 30, 329-334. (1982)

Griffiths, T., Evans, M.C. and Meldrum, B.S. The role of calcium in selective neuronal loss in status epilepticus — an experimental study in the rat hippocampus. In: Cerebral blood flow, metabolism and epilepsy. edit. N. Baldy-Moulinier, D. Ingvar and B.S. Meldrum, J. Libbey and Co., London. (1983a)

Griffiths, T., Evans, M.C. and Meldrum, B.S. Intracellular calcium accumulation in rat hippocampus during seizures induced by bicuculline or L-allyglycine. Neuroscience, 10, 385-395. (1983b)

Griffiths, T., Evans, M.C. and Meldrum, B.S. Status epilepticus: the reversibility of calcium loading and acute neuronal pathological changes in the rat hippocampus. Neuroscience (in press). (1984)

Haack, D.W., Abel, J.H. and Jaenke, R.S. Effects of hypoxia on the distribution of calcium in arterial smooth muscle cells of rats and swine. Cell Tiss. Rev., 157, 125-140. (1975)

Harris, R.J., Symon, L. Branston, N.M., Bayhan, M. Changes in extracellular calcium activity in cerebral ischaemia. J. Cerebr. Blood flow and metabol., 1, 203-210. (1981)

Henkart, MPP., Reese, T.S. and Brinley, F.J. Endoplasmic reticulum sequesters calcium in the squid giant axon. Science, 202, 1300-1303. (1978)

Hof, R.P.. Calcium antagonist and the peripheral circulation: differences and similarities between PY 108-068, nicardipine, verapamil and diltiazem. Brit. J. Pharmacol., 78, 375-394. (1983)

Hossmann, K-A, Paschen, W. and Csiba, L. Relationship between calcium accumulation and recovery of cat brain after prolonged cerebral ischaemia. J. Cerebr. Blood flow metabol., 3, 346-353. (1983)

Jande, S.S., Maler, L. and Lawson, D.E.M. Immunohistochemical mapping of vitamin D-dependent calcium-binding protein in brain. Nature, 294, 765-767 (1981)

Jenkins, L.W, Povlishoch, J.T., Becker, D.P., Miller, J.P., and Sullivan, H.G. Complete cerebral ischaemia. An ultrastructural study. Acta Neuropathol. (Berl.), 48, 113-125. (1979)

Kazda, S., Hoffmeister, F., Garthoff, B., Towart, R. Prevention of post-ischaemic impaired reperfusion of the brain by nimodipine (Bay e 9736). Acta Neurol. Scand., 60 (Suppl 72), 302-303. (1979)

Leonard, J.P. and Salpeter, M.M. Agonist induced myopathy at the neuromuscular junction is mediated by calcium. J Cell. Biol., 82, 811-819. (1979)

Levy, D.E. and Duffy, T.E. Cerebral energy metabolism during transient ischaemia and recovery in the gerbill. J. Neurochem., 28, 63-70. (1979)

Llinàs, R. and Hess, R. Tetrodoxin-resistant dendritic spikes in avian Purkinje cells. Proc. Nat. Acad. Sci. (Wash.), 73, 2520-2523. (1976)

Marciani, M.G, Louvel, J. and Heinemann, U. Aspartate-induced changes in extracellular free calcium in in vitro hippocampal slices of rats. Brain Res., 238, 272-277. (1982)

Meldrum, B.S. Metabolic effects of prolonged epileptic seizures and the causation of epileptic brain damage. In: Metabolic disorders of the nervous system. edit. F.C. Rose, Pitman Medical, pp 175-187. (1981)

217

Meldrum, B.S. Metabolic factors during prolonged seizures and their relation to nerve cell death. In: Advances in Neurology, Vol. 34, Status Epilepticus: Mechanisms of Brain Damage and Treatment. edits. A.V. Delgado-Escueta, C.G. Wasterlain, D.M. Treiman and R.J. Porter. Raven Press, New York, pp 261-276. (1983)

Meldrum, B., Griffiths, T. and Evans, M. Hypoxia and neuronal hyperexcitability — a clue to mechanisms of brain protection. In: Protection of Tissues against Hypoxia. edits. A. Wauquier, M. Borgers and W.K. Amery, Elsevier, Amsterdam, pp 275-286. (1982)

Müller-Schweinitzer, E. and Neumann, P. *In vitro* effects of calcium antagonists PN 200-110, Nifedipine and Nimodipine on human and canine cerebral arteries. *J. Cereb. Blood Flow Metabol.*, **3**, 354-361. (1983)

Naquet, R. Epileptic activity evoked by air embolism in cat, monkey and man. In: Z Servit (ed.) Proc. Int. Symp. Comp. Cell. Pathophysiol. Epilepsy. Excerpta Medica, Amsterdam pp 89-102. (1966)

Nayler, W.G., Fassgold, E., Yepez, C. Pharmacological protection of mitochondrial function in hypoxic heart muscle: effect of verapamil, propranolol and methylprednisolone. *Cardiovascular Res.*, **12**, 152-161. (1978)

Nicholls, D. and Åkerman, K. Mitochondrial calcium transport. *Biochem. Biophys. Acta*, **683**, 57-88. (1982)

O'Hara, P.T., Wade, C.R. and Lieberman, A.R. Calcium storage sites in axon terminals and other components of intact C.N.S. tissue: studies with a modified pyroantimonate technique. *J. Anat.*, **129**, 869-870. (1979)

Publicover, S.J., Duncan, C.J. and Smith, J.L. The use of A23187 to demonstrate the role of intracellular calcium in causing ultrastructural damage in mammalian muscle. *J. Neuropathol. exp. Neurol.*, **37**, 554-557. (1978)

Reedy, D.P., Little, J.R., Capraro, J.A., Slugg, R.M. and Lesser, R.P. Effects of verapamil on acute focal cerebral ischaemia. *Neurosurgery*, **12**, 272-276. (1983)

Rubinson, K.A. and Baker, P.F. The flow properties of axoplasm in a defined chemical environment: influence of anions and calcium. *Proc. Roy. Soc. B. Lond. B.*, **205**, 323-345. (1979)

Schanne, F.A.X., Kane, A.B., Young, E.E. and Farber, J.L. Calcium dependence of toxic cell death: a final common pathway. *Science*, **206**, 700-702. (1979)

Schmidt, R. and Zimmerman, H. Mitochondrial release of Ca^{2+} during sustained nerve activity in the electric organ of Torpedo Marmorata. *Exp. Brain Res.*, **38**, 405-417. (1980)

Schwartzkroin, P.A. and Wyler, A.R. Mechanisms underlying epileptiform burst discharges *Ann. Neurol.*, **7**, 95-107 (1979)

Sloper, J.J., Johnson, P. and Powell, T.P.S. Selective degeneration of interneurons in the motor cortex of infant monkeys following controlled hypoxia. A possible cause of epilepsy. *Brain Res.*, **198**, 204-209. (1980)

Sloviter, R.S. "Epileptic" brain damages in rats induced by sustained electrical stimulation of the perforant path. I. Acute electrophysiological and light microscopic studies. *Brain Res. Bull.* **10**, 675-697. (1983)

Sloviter, R.S. and Damiano, B.P. On the relationship between kainic acid-induced epileptiform activity and hippocampal neuronal damage. *Neuropharmacology*, **20**, 1003-1011. (1981)

Snyder, B.D., Haused, W.A., Loewnson, R.B., Leppik, I.E., Ramirez-Lasspas, M. and Gumnit, R.J. Neurologic prognosis after cardiopulmonary arrest: III. Seizure activity. *Neurology*, **30**, 1292-1297. (1980)

Steen, P.A., Newberg, L.A., Milde, J.H. and Michenfelder, J.D. Nimodipine improves cerebral blood flow and neurologic recovery after complete cerebral ischaemia in the dog. *J. Cerebr. Blood Flow and Metabol.*, **3**, 38-43. (1983)

Stoclet, J-C. Calmodulin. An ubiquitous protein which regulates calcium-dependent cellular functions and calcium movements. *Biochem. Pharmacol.*, **30**, 1723-1729. (1981)

Towart, R. The pathophysiology of cerebral vasospasm, and pharmacological approaches to its management. *Acta Neurochirurgica*, **63**, 253-258. (1982)

Towart, R., Wehinger, E., Meyer, H. and Kazda, S. The effects of nimodipine, its optical isomers and metabolites on isolated vascular smooth muscle. *Arzneimittel-Forsch.*, **32**, 338-346. (1982)

Van Nueten, J.M. and Vanhoutte, P.M. Improvement of tissue perfusion with inhibitors of calcium ion influx. *Biochem. Pharmacol.*, **29**, 479-481. (1980)

Van Reempts, J. and Borgers, M. Morphological assessment of pharmacological brain protection. In: Protection of Tissues against Hypoxia. edit. A. Wauquier, M. Borgers and W.K. Amery, Elsevier Biomedical Press, Amsterdam pp 263-274. (1982)

Van Reempts, J. and Borgers, M. Morphological aspects of brain protection in experimentally induced hypoxia. In: Problems and Perspectives of Brain Protection. Edit. S. Hoyer. Springer Verlag Berling (in press). (1983)

White, B.C., Gadzinski, D.S., Hohner, P.J., Krone, C., Hoehner, T., White, J.D. and Trombley, J.H. Jr. Effects of flunarizine on canine cerebral cortical blood flow and vascular resistance post cardiac arrest. *Ann. Emerg. Med.*, **11**, 119-126. (1982)

Wong, R.K.S., Prince, D.A. and Basbaum, A.I. Intradenditic recordings from hippocampal neurons. *Proc. Nat. Acad. Sci.* (Wash.), **76**, 986-990. (1979)

Wrogemann, K. and Pena, S.D.J. Mitochondrial calcium overload: a general mechanism for cell-necrosis in muscle diseases. *Lancet*, **1**, 672-674. (1976)

Calcium entry blockers and cerebral resuscitation

B.C. White, C.D. Winegar, P.J. Hoehner,
D.S. Gadzinski, T. Hoehner, J. Trombley Jr.

Summary

Our work, the data from Hoffmeister et al. (1979) and review of pathologic mechanisms suggest that calcium entry blockers are an effective and critical part of our rapidly expanding ability to protect the brain following anoxic or ischemic insults. Calcium is implicated in the genesis of all the injury mechanisms which we have discussed. A number of critical questions need to be pursued and answered promptly. They include the following:

1. A prospective blind trial of selective calcium blockers needs to be done in patients following successful resuscitation from cardiac arrest. The test in this trial is clearly the recovery of functional neurological status.

2. Cerebral energy studies need to be done following arrest and resuscitation in experimental animals with calcium blockers.

3. The question of whether the calcium blockers are able to inhibit the burst of FFA which has been seen following cerebral anoxia needs to be examined.

4. The controversy surrounding the putative role of superoxide and free radicals in neuron damage needs to be resolved, and studies need to be designed to examine the possibility that calcium entry blockers may interfere with the production of these oxidants.

5. The question of whether the calcium blockers will be more effective when used together with a therapeutic regimen including other interventions in the processes that we have reviewed, such as indomethacin, the barbiturates, and free radical scavengers, needs to be examined.

Résumé

Notre travail, les données de Hoffmeister et al. (1979) et une revue des mécanismes pathologiques suggèrent que les inhibiteurs calciques constituent une part efficace et critique de notre faculté rapidement croissante de protection du cerveau suite à des agressions anoxiques ou ischémiques. Le calcium joue un rôle dans la genèse de tous les mécanismes de lésion dont nous avons parlé. Plusieurs questions critiques doivent être explorées davantage et résolues rapidement. Elles englobent:

1. Une étude prospective à double insu d'inhibiteurs calciques sélectifs doit être effectuée chez des patients après une ressuscitation fructueuse d'un arrêt cardiaque. Le test dans cette étude porte clairement sur le retour à un statut neuroleptique fonctionnel.

2. Les effets des inhibiteurs calciques sur l'énergie cérébrale doivent être étudiés après arrêt et ressuscitation chez des animaux de laboratoire.

3. Il convient d'examiner la question de savoir si les bloqueurs de calcium sont en mesure d'inhiber l'augmentation des FFA observée après une anoxie cérébrale.

4. La controverse entourant le rôle putatif du superoxyde et des radicaux libres dans la détérioration neuronale doit être résolue et il convient d'entreprendre des études destinées à examiner la possibilité selon laquelle les inhibiteurs calciques peuvent interférer avec la production de ces oxidants.

5. Il est nécessaire d'examiner la question de savoir si les inhibiteurs calciques seront plus efficaces lorsque combinés avec d'autres interventions thérapeutiques dans les processus déjà passés en revue, telles qu'administration d'indometacine, de barbituriques et de produits neutralisant les radicaux libres.

Resumen

Nuestros datos, así como los de Hoffmeister, et al. (1979) y la reseña de los mecanismos patológicos, sugieren que los inhibidores de la penetración intracelular de calcio forman una parte efectiva e importante de las crecientes posibilidades de la protección del cerebro después de lesiones provocados por anoxia o isquemia. El calcio va implicado en la génesis de todos los mecanismos lesivos que hemos discutido. Hace falta considerar y resolver un número de problemas que se plantean, tales como siguen:

1. Un prospectivo ensayo a ciegas de bloqueadores de calcio selectivos tiene que hacerse en pacientes que siguen una recuperación exitosa de un paro cardíaco. La prueba en este ensayo es claramente el restablecimiento de la condición funcional neurológica.

2. Los efectos de los bloqueadores de calcio sobre la energía cerebral tienen que estudiarse en animales experimentales, después de un paro cardíaco y resuscitación.

3. Se necesita considerar la cuestión de si los inhibidores de la penetración intracelular de calcio son capaces de inhibir el desencadenamiento de la acción de los ácidos grasos libres que se ha notado en anoxia cerebral.

4. Se necesita resolver la polémica en cuanto al papel supuesto de superóxido y los radicales libres en afecciones neurónicas. Queda por estudiar si los inhibidores de la penetración intracelular de calcio pueden interferir en la producción de estos oxidantes.

5. Hace falta examinar si los inhibidores de calcio serán más eficaces, cuando son empleados junto con un régimen terapéutico que incluye otras intervenciones en los procesos que hemos examinado, tales como indometacina, barbitúricos y productos recogedores de radicales libres.

Zusammenfassung

Unsere Arbeit, die Ergebnisse von Hoffmeister et al. (1979) und ein Überblick über die pathologischen Mechanismen führen zur Auffassung, daß Kalziumeinstromhemmer im Zusammenhang mit unserer schnell zunehmenden Fähigkeit, das Gehirn nach anoxischen bzw. ischämischen Anfällen zu schützen, eine effektive und entscheidende Rolle spielen. Kalzium ist beim Entstehen aller dargelegten Schädigungsmechanismen einbezogen. Einige wichtige Fragen, die sich dabei stellen, fordern eine Antwort. So u.a.:

1. Bei Patienten mit erfolgreicher Hirnreanimation nach Herzstillstand ist ein orientierender Blindversuch mit selektiven Kalziumhemmern durchzuführen. Als Erfolgskriterium ist ein Test zur Wiederherstellung des funktionellen neurologischen Status zu verwenden.

2. Bei Versuchstieren sind Gehirnenergiestudien mit Kalziumhemmern durchzuführen, wobei die Tiere nach Herzstillstand reanimiert werden.

3. Die Frage, ob Kalziumhemmer imstande sind, die einer Hirnanoxie folgende Freisetzung freier Fettsäuren zu hemmen, ist zu untersuchen.

4. Die Kontroverse über die mutmaßliche Rolle von Peroxyden und freien Radikalen bei Neuronen-schäden muss gelöst werden. Studienmodelle sind zu entwerfen um feststellen zu können, ob Kalzium-einstromhemmer die Erzeugung dieser Oxydantien beeinflussen.
5. Die Frage ist zu lösen, ob Kalziumhemmer im Anschluss an andere therapeutische Maßnahmen, welche die diskutierten Stoffe, Indomethacin, Barbiturate und Fänger freier Radikale umfassen, wirkungs-voller werden.

Introduction

Permanent functional neurological disability occurs in over 50% of patients surviving cardiac arrest outside the hospital (Myerburg *et al.*, 1980). In view of the amount of time, money, and other resources expended on resuscitation, this outcome data reflects a terrible failure of medical efforts. Thus, the rapidly advancing studies of the mechanisms of cerebral injury and the rapid clinical application of this information for effective cerebral resuscitation are of utmost importance.

Based on studies done in the 1940's (Heymans, 1950, Weinberger *et al.*, 1940), it has been widely believed that permanent cerebral injury is the inevitable result of more than 4 to 6 minutes of normothermic cerebral anoxia. It had been hoped that the rapid application of effective cardiopulmonary resuscitation (CPR) after witnessed cardiac arrest would protect the brain for substantially longer periods of time. However, recent reports indicate that basic CPR produces little arteriovenous pressure gradient (Rogers *et al.*, 1981), and is of limited effectiveness in prolonging cerebral survival during cardiac arrest (Rogers *et al.*, 1981, Holder *et al.*, 1977). Indeed, if definitive resuscitation and spontaneous perfusion are not achieved within 15 minutes after cardiac arrest, neurologic prognosis is poor.

Evidence has accumulated during the last 20 years indicating that this neurologic injury after periods of anoxia does not reflect immediate neuronal death. Ames and Guarian (1963) reported prolonged retinal neuronal survival in anoxic tissue baths. Hossmann and Kleihues (1973) did extensive biochemical studies on cat and monkey brain anoxia preparations, and reported recovery of high energy metabolism, enzymatic functions, and action potential generation after 60 minutes of anoxia. This evidence shows there is no "four minute barrier" of certain anoxic neuronal death. Rather, neuronal death probably occurs later, and post resuscitation brain death may be a result of neuronal injuries occurring after resuscitation. Based on the evidence for persistant neuronal viability and Goldstein's observation of pentobarbital's ability to improve cerebral toleration of prolonged anoxia, extensive laboratory and clinical studies continue with pentobarbital for amelioration of anoxia encepholapathy (Safar, 1982).

Living tissue is a thermodynamically highly ordered system. The process of death is a process in which living tissue undergoes a set of reactions which decrease total order and increase free heat. Data accumulated within the last 5 years, which we will review, implicates the calcium ion (Ca^{2+}) as a triggering element in a number of these reactions in brains after anoxia. Shifts of this ion have also been implicated in capillary hypoperfusion in organ systems following resuscitation from anoxic or ischemic insults.

Our purpose is to:
1. Review the evidence for calcium ion shifts during anoxia and ischemia.
2. Review the relationship of energy metabolism and calcium handling by intracellular organelles.
3. Review the evidence for calcium involvement in the intracellular increase in free fatty acids which occur simultaneously with a decrease in plasma membrane order.
4. Review the evidence implicating calcium as a triggering element in the production of oxidative free radicals which may be involved in continuing cellular injury.
5. Review the "No Reflow Phenomenon" in the brain following cardiac arrest, and the evidence implicating calcium in this phenomenon.
6. Present the evidence indicating that the calcium blocking agents have a major role as therapeutic intervention to modify these pathological processes.

Anoxia-ischemia and calcium shifts

Calcium ion is actively maintained out of the cell with a gradient of 10,000 to 1 across the plasma membrane (Katz and Reuter, 1979). There are at least 2 ionic pumps responsible for the maintenance of this gradient. One, is an ATP and Mg^{2+} dependent pump which is unidirectionally committed "out", first characterized in squid axons (Dipolo, 1978). This pump has subsequently been identified in human red cells (Penniston et al., 1980), neutrophils (Schneider et al., 1974), neurons (Sobue et al., 1979), and myocardium (Caroni and Carafoli, 1980).

According to Penniston et al. (1980), this carrier system, reacts with and pumps intracellular calcium in both a low affinity slow pumping mode, and also in a high affinity rapid pumping mode. The change in mode of this system, which has been highly purified by these investigators, is induced by calcium activated calmodulin. When calcium activated calmodulin binds to this carrier, there is an increase in the maximum velocity of transport and fourfold increase in the binding affinity for calcium. Thus, this ATP dependent carrier functions maximally if there are significant increases in intracellular calcium at the same time that adequate ATP levels are maintained.

The other membrane pump is a sodium-calcium exchange-pump which will move one calcium out of the cytosol and into the interstitial fluid at the same time that it moves 3 sodiums into the cell (Blaustein, 1974; Carafoli and Crompton, 1978). This pump may also be partially ATP dependent (Carafoli and Crompton, 1978).

The precise characteristics of the systems controlling Ca^{2+} entry into excitable cells need further experimental clarification. Early work suggested that Ca^{2+} entry was ATP dependent (Hofer and Kleinzeller, 1963; Janda, 1969). However, when the magnitude of the gradient across the cell membrane was recognized, thermodynamic objections to the concept of ATP dependent influx became evident (Borle, 1981). Current hypotheses suggest the following mechanisms of influx:
1. Depolarization dependent entry activated by increased extracellular K^+ (Blaustein et al., 1972; Van Breemen et al., 1973) and intracellular Na^+ (Blaustein, 1974; Blaustein and Weismann, 1970).
2. Depolarization independent steady state entry systems (Dipolo, 1979).

3. Changes in membrane fluidity related to shifts in membrane phospholipid content induced by adrenergic agonists (Hirata and Axelrod, 1980; Toyoshma and Osawa, 1975).

During anoxia or ischemia in the brain, as in other organs, the failure of oxidative metabolism results in rapid depletion of cellular ATP stores (Ljunggren et al., 1974). Moreover, the brain has very little substrate reserve for anerobic metabolism and is not as able to maintain residual ATP by glycolysis. The precipitous reduction of high energy compounds would be expected to adversely affect the cells' ability to maintain ionic gradients across the plasma membrane. The validity of this assumption has been confirmed in the laboratory (Vyskocil et al., 1972; Nicholson, 1980; Nicholson et al., 1977; Siemkowicz and Hansen, 1981). These investigators have shown that after 1 to 2 minutes of cerebral anoxia there is a massive potassium efflux from the cells and marked sodium and calcium influx into the cells accompanied by a 90% reduction in the extracellular calcium concentrations in interstitial fluid. Further evidence for the massive calcium influx into neurons is the rapid accumulation of this ion in pathologic concentrations in their mitochondria (Strosnajder, 1980).

This phenomenon of massive calcium influx down the concentration gradient during anoxic or ischemic insults is not confined to neurons. Van Nueten and Vanhoutte (1980) have demonstrated that this occurs in the media of vascular walls. It also occurs in myocardium and is associated with an increase in resting tension (Nayler et al., 1979; Poole-Wilson, 1980). The early evidence developed by Trunkey et al. (1976; 1978) demonstrated reductions in serum calcium concentrations in baboons subjected to 2 different models of shock. This suggests that Ca^{2+} entry during ischemia is in fact a generalized phenomenon in cells throughout the body.

Siesjo (1981) suggests that Ca^{2+} entry also accompanies other global cerebral insults (i.e., hypoglycemia and status epilepticus) which may result in permanent brain injury. Happel et al. (1981) have also demonstrated that massive calcium influx into contused spinal cords results in a four-fold increase in calcium content.

Organell calcium handling

The elucidation of the large (10^4) ionic calcium gradient across plasma membranes and the shifts in that gradient occurring during anoxia or ischemia have been accompanied by a rapid expansion of our understanding of calcium handling by cellular substructures.

Mitochondria are the organelles responsible for oxidation of energy substrates and for the conversion of the energy derived from these "burns" into the high energy bonds of ATP. The mechanism of this conversion was outlined in the "chemiosmotic hypothesis" developed by Mitchell and Moyle (1967). In this system, NADH derived from the reduction of NAD in the Krebs cycle is oxidized by the cytochrome system on the inner surface of the mitochondrial membrane.

The oxidation sites are intimately associated with proton pumping in the membrane. The energy from oxidation is directly harnessed to pump $H+$ out of the mitochondria, establishing an electrochemical energy gradient across the mitochondrial membrane. This gradient may be used by the mitochondria for 3 known processes: 1) ATP synthesis, 2) reverse electron transport resulting in the reduction of NAD or 3) active (osmotically uphill) transport of certain ions.

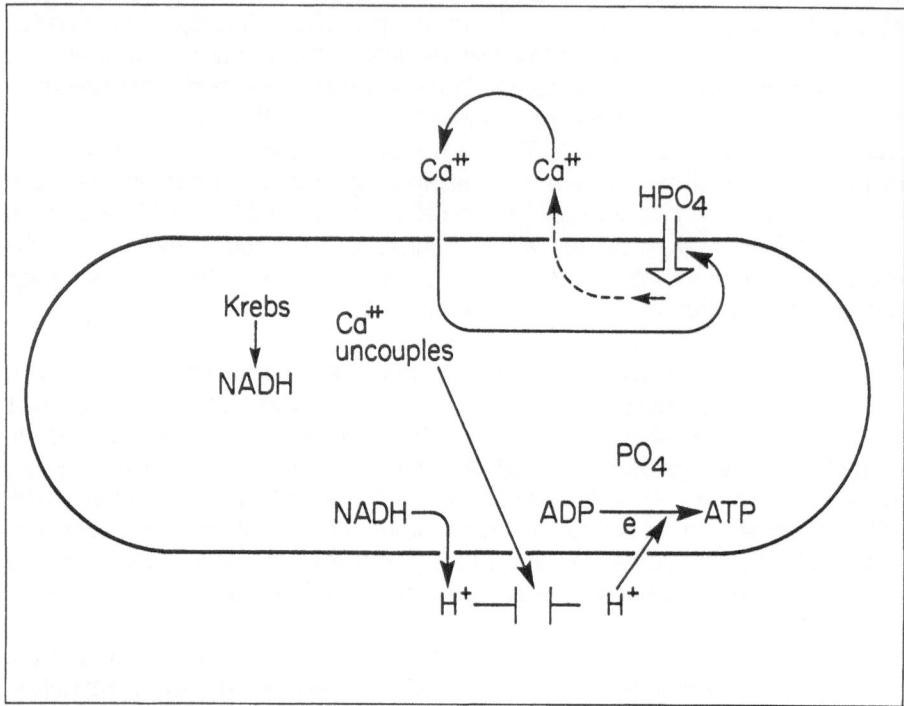

Figure 1: Schematic drawing of mitochondrial ATP production. The energy derived in the electron transport system from the oxidation of NADH is used to drive proton pumps which move $H+$ out, creating a chemiosmotic energy gradient. The readmission of $H+$ down this gradient provides the energy for ATP synthesis. Calcium uptake by the mitochondria directly uses the energy of the $H+$ gradient, which can then not be used for ATP synthesis. HPO_4^{2-} releases calcium from he mitochondria. Elevated $Na+$ and free fatty acid concentrations in the cytosol have similar calcium releasing effects.

Exposure of mitochondria to calcium and metabolic substrate results in a burst of oxygen consumption, accompanied by the pumping of protons out of the mitochondria and uptake of calcium (White *et al.*, 1980; Lehninger, 1974). Thus, the electrochemical gradient established from the energy of oxidation is directly used in mitochondrial uptake of calcium, without the intermediate production of ATP (Fig. 1). In the presence of physiologic concentrations of phosphate, the calcium pumped into the mitochondria is bound in the mitochondrial matrix. Thus, there exists in the mitochondrial membrane another mechanism by which the cell jealously guards against significant elevations of calcium concentration in the cytosol. Mitochondrial calcium pumping is obligatory, energy consuming, and uncouples the use of oxidation derived energy from the production of ATP (Fig. 2) (Toyoshma and Osawa, 1975; Ljunggren *et al.*, 1974).

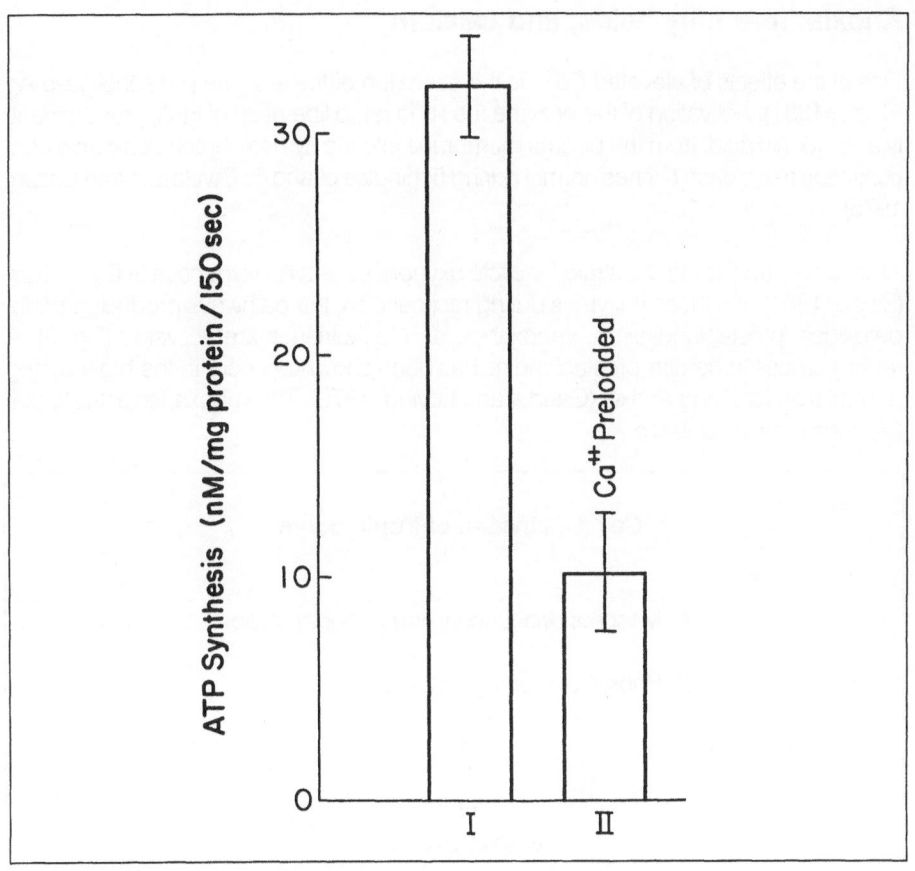

Figure 2: Mitochondrial ATP synthesis in control (I) mitochondria and in mitochondria pretreated for 2 minutes with 200 μM CaCl$_2$ and 1 mM K$_2$HPO$_4$ (II).

The exit channel for calcium out of the mitochondria is separate from the uptake system that we have just described (Peng *et al.*, 1977; Fiskum and Lehninger, 1979). There are a number of situations when the mitochondria are unable to retain the calcium cleared from the cytosol. Phosphate concentrations in the milimolar range, which quickly occur during anoxia (Kubler and Katz, 1977), will release the calcium from the mitochondria (Haugard *et al.*, 1964). Increases in the concentration of free fatty acids (FFA) and of Na$^+$ in the cytosol, which occur in global neuronal insults, will also release calcium from mitochondria (Harris, 1977; Crompton *et al.*, 1978). Clark and Roman (1980) have demonstrated that magnesium ions can depress the FFA stimulated release of calcium by mitochondria in the brain by as much as 70%.

Another subcellular structure that is active in the hemostasis of cellular calcium is the sarcoplasmic reticulum (Hasselbach, 1978). The sarcoplasmic reticulum will actively pump and bind calcium. This pumping requires magnesium and ATP, and is again accompanied by a burst of proton ejection from the sarcoplastic reticulum (Madeira, 1980).

Anoxia, free fatty acids, and calcium

One of the effects of elevated Ca^{2+} is the activation of the enzyme phospholipase A_2 (Siesjo, 1981). Activation of this enzyme results in rapid liberation of FFA, predominantly arachidonic acid, from the plasma membrane into the cytosol. Arachidonic acid concentration may reach 5 times normal during 5 minutes of anoxia (Aveldano and Bazan, 1975).

Arachidonic acid is the substrate for cyclo-oxygenase and lipoxygenase at O_2 12 Torr. (Siesjo, 1981). Via these enzymes during recirculation, the pathways producing endoperoxides, prostaglandins, thromboxanes, and leukotrienes are activated (Fig. 3). A rapid increase in cellular prostaglandins has been shown to occur in the brain during recirculation following anoxia (Gaudet and Leving, 1979). Thromboxanes activate platelets and are vasoplastic.

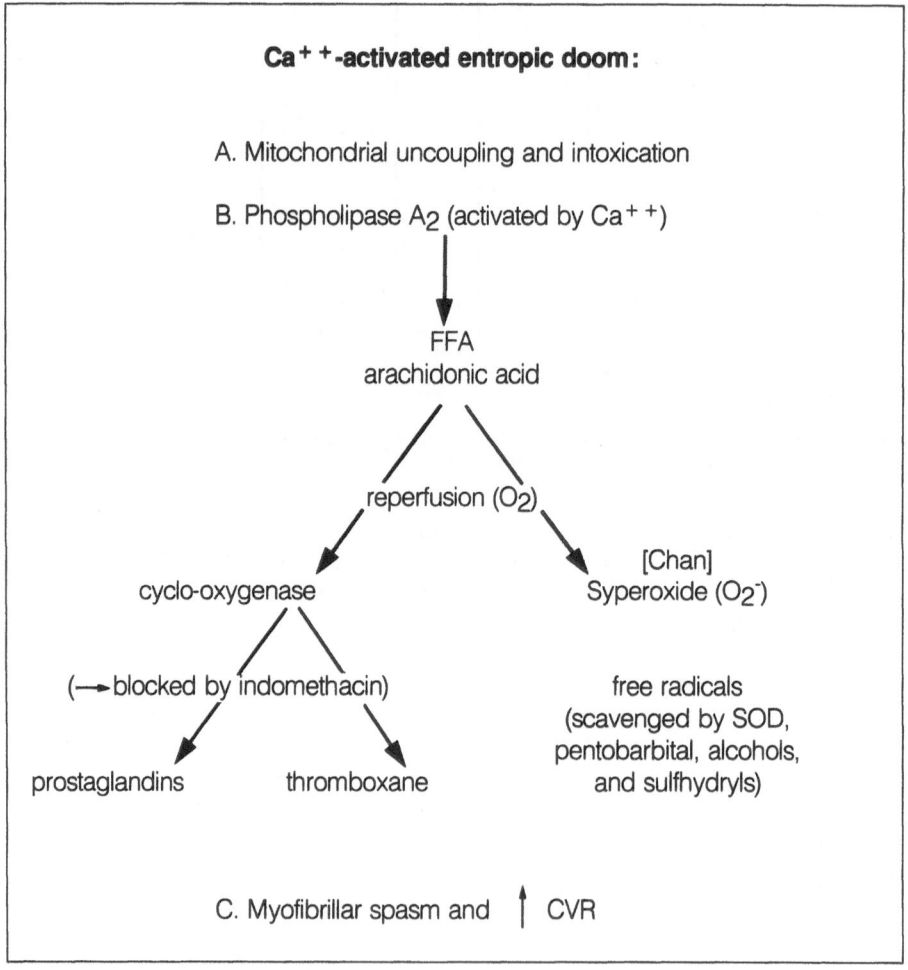

Figure 3: SOD = Superoxide-dismutase

228

Leukotrienes are implicated in the pathogenesis of anaphylaxis. Endoperoxides may have free radical oxidant characteristics (Siesjo, 1981). Thus, the increased concentration of arachidonic acid initiated by Ca^{2+} entry during anoxia or ischemia leads to the generation of several toxic compounds. The cyclo-oxygenase inhibitor indomethacin blocks the post anoxic prostaglandin surge (Flower, 1974; Hallenbeck and Furlow, 1979). There is evidence that this may improve the quality of neurologic survival in experimental animals (Hallenbeck and Furlow, 1979).

Nemoto et al. (1981) have noted the constancy of the sharp increase in concentration of FFA in neurons following anoxic insults in a variety of models. They reported the capacity of pentobarbital to depress both the concentrations of arachidonic acid and FFA in neurons after these insults. This report is very interesting in light of the evidence developed by Altura et al. (1980) that pentobarbital is a weak calcium entry blocker in arterioles. Blaustein and Ector (1975) and Elrod and Leslie (1980) found pentobarbital to be an inhibitor of calcium entry into neurons.

There is observational data, therefore, showing that the concentrations of FFA and arachidonic acid increase sharply in neurons during anoxia and reperfusion. The biochemical pathways outlined (Fig. 3) demonstrate that the calcium flux into neurons occurring during anoxia is potentially responsible for the activation of these pathways at phospholipase A_2. Moreover, two clinical pharmacologic agents which may be useful in preserving neuronal integrity and brain function following anoxic or ischemic insults have been shown to interfere in this sequence by calcium entry blocking activity or, in the case of indomethacin, by a direct inhibition of one of the enzymes. Thus, shift of calcium ion into neurons occurring during ischemia may be implicated as the primary pathologic event resulting in the liberation of FFA and their metabolites which may result in further neuronal damage.

Calcium, oxidative radicals, and post-anoxic damage

The superoxide radical (O_2^-) is generated by a number of oxidative enzymes and also by phagocytic leukocytes (Loschen et al., 1974; Babior, 1978). The classic reaction which results in the production of this radical is between the enzyme xanthine oxidase and its substrate xanthine. We have already seen how cerebral anoxia or ischemia results in a rapid rise in FFA. Chan and Fishman (1978) have reported that the high concentration of FFA in brain slices triggers the production of superoxide radicals. Superoxide has been shown to attack membrane proteins (Greenwald and Moy, 1979; Goldberg and Stern, 1977) and oxidise polyunsaturated lipids (Gutteridge, 1977; Thomas et al., 1978). The superoxide radical also reacts with hydrogen peroxide to produce extremely active oxidants including the hydroxyl radical (Brawn and Friedovich, 1980) which can attack and disrupt DNA.

Neutrophils can secrete substantial amounts of the superoxide radical (Brawn and Friedovich, 1980). In circulating blood and in cells, the radical is normally controlled by the enzyme superoxide dismutase. This enzyme catalyzes a reaction in which 2 superoxide radicals are combined with a hydrogen ion to produce hydrogen peroxide and molecular oxygen.

$$2\,O_2^- + 2H^+ \xrightarrow{\text{superoxide dismutase}} H_2O_2 + O_2$$

Hydrogen peroxide can be eliminated from the system, either by catalase or by glutathione peroxidase. In the catalase reaction, 2 molecules of hydrogen peroxide are converted into water and molecular oxygen.

$$2H_2O_2 \xrightarrow{\text{catalase}} 2H_2O + O_2$$

In the glutathione peroxidase reaction (Siesjo, 1981), 2 glutathiones react with hydrogen peroxide to produce sulfhydryl polimerized glutathione and water.

$$2GSH + H_2O_2 \xrightarrow{\text{glutathione peroxidase}} GS\text{-}SG + 2H_2O$$

Del Maestro et al. (1980) and Demopoulos et al. (1980) suggested that superoxide production and the subsequent generation of free radicals, such as the hydroxyl radical, may be involved in final irreversible neuronal injury. Ascorbic acid, normally found in high concentrtion in the central nervous system reacts readily with the hydroxyl free radical. Demopoulos et al. (1980) reported data from both ischemic brain and spinal cord contusion models demonstrating a reduction in the concentration of ascorbic acid after the insult. They suggested that this is direct evidence for activity of superoxide and hydroxyl free radicals. Thiopental has been shown to have free radical scavenging activity (Rehncrona et al., 1980).

However, Siesjo et al. (1980) have been unable to demonstrate a decrease in the ratio of glutathione to glutathione-polymer in the brain during complete anoxia, incomplete ischemia, hypoglycemia, or status epilepticus. Cooper et al. (1980) have confirmed this data. Rehncrona et al. (1980) have also failed to find evidence for lipid peroxidation by oxidative radicals during ischemia.

Thus the evidence for the putative role of superoxide and/or free radicals in the mechanism of definitive cerebral injury is unclear. The fact that the reaction sequence to produce these potent oxidants can be ignited by the observed increase in FFA content of neurons during ischemia is, however, clear. Moreover, the role of ionized calcium in triggering the surge in FFA content seems clear, as we have already discussed. The demonstration of the ability of the barbiturates to block calcium entry into vascular cells and neurons (Altura et al., 1980; Elrod and Leslie, 1980) also raises the question of whether the reduction in FFA content and the evidence for free radical quenching seen in the model systems treated with thiopental may not be a secondary effect related to primary modulation of cellular Ca^{2+} by this drug.

The no-reflow-phenomenon

Organ perfusion is mandatory for maintenance of high energy metabolism and thermodynamic order. During the last 20 years, studies of cerebral perfusion after anoxia or ischemia have provided uniform evidence of disturbances in blood flow during reperfusion (Ames et al., 1968).

Drewes et al. (1973) reported that cerebrovascular resistance is massively increased after 2 hours of reperfusion following a 30 minute anoxic cerebral insult. Rehncrona et al. (1979) and Snyder et al. (1975) reported evidence that perfusion deteriorates progressively following cerebral anoxia. Evidence from our laboratories has confirmed this phenomenon (Gadzinski et al., 1982). Moreover, we have now followed blood flow rates in the cerebral cortex for 18 hours following resuscitation after a 20 minute cardiac arrest in dogs. Not only is the flow rate in the cortex near zero after 90 minutes of reperfusion at good blood pressure, but deep hypoperfusion persists for at least 18 hours post arrest. There is, therefore, a progressive and deep depression of cerebral blood flow in the cortex following cardiac arrest, which is prolonged.

There were 2 early explanations for this phenomenon. It was first thought that cellular swelling following the anoxic insult might produce an increase in intracranial pressure to levels high enough to depress perfusion. This is not the case in cerebral injury models which do not involve trauma (Snyder et al., 1975; Gadzinski et al., 1982).

The second hypothesis that was offered to explain the "No-Reflow-Phenomenon" was that platelet aggregation and intravascular coagulation obstructed cerebral blood flow in the small vessels. According to Hossman et al. (1980), platelet trapping is increased 3 to 4 fold in the brain after a 1 hour ischemic insult. Platelet aggregation is stimulated by arachidonic acid and blocked by calmodulin inhibitors (Suda and Aoki, 1981). However, Chiang et al. (1968) using light and electron microscopy studies after anoxic cerebral insults in rabbits, found no evidence of fibrin or platelet thrombi in the vessels. Moreover, clinical trials of heparin have been unsuccessful in changing the functional neurologic outcome following cerebral anoxic insults in patients (Fischer and Ames, 1972). Heparinization also did not protect cortical flow following arrest in our studies (Gadzinski et al., 1982).

Recent work has drawn attention to the importance of the calcium influx during anoxia or hypoperfusion in the development of myofibrillar contracture. Henry et al. (1977) have shown that hypoperfusion of the myocardium is quickly followed by:
1. Elevated calcium in the cells
2. Elevated calcium in the mitochondria
3. Contracture of the myofibrills

Nayler et al. (1980) have confirmed these findings and the uncoupling of oxidation from phosphorilation which accompanies this process. Van Nueten and Vanhoutte (1980) have demonstrated arterial spasm in response to calcium influx during anoxia. It is reasonable to suggest that once the actinomyosin complex is formed, high concentrations of calcium in the cell would discourage relaxation. We have, therefore, argued that the no-reflow-phenomenon is directly and primarily related to increased vascular resistance in the brain following ischemic insults (Gadzinski et al., 1982), accompanied as they are by massive calcium influx in both neurons and vascular cells. Betz et al. (1973) demonstrated that elimination of Ca^{2+} from the fluid bathing pia halted arterial spasm. Edvinson et al. (1970) have reported the efficacy of nifedipine against norepinephrine or 5-hydroxytryptamine induced vasospasm of the pial arteries.

Summary and synthesis: calcium and hypoxic encephalopathy

We have reviewed data on anoxic-ischemic brain injury showing that:

1. Neurons do not irreversibly die during periods of anoxia up to about 1 hour.

2. There is a massive shift of Ca^{2+} from extracellular fluid to the intracellular space during anoxia. This occurs with the precipitous fall of ATP required to drive the pumps which maintain calcium homeostasis at the plasma membrane.

3. In addition to homeostatic pumps in the plasma membrane, mitochondria and sarcoplasmic reticulum are involved in calcium homeostasis in the cytosol. Mitochondria pump calcium in by using the chemiosmotic gradient generated by oxidative metabolism. This activity is obligatory, uncouples oxidation from phosphorylation, and in the presence of elevated free HPO_4^{2-} can FFA, or Na^+ in irreversible mitochondrial damage. The sarcoplasmic reticulum sequesters Ca^{2+} using an ATP consuming H^+ antiport pump. Mitochondria and sarcoplasmic reticulum from neurons injured by anoxia are Ca^{2+} overloaded.

4. The enzyme phospholipase A_2 is calcium activated and releases FFA from membranes. A large and rapid increase in neuronal FFA content, especially of arachidonic acid, is a constant feature of anoxic-ischemic neuronal injury. As oxygen becomes available during reperfusion, the activation of cyclo-oxygenase and lipoxygenase produces a burst of prostaglandin and leukotriene synthesis. Drug inhibition of the cyclo-oxygenase reaction improves functional neurologic recovery. Pentobarbital is a weak calcium entry blocker, and it depresses arachidonic acid production during anoxia, and improves functional neurologic recovery.

5. Elevated FFA in neurons trigger the production of superoxide (O_2^-) radical. This radical may directly attack lipoproteins, or it may react with hydrogen peroxide to produce hydroxyl radical that can attack nucleic acids. The evidence for an *in vivo* role for these oxidative radicals in definitive neuronal injury is controversial and unsettled; however, the entropic threat posed by the potential reaction cascades from these oxidants is so great that they cannot be lightly dismissed. Pentobarbital is an effective oxidative radical scavenger, as are sulfhydrylamino acids.

6. Delayed hypoperfusion during reperfusion is a constant finding following cerebral anoxia-ischemia. This hypoperfusion is characterized as deep (at least a 50-90% flow reduction in the outer cortex 90 minutes post resuscitation) and prolonged. This phenomenon is directly related to vascular resistance. There is no clear evidence supporting roles for increased ICP or intravascular coagulation in its genesis. Ca^{2+} overload during ischemia has been implicated in myofibrillar contracture and increased vascular resistance.

Schanne *et al.* (1979) have reported that in the absence of Ca^{2+}, hepatocytes were protected from 12 different membrane active toxins. In the presence of Ca^{2+}, all cells died. This report and the data we have reviewed strongly support the thesis advanced by Hass (1981) and Siesjo (1981) that the critical triggering event for neuronal death following anoxia-ischemia is increased Ca^{2+} in the cytosol.

Protection with calcium blocking agents

We have recently reported protection by the calcium antagonist flunarizine of cerebral cortical blood flow and cerebral oxygen consumption during reperfusion following a 20 minute cardiac arrest (White *et al.*, 1982). Both blood flow and oxygen consumption were protected at normal levels for the 2 hours of study post resuscitation (Fig. 4).

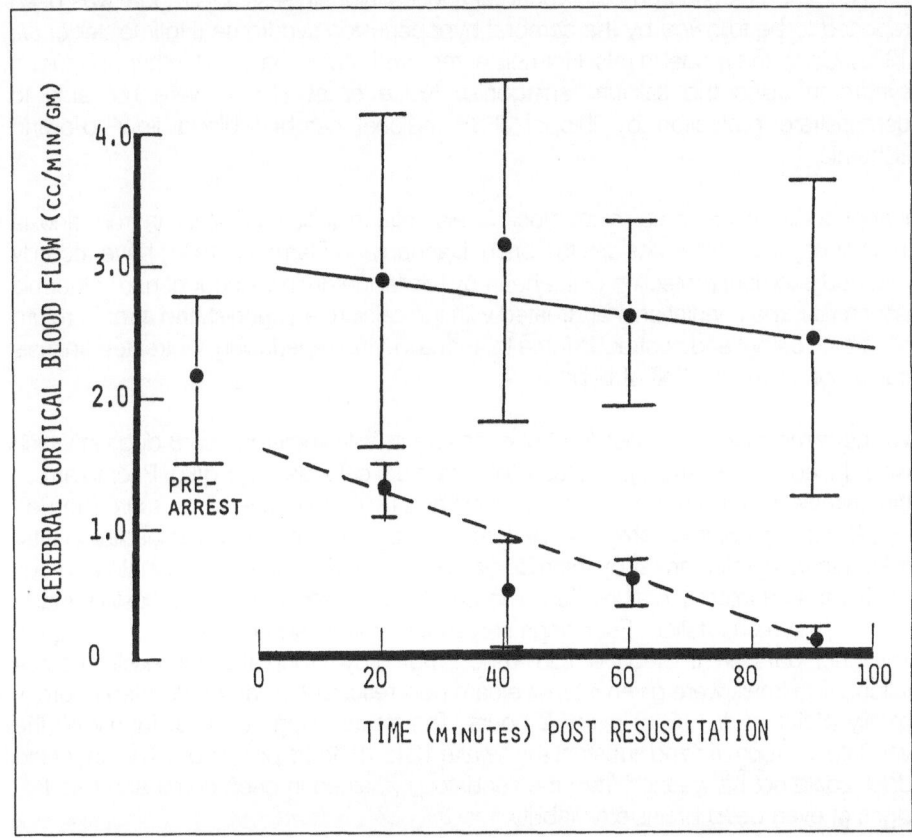

Figure 4: Flunarizine (6 µg/kg IV post resuscitation): protection of cerebral cortical blood flow in dogs following resuscitation from a 20 minute cardiac arrest.
Upper solid line: treated with flunarizine (n = 5)
Lower dotted line: untreated (n = 5)

We have also studied the effectiveness of verapamil (0.1 mg/kg IV) and magnesium sulfate (used as a Ca^{2+} blocker (Turlapaty and Altura, 1978)) in preserving cerebral blood flow using the cardiac bypass model post 20 minute arrest in dogs. Both of these agents are effective in preserving cerebral blood flow and oxygen consumption following cardiac arrest and resuscitation.

Hofmeister *et al.* (1979) have reported similar data with the calcium antagonist nimodipine administered to rats following a cerebral ischemic insult produced by circumferential neck pressure and simultaneous reduction of systemic blood pressure. This model, used by Hofmeister and many others (Nemoto *et al.*, 1977; Kowada *et al.*, 1968), is probably somewhat different from a true cardiac arrest model. We have attempted to use this model in dogs in our laboratories, and have been unable to produce a complete cessation of blood flow to the cortex of the brain. This remained the case when the circumferential neck pressure was accompanied by cross clamping of both common carotid and both vertebral arteries. Nonetheless, this model was been reported to be followed by the cerebral hypoperfusion syndrome (Hoffmeister *et al.*, 1979). Using this model in rats, Hofmeister reported protection from the hypoperfusion syndrome using the calcium antagonist. Kofke *et al.* (1979) were not able to demonstrate protection by thiopental of regional cerebral blood flow following ischemia.

It appears likely that the calcium blockers also offer significant protection from anoxia in other organ systems besides the brain. Daenen and Flameng (1981) have recently reported excellent protection of the heart by lidoflazine during 1 hour of normothermic ischemia. Experimental animals treated with the calcium antagonist had a rapid return of cardiac output and contractile force to normal during reperfusion. Untreated animals could not be weaned off of bypass.

We have recently carried out a set of experiments with lidoflazine on 8 dogs in which we induced cardiac arrest by injection of potassium chloride, 1 mEq/kg. Prior to arrest, the animals were instrumented for systemic and pulmonary arterial pressure monitoring. A sterile left thoracotomy was performed and the animals were resuscitated after a 25 minute cardiac arrest by internal massage, use of sodium bicarbonate and epinephrine, and internal defibrillation. The chest was closed and a thoracostomy tube placed post resuscitation. Four dogs served as controls and received no lidoflazine. The other four were treated with lidoflazine 1 mg/kg by IV drip after successful resuscitation. All animals were given intensive care post resuscitation and evaluated neurologically (Safar *et al.*, 1976) every 2 hours. The treated dogs were uniformly off the ventilator on room air and substantially awake 12 to 18 hours post arrest. The untreated dogs could not be weaned from the ventilator, remained in deep coma and had few signs of even deep brainstem viability.

References

Altura, B.T., Turlapaty, P.D. and Altura, B.M. Pentobarbital sodium inhibits calcium uptake in vascular smooth muscle. *Biochem. biophys. Acta*, **595**, 309 (1980).

Ames, A. and Guarian, B.S. Effects of glucose deprivation on function of isolated mammalian retina. *J. Neurophysiol.*, **26**, 617 (1963).

Ames, A., Wright, R L , Kowada, M et al. Cerebral ischemia, II: the no-reflow-phenomenon. *Am. J. Pathol.*, **52**, 437 (1968).

Aveldano, M.I. and Bazan, N.G. Rapid production of diacylglycerols enriched in arachidonat and stearate during early brain ischemia. *J. Neurochem.*, **25**, 919 (1975).

Babior, B.M. O_2 dependent microbrial killing by phagocytes. *New Engl. J. Med.*, **298**, 659 (1978).

Betz, E., Enzenrob, H.G and Vlahov, V Interaction of H^+ and Ca^{2+} in the regulation of local pial vascular resistance. *Pflügers Arch.*, **343**, 79 (1973).

Bilexikian, J.P., Spiegel, A.M., Gammon, G.D. and Aurbach, G.D. Identification and persistance of beta adrenergic receptors during maturation of the rat reticulocyte. *Mol. Pharmacol.*, **13**, 786 (1977).

Blaustein, M.P. The interrelationship between sodium and calcium fluxes across cell membranes. *Rev. Physiol. Biochem. Pharmacol.*, **70**, 33 (1974).

Blaustein, M P. and Ector, A.C. Barbiturate inhibition of calcium uptake in depolarized nerve terminals in vitro. *Mol. Pharmacol.*, **22**, 369 (1975).

Blaustein, M.P., Johnson, E.M. and Needleman, P. Calcium dependent norepinephrine released from synaptic terminals. *Proc. Nat. Acad. Sci.*, **69**, 2237 (1972).

Blaustein, M.P. and Weismann, W.P. Effect of sodium ions on calcium movements in isolated synaptic terminals. *Proc. Nat. Acad. Sci.*, **66**, 664 (1970).

Borle, A. Control, modulation and regulation of cell calcium. *Rev. Physiol. Biochem. Pharmacol.*, **90**, 14 (1981).

Brawn, K. and Friedovich, I. Superoxide radical and superoxide dismutases: threat and defense. *Acta Physiol. Scand.*, **Suppl. 492**, 9 (1980).

Carafoli, E. and Crompton, M. The regulation of intracellular Ca^{2+}. *Current topics in membrane transport*, **10**, 151 (1978).

Caroni, P. and Carafoli, E. An ATP dependent Ca^{2+} pumping system in dog heart sarcolemma. *Nature*, **283**, 765 (1980)

Chan, P.H. and Fishman, R.A. Transient formation of superoxide radicals in polyunsaturated fatty acid induced brain swelling. *J. Med.*, **298**, 659 (1978).

Chiang, J., Kowada, M., Ames, A., Wright, R.L. and Najno, G. Cerebral ischemia III: vascular changes, *Am. J. Pathol*, **52**, 455 (1968).

Clark, A F. and Roman, I.J Mg^{2+} inhibition of Na^+ stimulated Ca^{2+} release from brain mitochondria. *J. Biol. Chem.*, **255**, 6556 (1980)

Cooper, A.J., Pulsineli, W.A. and Duffy, T.F. Glutathione and ascorbate during ischemia and postischemic reperfusion in the rat brain. *J. Neurochem.*, **35**, 1242 (1980).

Crompton, M., Moser, R., Ludi, H. and Carafoli, E. The interrelation between the transport of Na^+ and Ca^{2+} in mitochondria of various mammalian tissues. *Eur. J. Biochem.*, **82**, 25 (1978).

Daenen, W. and Flameng, W. Myocardial protection by lidoflazine during one-hour normothermic global ischemia. *Angiology*, **32**, 543 (1981).

Del Maestro, R.F , Thaw, H.H., Bjork, J. et al. Free radicals as mediators of tissue injury. *Acta Physiol. Scand.*, **Suppl. 492**, 43 (1980).

Demopoulos, H.B., Flamm, E.S., Pictronigro, D.D. and Seligman, M.D. The free radical pathology and the microcirculation in the major CNS disorder. *Acta Physiol. Scand.*, **Suppl. 492**, 91 (1980)

Dipolo, R. Ca^{2+} pump driven by ATP in squid axons *Nature*, **274**, 390 (1978).

Dipolo, R. Calcium influx in internally dialyzed giant squid axons. *J. Gen. Physiol.*, **73**, 91 (1979).

Drewes, L R., Golboe, D.D. and Betz, A.L. Metabolic alterations in brain during anoxic-anoxia and subsequent recovery. *Arch. Neurol.*, **29**, 385 (1973).

Edvinson, L., Brandt, L., Anderson, K.E. and Bengtsson, B. Effects of Ca^{2+} antagonist on experimental constriction of human brain vessels. *Surgical Neurol.*, **11**, 327 (1970).

Elrod, S.V. and Leslie, S.W. Acute and chronic effects of barbiturates on depolarization-induced calcium influx into synaptosomes from rat brain regions. *J. Pharmacol. exp. Therap.*, **212**, 313 (1980).

Fischer, E.G. and Ames, A. Studies on mechanisms of impairment of cerebral circulation following cerebral ischemia: effect of hemodilution and perfusion pressure. *Stroke*, **3**, 538 (1972).

Fiskum, G. and Lehninger, A.L. Regulated release of Ca^{2+} from mitochondria by $Ca^{2+}/2H^+$ antiport. *J. Biol. Chem.*, **254**, 6236 (1979).

Flower, R.J. Drugs which inhibit prostaglandin biosynthesis. *Pharmacol. Rev.*, **26**, 33 (1974).

Gadzinski, D.S., White, B.C., Hoehner, P.J., Hoehner, T., Krome, C., White, J.D. Alterations in canine cerebral cortical blood flow and vascular resistance post cardiac arrest. *Ann. Emerg. Med.*, **99**, 58 (1982).

Gaudet, R.J. and Leving, L. Transient cerebral ischemia and brain prostaglandins. *Biochem. Biophysic. Res. Comm.*, **6**, 893 (1979).

Ginsberg, M.D., Reivich, M. and Frank, S. Pyridine nucleotide redox state and blood flow in the cerebral cortex following middle cerebral artery occlusion in the cat. *Stroke*, **7**, 125 (1976).

Ginsberg, M.D., Welsh, F.A. and Budd, W.W. Abnormalities of brain blood flow and metabolism during recovery from diffuse cerebral ischemia: dependence upon duration of ischemia. *Acta Neurol. Scand.*, **56** (Suppl. 64), 210 (1977).

Ginsberg, M.D. and Meyers, R.E. The topography of impaired microvascular perfusion in the primate brain following total circulatory arrest. *Neurol.*, **22**, 998 (1972).

Goldberg, B. and Stern, A. The role of the superoxide anion as a toxic species in the erythrocyte. *Arch. Biochem. Biophys.*, **178**, 218 (1977).

Goldstein, A., Wells, B.A. and Keats, A.S. Increased tolerance to cerebral anoxia by pentobarbital. *Arch. Int. Pharmacodyn. Ther.*, **161**, 138 (1966).

Greenwald, R.A. and Moy, W.W. Inhibition of collagen gellation by action of the superoxide radical. *Arthritis and rheumatism*, **22**, 251 (1979).

Gutteridge, J.M. The protective action of superoxide dismutase on metal ion catalysed peroxidation of phospholipids. *Biochem. Biophys. Res. Comm.*, **77**, 379 (1977).

Hallenbeck, J.M. and Furlow, T.W. Prostaglandin I_2 and Indomethacin prevent impairment of post-ischemic brain reperfusion in the dog. *Stroke*, **10**, 629 (1979).

Happel, R.D., Smith, K.P., Banik, N.L. et al. Ca^{2+} accumulation in experimental spinal cord trauma. *Brain Res.*, **211**, 476 (1981).

Harris, E.J. The uptake and release of Ca^{2+} by heart mitochondria. *Biochem. J.*, **168**, 447 (1977).

Hass, W.K. Beyond cerebral blood flow, metabolism, and ischemic thresholds: an examination of the role of Ca^{2+} in the initiation of cerebral infarction. In: Cerebral vascular disease, Vol. 3, Proceedings of the Salzburg conference on cerebral vascular disease (Amsterdam), *Excerpta Medica*, pp. 3-17 (1981).

Hasselbach, W. The reversibility of the sarcoplasmic calcium pump. *Biochem. Biophys. Acta*, **515**, 23 (1978).

Haugard, N., Haugaard, E., Lee, N. et al. Possible role of mitochondrial Ca^{2+} transport in cardiac contractility. *Fed. Proc.*, **28**, 1657 (1964).

Henry, P.D., Shuchleid, R., Davis, J. et al. Myocardial contracture and accumulation of mitochondrial calcium in ischemic rabbit heart. *Am. J. Physiol.*, **233**, H677 (1977).

Hesse, B., Jensen, G., Sigurg, B. Emergency room patients with cardiac arrest, a prognostic-prospective study. *Danish Med. Bull.*, **20**, 23 (1973).

Heymans, C. Survival and revival of nervous tissue after arrest of circulation. *Physiol. Rev.*, **30**, 375 (1950).

Hirata, F. and Axelrod, J. Enzymatic methylation of phosphatidylethanolamine increases erythrocyte membrane fluidity. *Nature*, **275**, 219 (1978).

Hirata, F and Axelrod, J. Phospholipid methylation and biological signal transmission. *Science*, **209**, 1082 (1980).

Hirata, F., Strittmatter, W.J. and Axelrod, J. Beta adrenergic receptor increases phospholipid methylation, membrane fluidity, and beta adrenergic receptor-adenylate cyclase coupling. *Proc. Nat. Acad. Sci.*,**76**, 368 (1979).

Hirata, F.V., Viveros, O H., Doliberto, E.J. and Axelrod, J. Identification and properties of two methyltransferases in conversion of phosphatidylethanolamine to phosphatidyl choline. *Proc. Nat. Acad. Sci.* **75**, 1718 (1978).

Hofer, M. and Kleinzeller, A. Calcium transport in slices of rabbit kidney cortex: the uptake and distribution of calcium. *Physiol. Bohemoslov.*, **12**, 405 (1963).

Hoffmeister, F., Kazda, S. and Krause, H.P. Influence of nimodipine on the postischemic changes of brain function. *Acta Neur. Scand.*, **60** (Suppl. 72), 358 (1979).

Holder, D., Sniderman, A. and Fraser, G. Experience with Bretylium tosylate by a hospital cardiac arrest team. *Circulation*, **5**, 541 (1977).

Hossman, V., Hossman, K.A. and Takagi, N. Effect of intravascular platelet aggregation on blood recirculation following prolonged ischemia of the cat brain. *J. Neurol.*, **222**, 159 (1980).

Hossmann, K.A. and Kleihues, P. Reversibility of ischemic brain damage. *Arch. Neurol.*, **29**, 375 (1973).

Janda, S. Mechanism of calcium transport in kidney cortex slices. *Physiol. Bohemoslov*, **18**, 413 (1969).

Katz, A.M. and Reuter, H. Cellular calcium and cardiac cell death. *Am. J. Cardiol.*, **44**, 188 (1979).

Kofke, W.A., Nemoto, E.M., Hossman, K.A. et al. Brain blood flow and metabolism after global ischemia and post-insult thiopental therapy in monkeys. *Stroke*, **10**, 554 (1979).

Kowada, M., Ames, A., and Majno, G. Cerebral ischemia I: An improved experimental method for study: cardiovascular effects and demonstration of an early vascular lesion in the rabbit. *J. Neurosurgery*, **28**, 150 (1968).

Kubler, W. and Katz, A.M. Mechanism of early pump failure of the ischemic heart: possible role of ATP depletion and inorganic HPO_4^{2-} accumulation. *Am. J. Cardiol.*, **40**, 467 (1977).

Lehninger, A.L. Role of phosphate and other proton donating cations in respiration-coupled transport of Ca^{2+} by mitochondria. *Proc. Nat. Acad. Sci.*, **71**, 1520 (1974).

Ljunggren, B., Schutz, H. and Siesjo, D.K. Changes in energy state and acid-base parameters of the rat brain during complete compression ischemia. *Brain Res.*, **73**, 277 (1974)

Loschen, G., Azzi, A., Richler, C. and Flohe, L. Superoxide radical as precursor of mitochondrial hydrogen peroxide. *FEBS Letters*, **42**, 68 (1974).

Madeira, V.M.C. Proton movements across the membranes of sarcoplasmic reticulum during the uptake of Ca^{2+}. *Arch. Biochem. Biophys.*, **200**, 319 (1980).

McCord, J.M. and Fridovich, I. The reduction of cytochrome C by xanthine oxidase. *J. Biol. Chem.*, **243**, 5753 (1968).

Mitchell, P. and Moyle, J. Chemiosmotic hypothesis of oxidative phosphorylation. *Nature*, **213**, 137 (1967).

Myerburg, R.J., Conde, C.A , Sung, R.J., Mayorga-Cortez, A., Mallon, S.M., Sheps, D.S., Appel, R.A. and Castellanos, A. Clinical, electrophysiologic and hemodynamic profiles of patients resuscitated from prehospital cardiac arrest. *Am. J. Med.*, **68**, 568 (1980).

Nayler, W.G., Mas-Oliva, J. and Williams, A.J. Cardiovascular receptors and calcium. *Circulat. Res.*, **46** (Suppl. I), I-161 (1980).

Nayler, W.G., Poole-Wilson, P.A. and Williams, A. Hypoxia and calcium. *J. Mol. Cell. Cardiol.*, **11**, 683 (1979).

Nemoto, E.M., Bleyaert, A.L. and Stezoski, S.W. Global brain ischemia: a reproducible monkey model. *Stroke*, **8**, 558 (1977).

Nemoto, E.M., Shiu, G.K., and Bleyaert, A.L. Efficacy of therapies and attention of brain free fatty acid liberation during global ischemia. *Critical Care Med.*, **9**, 397 (1981).

Nicholson, C. Measurement of extracellular ions in the brain. *Trends in neurosciences*, **3**, 216 (1980).

Nicholson, C., Ten Bruggencate, G., Steinberg, R. et al. Calcium modullation in brain extracellular microenvironment demonstrated with ion-selective micropipette. *Proc. Nat. Acad. Sci.*, **74**, 1287 (1977).

Nordstrom, C.H., Rehncrona, S. and Siesjo, B.K. Restitution of cerebral energy state after complete incomplete ischemia of 30 minutes duration. *Acta Physiol. Scand.*, **97**, 270 (1976).

Peng, C.F., Straub, K.D., Kane, J.J. et al. Effects of adenine translocase inhibitors on dinitrophenol induced Ca^{2+} efflux from pig heart mitochondria. *Biochem. Biophys. Acta*, **462**, 403 (1977).

Penniston, J.T., Graf, E. and Itano, T. Calmodulin regulation of the Ca^{2+} pump of erythrocyte membranes. *Ann. N.Y. Acad. Sci.*, **356**, 245 (1980).

Poole-Wilson, P.A. Continuous measurement of $^{47}Ca^{2+}$ uptake during and after hypoxia in rabbit myocardium. *Adv. Myocardiol.*, **2**, 285 (1980).

Rehncrona, S., Abdul-Rahman, A. and Siesjo, B.K. Local cerebral blood flow in the post ischemic period. *Acta Neurol. Scand.*, **60** (Suppl. 72), 294 (1979)

Rehncrona, S., Siesjo, B.K. and Smith, D.S. Barbiturates as protective agents in brain ischemia and as free radical scavengers in vitro. *Acta Physiol. Scand.* **Suppl. 492**, 129 (1980).

Rehncrona, S., Smith, O.S., Akesson, B. et al. Peroxidative changes in brain cortical fatty acids phospholipids, as characterized during Fe^{2+} and ascorbic acid-stimulated lipid peroxidation in vitro. *J. Neurochem.*, **24**, 1630 (1980).

Rogers, M.C., Weisfeldt, M.L. and Traystan, R.J. Cerebral blood flow during CPR. *Anesth. Analg.*, **60**, 73 (1981).

Safar, P., Stezoski, W. and Nemoto, E.M. Amelioration of brain damage after 12 minutes cardiac arrest in dogs. *Arch. Neurol.*, **33**, 91 (1976).

Safar, P. Cerebral resuscitation: current state of the art. *Ann. Emerg. Med.*, **11** (162) (1982).

Schanne, F.A., Kane, A.B. and Young, E.E. Calcium dependence of toxic cell death: a common pathway. *Science*, **206**, 700 (1979).

Schneider, C., Mottola, C. and Romeo, D. Ca^{2+} dependent ATPase activity and plasma membrane phosphorylation in the human neutrophil. *Biochem. J.*, **182**, 655 (1974).

Siemkowicz, E., and Hansen, A.J. Brain extracellular ion composition and EEG activity following 10 minutes ischemia in normo- and hyperglycemic rats. *Stroke*, **12**, 236 (1981).

Siesjo, B.K. Cell damage in the brain: a speculative synthesis. *J. Cer. Blood Flow and Metabol.*, **1**, 155 (1981).

Siesjo, B.K., Rehncrona, S. and Smith, D.S. Neuronal cell damage in the brain: possible involvement of oxidative mechanisms. *Acta Physiol. Scand.* **Suppl. 492**, 121 (1980).

Snyder, J.V., Nemoto, E.M, Carrol, R.G. and Safar, P. Global ischemia in dogs: intracranial pressure, brain blood flow and metabolism. *Stroke*, **6**, 21 (1975)

Sobue, K., Ichida, S., Yoshida, H. et al. Occurrence of a Ca^{2+} and activator protein-activatable ATPase in the synaptic plasma membrane. *FEBS Letters*, **99**, 199 (1979).

Strosnajder, J. Role of phospholipids in calcium accumulation in brain mitochondria from adult rat after ischemia-anoxia and hypoxic-hypoxia. *Bull. Acad. Pol. Sci. Biol.*, **27**, 683 (1980).

Suda, J. and Aoki, N. Inhibition of platelet function by a calmodulin interacting agent, W-7 *Thrombosis Res.*, **21**, 447 (1981).

Thomas, M.J., Mehl, K.S. and Pryor, W.A. The role of the superoxide anion in the xanthine oxidase induced autoxidation of linoleic acid. *Bioch. Biophys. Res. Comm.*, **83**, 927 (1978).

Toyoshma, S. and Osawa, T Lectins from *Wisteria floribunda* seeds and their effect on membrane fluidity of human peripheral lymphocytes. *J. Biol. Chem.*, **250**, 1655 (1975).

Trunkey, D.D., Holcroft, J. and Carpenter, M.A. Calcium flux during hemorrhagic shock in baboons. *J. Trauma*, **16**, 633 (1976).

Trunkey, D., Holcroft, J. and Carpenter, M.A. Ionized calcium and magnesium : the effect of septic shock in baboons. *J. Trauma*, **18**, 166 (1978).

Turlapaty, P.D. and Altura, B.M. Extracellular magnesium ions control calcium exchange and content of vascular smooth muscle. *Eur. J. Pharmacol.*, **52**, 421 (1978).

Van Breemen, C., Forinas, B.R , Casteels, R. et al. Factors controlling cytoplasmic Ca^{2+} concentration. *Phil. Trans. Res. Soc. London*, **265**, 57 (1973).

Van Nueten, J.M. and Vanhoutte, P.M Improvement of tissue perfusion with inhibitors of calcium ion influx. *Biochem. Pharmacol.*, **29**, 479 (1980).

Vyskocil, F., Kritz, N. and Bures, J. Potassium selective microelectrodes used for measuring the extracellular brain potassium during spreading depression and anoxic depolarization in rats. *Brain Res.*, **39**, 255 (1972).

Weinberger, L.M., Gibbon, M.H. and Gibbon, J.H. Temporary arrest of the circulation to the central nervous system · I. Physiologic effects. *Arch. Neurol. Psychiatry*, **43**, 615 (1940).

White, B.C., Gadzinski, D.S., Hoehner, P.N. et al. Correction of canine cerebral cortical blood flow and vascular resistance after cardiac arrest using flunarizine, a calcium antagonist. *Ann. Emerg. Med.*, **11**, 118 (1982).

White, B.C., Hoehner, P.J. and Wilson, R.F. Mitochondrial O_2 use and ATP synthesis : kinetic effects of Ca^{2+} and HPO_4^2 modulated by glucocorticoids. *Ann. Emerg. Med.*, **9**, 396 (1980).

Effect of calcium entry blockers in models of brain hypoxia

A. Wauquier

Summary

The present paper summarizes experimental evidence on the protection against brain hypoxia using calcium entry blockers in a variety of animal models. It appears that they are not a homogeneous class of pharmacological substances. This is partly due to the fact that the models used do not measure one particular causal factor related to hypoxia. The reasons for the final brain hypoxia are often multiple, originating from ischaemia (cardiovascular effects), respiratory problems, hypothermia, etc. However, the final outcome, independent of the original causes might be cellular toxicity by transmembrane calcium influx beyond physiological limits. Further studies are required to determine whether the protective action of calcium entry blockers resides primarily in their action on cerebral vessels and/or neurons. In view of the postulated role for calcium entry as the trigger of the events leading to cellular toxicity, it might be that calcium entry blockers will become important tools in preventing neuronal damage. Further emphasis will have to be given to physiologically controlled models of hypoxia and studies combining various techniques, including direct measures of ion fluxes through the membrane in order to achieve the final goal: brain protection.

Résumé

Le présent dossier résume les preuves expérimentales sur la protection contre l'hypoxie cérébrale, basée sur l'utilisation de bloqueurs de l'entrée de calcium chez une série d'animaux-modèles. Il en ressort que ceux-ci ne constituent pas une classe homogène de substances pharmacologiques. Ceci est dû en partie au fait que les modèles utilisés ne mesurent pas un facteur causal particulier lié à l'hypoxie. Les causes de l'hypoxie cérébrale engendrée sont souvent multiples, trouvant leur source dans l'ischémie (effets cardio-vasculaires), les problèmes respiratoires, l'hypothermie, etc. Cependant, le résultat final, indépendamment des causes initiales, peut être une toxicité cellulaire due à un influx de calcium transmembraneux passant outre les limites physiologiques. De nouvelles études sont nécessaires afin de préciser si l'action protectrice des bloqueurs d'entrée de calcium réside principalement dans leur action sur les vaisseaux cérébraux et/ou au niveau neuronal. Compte tenu que le rôle admis de l'entrée de calcium consiste à déclencher les circonstances conduisant à une toxicité cellulaire, il se pourrait que les bloqueurs de l'entrée de calcium deviennent d'importants instruments dans la prévention de la détérioration neuronale. Il faudra mettre l'accent sur les modèles d'hypoxie contrôlés physiologiquement et sur des études combinant diverses techniques englobant des mesures directes des flux d'ions au niveau de la membrane afin d'atteindre le but final, à savoir une protection cérébrale.

Resumen

Se resume la evidencia experimental, en cuanto a la protección contra hipoxia del cerebro, usando inhibidores de la penetración intracelular de Ca^{2+}, en una variedad de modelos animales. Estas substancias farmacológicas no parecen ser una clase homogénea. Esto es parcialmente debido al hecho de que los modelos empleados no dependen de un solo y específico factor causante de hipoxia. Las razones de la hipoxia cerebral final son a menudo múltiples, teniendo su origen en isquemia (efectos cardiovasculares) problemas respiratorios, hipotermia etc. Sin embargo, el resultado final, independiente de las causas originales, puede ser toxicidad celular por entrada transmembranosa de calcio más allá de los límites fisiológicos. Se requieren más estudios para saber si la acción protectora de los inhibidores de la penetración intracelular de Ca^{2+} reside esencialmente en su acción en vasos cerebrales y/o al nivel de las neuronas. Dado el papel supuesto que juega el acceso de calcio como provocador de los acontecimientos que conducen a la toxicidad celular, podría ser que los inhibidores de la penetración intracelular del calcio se hicieran importantes instrumentos que impiden la lesión neurónica. Se necesitará más insistencia en modelos de hipoxia controlados fisiológicamente y estudios que combinan técnicas distintas, incluyendo directas medidas de flujos de iones a nivel de la membrana para poder alcanzar el objetivo final: la protección del cerebro.

Zusammenfassung

Die Studie faßt das experimentelle Beweismaterial über den Schutz vor Gehirnhypoxie, das nach Gabe von Kalziumeinstromhemmern in verschiedenen Tiermodellen gesammelt wurde, zusammen. Die Arzneimittelgruppe ist in dieser Hinsicht nicht homogen. Dies ist teilweise darauf zurückzuführen, daß die verwendeten Modelle sich nicht auf die Messung des gleichen hypoxieauslösenden Faktors beziehen. Die Gründe für die resultierende Hirnhypoxie sind öfters vielfach: Ischämie (kardiovaskuläre Wirkungen), Atemschwierigkeiten, Hypothermie usw. Unabhängig von den auslösenden Ursachen kann jedoch das Endergebnis in einer durch Kalziumeinstrom hervorgerufenen Zelltoxizität bestehen, die eine umfassendere als nur physiologische Auswirkung hat. Weitere Untersuchungen müssen zeigen, ob die Schutzwirkung von Kalziumeinstromhemmern hauptsächlich auf die Beeinflussung der Hirngefäße und/oder des Neuronalbereichs zurückzuführen ist. Im Hinblick auf die für Kalzium postulierte Rolle als Auslöser von Ereignissen, die zu Zelltoxizität führen, ist anzunehmen, daß Kalziumeinstromhemmer bei der Vorbeugung von Neuronalschäden in Zukunft eine wichtige Schutzrolle spielen werden. Um das Endziel, d.h. den Hirnschutz zu erreichen, sind weitere, physiologisch kontrollierte Hypoxiemodelle ebenso wie Versuche, in denen verschiedene Techniken, u.a. solche, welche die Ionenströme auf Membranebene direkt beeinflussen, kombiniert erforderlich.

Introduction

The aim of this paper is to review in a summarized form the presently available data on the efficacy of calcium entry blockers in various models of brain hypoxia. The drugs used are (in alphabetical order): cinnarizine, D-600, flunarizine, lidoflazine, nifedipine, nimodipine and verapamil. The models used range from simple basic tests to complicated physiologically controlled experimental situations. Finally, a description of protection against calcium overload in the cell is given.

1. Calcium in the brain

When applied extracellularly to neurons of cortex or other brain structures, Ca^{2+} has an important inhibitory effect on neuronal firing, without changing membrane potential or resistance. Intracellularly applied, calcium reduced cellular excitability in association with a decreased membrane resistance (Phillis, 1974). The effects of extracellularly and intracellularly applied calcium are respectively linked to an increased sodium and potassium permeability. These experiments illustrate the relationship between the relative concentrations of Ca^{2+} on both sides of cellular membranes and neuronal activity.

The extracellular milieu is much richer in Ca^{2+}-ions than the intracellular milieu. There is a concentration gradient of about 10^4 across the cell membrane and an electrochemical gradient tending to move Ca^{2+} within the cell. Various organelles within the cell are able to load and unload calcium (Henkart, 1980) in order to bring about calcium homeostasis in the cytoplasm.

According to Joó et al. (1980) mitochondria have a large capacity, but low affinity for Ca^{2+}, whereas non-mitochondrial ATP-dependent systems have a smaller capacity but high affinity for Ca^{2+}. An important ATP-dependent system involved in the sequestration of Ca^{2+} is the endoplasmatic reticulum, as has been shown in presynaptic terminals by Blaustein et al. (1978) for instance.

Calcium influx is an essential part of neurotransmission. It enters nerve cell bodies, axons, presynaptic terminals and dendrites during stimulation or depolarization (Joc et al., 1980). At the presynaptic endings Ca^{2+}-entry is a prerequisite for quantal transmitter release (Katz, 1964; Katz and Miledi, 1975. Miledi, 1973). Following influx there are two mechanisms involved in restoring the Ca^{2+}-gradients. One is the already mentioned sequestration by mitochondria and endoplasmatic reticulum, and one is ion-exchange. Though obviously important during neuronal activity and in pathological conditions, the relationships between the ion fluxes will not be further dealt with herein.
At the level of the postsynaptic membrane, a slow transition from Ca^{2+}-dependent electrogenesis develops to spike generation. Dendritic spikes are present in the cerebellum (Llinàs and Hess, 1978), hippocampus (Schwartzkroin and Slawsky, 1977) and possibly also in the cortex (Traub, 1979). These spikes are Ca^{2+}-dependent since they are resistant to tetrodoxin application. In hippocampal neurons (Wong et al., 1979), two kinds of spikes were recorded from dendrites: small short-lasting spikes, probably mediated by Na^+ and tetrodoxin-resistant spikes, which were of a larger amplitude in dendrites than in cell bodies.

There is thus an active spike generation originating largely in dendrites, and it has been suggested that these may be of importance in dendro-dendritic interaction (Llinàs and Hess, 1978).

Thus, two important features of the role of calcium in brain are apparent: brain functioning through neuronal transmission for which Ca^{2+}-entrance at presynaptic terminals is essential and the occurrence of dendritic Ca^{2+}-mediated spikes in particular brain regions. In pathological conditions, such as hypoxia, Ca^{2+}-influx exceeding the sequestration capacity appears to be toxic to the cell. This has been firmly established for liver cells (Schanne et al., 1979), for the heart (e.g. Flameng et al., 1980) and is postulated for brain cells as well (Siesjö, 1981; Wauquier et al., 1981). Further, it appears that brain regions in which Ca^{2+}-dendritic spikes occur are those which show a selective vulnerability to hypoxia-induced cellular damage (Meldrum, 1981).

Taking the above into account it appears logical to assume that inhibitors of calcium influx might be important tools to prevent the cellular alterations leading to a destruction of cellular integrity for which calcium appears to be the trigger. Many drugs appear to have some calcium antagonistic properties (Rhawan et al., 1979). Since Ca^{2+} is present extra- and intracellularly and drugs may either preferentially act at one of these levels, they can be classified according their site of action. To those interfering with intracellular calcium belong magnesium and sodium nitroprusside; to those acting on extracellular shifts belong those which have effects on both sodium and calcium (i.e. local anaesthetics, hypnotics) and those which have a specific effect on Ca^{2+}-transmembrane influx. Specifically the latter compounds, to which belong flunarizine, cinnarizine and nifedipine for instance, appear of interest in studying brain protection.

2. Calcium entry blockers in models of brain hypoxia

2.1. Survival models

For comparative pharmacological research various models exist in which small animals such as mice or rats are used and in which the criteria for protection are either prolongation of survival or prevention of lethality. These models do not aim to mimic a clinical situation, but the models are quite selective in finding chemical substances which do have antihypoxic properties. For instance, we studied the hypnotic etomidate as compared with barbiturates (Wauquier et al., 1980 a, b) and Nugent et al. (1982) studied some benzodiazepines in such simple models, demonstrating that a number of these compounds might be useful for cerebral protection. Obviously, supplementary studies aiming at proving protection of the cell by using histological techniques (Ashton et al., 1982, 1983; Van Reempts et al., 1982, 1983; Wauquier et al., 1982) or by clinically oriented experiments (Mullie et al., 1981; Nugent et al., 1982) are required. Hereafter, some of these basic tests are described and the activity of a number of calcium entry blockers in these tests. The tests used were: hypobaric hypoxia in mice, hypoxic hypoxia in rats by exposure to 100% nitrogen and histotoxic hypoxia by injecting potassium cyanide (KCN) in rats. Table 1 shows the effects of the compounds tested in these situations: verapamil, D-600, flunarizine, cinnarizine, nifedipine, nimodipine and lidoflazine.

Table 1: ED_{50}-values (mg/kg) and limits of the activity of calcium entry blockers in three different models of hypoxia. For details see text.

Test	Hypobaric hypoxia (mice)			Nitrogen hypoxia (rats)			Histotoxic hypoxia (rats)		
Compound	Rte	Time (min)	ED_{50} (limits)	Rte	Time (min)	ED_{50} (limits)	Rte	Time (min)	ED_{50} (limits)
Verapamil	i.p.	- 30	> 160	i.p.	- 60	84.2 (48.8 - 145)	s.c.	- 60	> 40
D-600	i.p.	- 30	2.33* (1.55 - 4.01)	i.p.	- 60	9.31* (5.39 - 16.1)	s.c.	- 60	> 40
Flunarizine	or.	-240	> 80	or.	-240	14.0 (8.83 - 22.3)	or.	- 60	23.6 (7.34 - 75.9)
								-120	16.8 (3.20 - 88.2)
								-240	12.4 (3.28 - 47.1)
Cinnarizine	i.p.	- 30	80.8 (46.8 - 199)	or.	- 60	25.0 (14.5 - 43.2)	or.	- 60	34.3 (14.2 - 82.9)
Nifedipine	i.p.	- 30	71.7 (54.9 - 93.7)	i.p.	- 60	41.7 (31.7 - 54.1)	or.	- 60	> 40
Nimodipine	i.p.	- 30	> 80	i.p.	- 60	10.8 (6.27 - 18.7)			
Lidoflazine	i.p.	- 30	2.39 (1.39 - 4.13)	i.p.	- 60	> 80	s.c.	- 60	> 40
							i.v.	- 30	3.22 (1.77 - 5.87)

* Inverted U-shape dose response curve: doses $\geq$ 40 mg/kg are less active than 10 mg/kg or lethal.

In the hypobaric hypoxia test, mice are enclosed in a container and brought to a simulated height of 35,000 ft. (barometric pressure < 200 mm Hg, O_2-concentration 2 - 3%). Saline-treated mice do not survive longer than 4 min in this condition. Mice pretreated with hypnotics do survive longer in this condition (Wauquier et al., 1981 a, b). A similar effect (Table 1) is obtained with (in order of decreasing potency) D-600, lidoflazine, nifedipine and cinnarizine; flunarizine, nimodipine and verapamil were inactive (doses > 2.5 and < 160 mg/kg).

In the nitrogen hypoxia test, rats are exposed to 100% nitrogen in a closed chamber for 1 min, then they are rapidly removed, placed in an observation cage and scored for survival 1 h after exposure (Wauquier et al., 1980 a, 1981 a). None of the control rats survive this condition, unless they are ventilated following exposure (Van Reempts et al., 1982). The following compounds (in decreasing order of potency) were active (Table 1): D-600, nimodipine, cinnarizine, nifedipine, verapamil. Lidoflazine was inactive in this test (dose > 80 mg/kg).

In the histotoxic hypoxia test (Ashton et al., 1981; Wauquier et al., 1980 a, 1981 a, b) rats are given a rapid intravenous injection of 5 mg/kg of potassium cyanide. In saline-treated rats this dose is lethal in 94% of the animals. The following compounds (in decreasing order of potency) were active (Table 1): lidoflazine (i.v.), flunarizine, cinnarizine. Following compounds were inactive (doses > 40 mg/kg): verapamil, D-600, nifedipine.

Inspite of the common denominator 'calcium entry blocker', the presently tested drugs behave differently in these tests. Unless the differences can be explained simply on the basis of the administration route used, or on the basis of pharmacokinetics for instance, there appear to be substantial differences between the compounds in the same test and between the compounds in different tests. It has to be realized, however, that in these models various factors occur in association with or as a consequence of hypoxia: seizure activity, cardiovascular complications (ischaemia), respiratory depression, etc. Thus the antihypoxic properties demonstrated may not be interpreted solely in terms of neuronal membrane stabilization for calcium. It is also clear, however, that the group as a whole shows potential antihypoxic activities, which was further investigated in a number of other models.

2.2. Functional models

Obviously in previous experiments, a functional evaluation of the outcome of brain hypoxia is limited since in all models the insults resulted in death. A first approach in assessing brain functioning consists in studying the electroencephalographic activity in animals submitted to hypoxic conditions. A second approach consists in studying the effects of hypoxia on learning tasks or on memory tests. An example of the first approach is an experiment on the effects of flunarizine on hypercapnic hypoxia (Wauquier et al., 1980 a, 1982). An example of the second approach is an experiment in which the effect of hypoxia induced after learning on a subsequent retention measure was studied (Wauquier et al., 1980, 1982).

2.2.1. Hypercapnic hypoxia
The electroencephalographic (EEG) activity from the sensorimotor area of the cortex was recorded in rats, curarized with succinylcholine and artificially ventilated. After stabilization of the EEG, the artificial air supply was cut-off for 2 min and again for 3 min, 10 min later.

Rats were pretreated orally about 3 h before the first hypercapnic period with solvent or flunarizine at a dose of 0.16, 0.63, 2.5 or 10 mg/kg. The following parameters were recorded: the time from cutting-off the air supply to the occurrence of EEG silence, the time from switching on the ventilation to the return of the EEG activity and the time between electrical silence and recovery.

In flunarizine-treated rats there was a higher resistance to hypoxia, since the time from switch-off to electrical silence was significantly longer than in control rats. The EEG activity also returned faster when the ventilation was switched on again after 2 min. However, there was no dose-related effect, since almost identical effects were obtained with all doses used. There was also no difference in survival rate following a 3-min ventilation stop. In an additional group of 6 rats, it was found that 5 out of 6 rats were protected against lethality, at a dose of 40 mg/kg of flunarizine. In this test, hypnotics such as etomidate are more potent drugs (Wauquier et al., 1981 a). Verapamil was found inactive (doses $\geq$ 40 mg/kg), possibly because this calcium antagonist does not easily penetrate the brain.

2.2.2. Retention deficit

Animals were trained and tested in a two-compartment box, the left compartment being a platform located 6 cm above an electrifiable grid (right compartment). During training the animals were placed in the left compartment and received an electric shock upon stepping down into the right compartment. Animals were trained in a single session to remain on the platform for 3 consecutive minutes.

Twenty-four hours after training animals were placed on the platform and retention was tested over 6 minutes with the electrifiable grid turned-off. The latency to step down was used as a measure of retention. Rats were made hypoxic by giving an i.v. injection of 30 mg/kg of metrazol immediately following the learning task. Rats (n = 10 in each group) were orally treated with solvent or flunarizine at a dose of 0.63, 2.5, 10 or 40 mg/kg 1 h before the metrazol challenge. The results are depicted in Fig. 1.

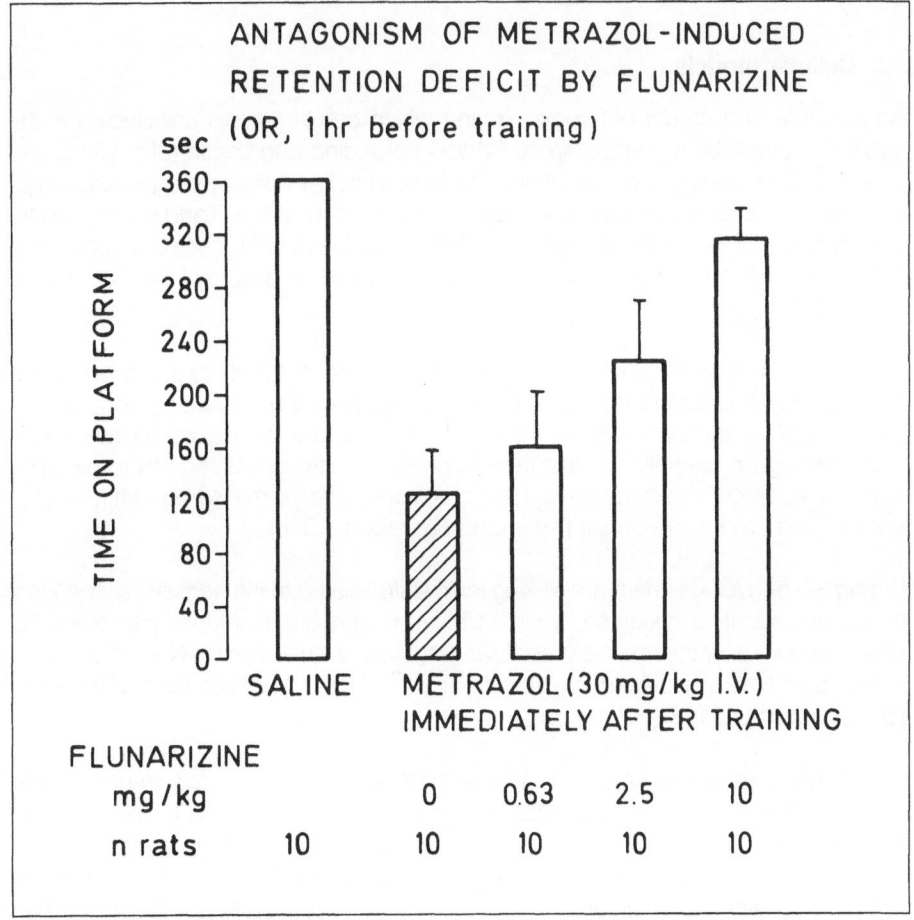

Figure 1: Passive avoidance retention test. Rats were trained to remain on a platform for 3 min in order to avoid an electrical paw shock upon stepping down on a grid. Rats given saline after training show a good retention. Rats given i.v. 30 mg/kg of metrazol after training show a retention deficit when tested 24 h later. Flunarizine given orally 1 h before training results in an antagonism of retention deficit.

As seen, in solvent-treated rats, an i.v. injection of metrazol immediately following training, caused a severe retention deficit when tested 24 h later. Flunarizine-treated rats showed a dose-related improved retention (they remain for progressively longer times on the platform). A one way analysis of variance showed a significant dose effect (df 1/3, $F = 4.83$, $p < .01$).

In the experimental set-up verapamil and papaverine were inactive (> 40 mg/kg). The possible anticonvulsant effect of flunarizine as a reason for improved retention was ruled out, because clonic seizures occurring following the s.c. metrazol injection were not prevented by flunarizine and treatment with the anticonvulsant diphenylhydantoin (> 80 mg/kg) did not prevent retention deficit. Massive energy and oxygen consumption in the brain during convulsions results in tissue hypoxia, and depletion of energy stores as reflected in a flat EEG. Flunarizine might reduce the exhaustion phase and preserve minimal cell functioning.

2.3. Cellular models

An example of a model of hypoxia during which cellular events are studied is the spreading depression phenomenon. Cortical spreading depression (SD), which can be elicited by a variety of chemical and electrical stimuli, is a slowly progressing negative wave of neuronal depolarization starting in the superficial layers and spreading into deeper layers of the cortex at a speed of 3 mm/min. During SD, there is a depression of EEG activity and a negative shift of the DC potential, a measure of the extracellular potential.

There are striking similarities between SD and the neuronal events following ischaemia (Hansen and Zeuthen, 1981): first at the start of SD there is excessive neuronal excitability possibly associated with an increase in extracellular potassium, followed by a longer-lasting inexcitability; second, there is initially an increased blood-flow followed by a decrease; thirdly, the extracellular ionic chain of events, as measured with ion-sensitive microelectrodes are similar (Kraig and Nicholson, 1978).

During SD or hypoxia, there are striking ionic shifts related to the negative shift in electrical potentials. It has been shown that Ca^{2+}-changes are an integral part of the SD phenomenon: after the rise in extracellular K^+, there is a decrease in Na^+ and Cl^- and at the same time a decrease in extracellular Ca^{2+} (Kraig and Nicholson, 1978; Hansen and Zeuthen, 1981).

The following experiment aimed to answer the question whether calcium entry blockers were able to antagonize SD, elicited by cortical application of KCl in rats. In curarized and artificially ventilated rats, the EEG was derived from 4 cortical screws; Ag-AgCl electrodes were used to measure DC-potential shifts via a differential amplifier. Successively, with an interval of at least 30 min, 1% and 2% of KCl was applied to a hole in the skull.

Figure 2 shows the effects of flunarizine (2.5, 10, 40 mg/kg), nifedipine (40 mg/kg) and verapamil (10 mg/kg). The depth of the spreading depression caused by 1% KCl or 2% KCl was only significantly reduced by the highest dose of flunarizine (40 mg/kg). The recovery time following spreading depression induced by 1% of KCl was significantly shortened by the three compounds, in order of potency: flunarizine, nifedipine, verapamil. The recovery time following spreading depression induced by 2% of KCl was only significantly shortened by flunarizine.

If calcium plays an important role in the spreading depression phenomenon, the following hypothesis might account for the effectiveness of some of the calcium entry blockers tested here. Due to the possible role of calcium-current in dendro-dendritic interaction (Llinàs and Hess, 1978), dendritic activity might be important in the spread of depolarization. The fact that the compounds tested did not prevent depolarization, but shortened the recovery time might give support to the idea that they more specifically inhibit the spread of depolarization, rather than the depolarization itself, provided that the recovery time is an index for spread. Further studies using direct measures of ion fluxes will be required to establish whether the Ca^{2+}-entry blockers used antagonize spread by preventing Ca^{2+}-influx involved in depolarization.

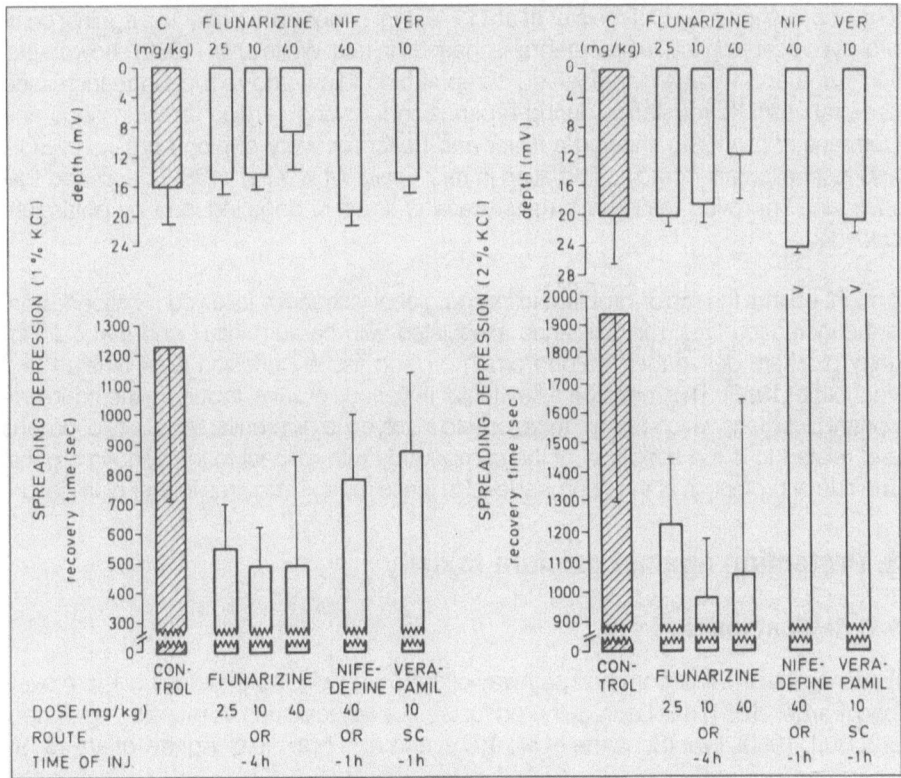

Figure 2: Spreading depression (SD) test. 1% (left) and 2% (right) KCl was applied to rat cortex inducing SD. In top: depth of SD, at the bottom: recovery time of the DC shift, in control ▨ and after flunarizine, nifedipine and verapamil, at the indicated doses, route and time of drug administration. N = 10

2.4. Resuscitation models

Using animals kept in physiologically controlled conditions, clinically oriented models aim to demonstrate the capacity of drugs to improve resuscitation by giving these drugs after the occurrence of a hypoxic insult as those found in man. Most of these models involve a complete global ischaemia or oligemia by applying a neck tourniquet preventing cerebral perfusion (e.g. Bleyaert et al., 1978), reducing arterial pressure (e.g. Hackel et al., 1979; Wauquier et al., 1980 b) or cardiac arrest (e.g. Hermans et al., 1982; Mullie et al., 1981; White et al., 1981).

Though the EEG changes found during haemorrhagic shock in dogs (for instance Wauquier et al., 1980 b) demonstrate that the brain is also involved, the beneficial effects of drugs are possibly the result of an improvement in the general circulation rather than the brain itself. It appears, nevertheless, important to find out whether calcium entry blockers are able to improve or restore cerebral hypoperfusion or improve disturbances in cerebral blood flow after reperfusion, especially in view of, at this moment rather circumstantial evidence, that cellular calcium influx might be largely responsible for disturbed cerebral perfusion (Rehncrona et al., 1979; White et al., 1982).

It has been shown by Hoffmeister et al. (1979) that nimodipine protected against cerebral hypoperfusion following cerebral ischaemia in rats; White et al. (1982) showed that flunarizine and verapamil preserved cerebral blood flow and reduced the increased cerebral vascular resistance during reperfusion following cardiac arrest in dogs and Hermans et al. (1982) showed a faster and better recovery of blood pressure, ECG and respiration after cardiac fibrillation in rats; finally White et al. (1982) described that lidoflazine improved resuscitation after cardiac arrest in dogs induced by potassium chloride.

It might be that the major problem following global ischaemia followed by reperfusion, is the increased vascular resistance associated with calcium influx and that calcium entry blockers derive their action from improving tissue perfusion (Van Nueten and Vanhoutte, 1980). This might be a key factor in various organs, including the brain. Important questions which remain to be solved involve the differential sensitivity of organs and related to it, the specificity of the compounds with respect to the various organs. The role of protection at the neuronal level in these models requires further clarification.

3. Protection against calcium toxicity

3.1. Calcium toxicity

Evidence that the final common pathway of cellular toxicity is intracellular calcium overload (Farber, 1981) has been gathered for various tissues, such as muscle (e.g. Emery and Burt, 1980), liver (Schanne et al., 1979) and also brain (e.g. Agnew et al., 1979).

A variety of experiments demonstrate that flunarizine protects against Ca^{2+}-overload in addition to the known antivasoconstrictive effects (Van Nueten, 1978; Van Nueten et al., 1978): it protects against myocardial ischaemia in dogs (Borgers, 1981); it protects against Ca^{2+}-overload in addition to the known antivasoconstrictive effects (Van Nueten, 1978; Van Nueten et al., 1978): it protects against myocardial ischemia in dogs (Borgers, 1981); it protects against endothelial cell injury in vivo (Hladovec and De Clerck, 1981); it protects against calcium-induced shape changes of erythrocytes (De Clerck et al., 1980). Furthermore, there exists histological evidence that the calcium distribution (cytochemically detected according to Borgers et al., 1977) in the brain of rats orally pretreated with 20 or 40 mg/kg of flunarizine and injected with potassium cyanide, was close to normal in contrast to the changes in untreated rats (Amery et al., 1981).

3.2. Protective effects of flunarizine

A histological study was carried out to find out whether flunarizine was able to protect against cellular damage caused by ischaemic hypoxia (Van Reempts et al., 1983). According to previous histological studies, some ischaemic neuronal cell changes have been differentiated, provided care is taken to avoid cytological artefacts (Brown, 1977): microvacuolization of neuronal cytoplasm, followed by progressive ischaemic cell changes up to irreversible cell loss. These stages can be seen both in experimental models of brain hypoxia, as well as in hypoxic brain damage in man (Graham, 1977); the exact localization, however, appears to be dependent on the kind of hypoxic insult. The hypoxic induced brain damage does not imply the presence of scattered neuronal lesions, but there exists a selective vulnerability of particular brain regions (Brierly, 1977). There are mainly the pyramidal cells of cortex, layers 3, 5 and 6, the Sommer sector and endfolium of hippocampus and Purkinje cells of cerebellum. Recent hypotheses propose that this selective vulnerability is associated with the presence of Ca^{2+}-sensitive dendritic regions (Meldrum, 1981; Siesjö, 1981).

One well studied model of ischaemic-hypoxic brain damage is the rat Levine preparation (Levine, 1960) which has only recently been introduced to study pharmacological protection (Van Reempts et al., 1982). In this model, cell ischaemic changes are produced by intermittent exposure of rats to a pure nitrogen environment for several periods of 1 min, each followed by artificial respiration; one hemisphere is made more vulnerable by a preceding unilateral carotid ligation. Twenty-four hours later, rat brains are perfused and histology carried out. This set-up was used to study whether flunarizine is capable of preventing cell ischaemic changes (Van Reempts et al., 1983; Wauquier et al., 1982). Rats were orally pretreated with 40 mg/kg, 5 h before the first nitrogen exposure. Samples from both hemispheres in control and in flunarizine-pretreated animals were taken and 2 μm sections were scored for the occurrence of microvacuolation, ischaemic cell change, severe cell change and cell loss.

In this model, cell ischaemic changes are restricted to one hemisphere and occur predominantly in cortical cells of the 3rd layer. In the control group, the 7 rats studied showed cerebral damage: microvacuolation in 4, ischaemic cell change in 7, severe cell change in 4 and cell loss in 4. In the flunarizine-treated rats only a moderate and limited ischaemic cell change was found in 4 out of 7 rats. It was thus convincingly demonstrated that flunarizine protected against neuronal cell damage and these results might support the hypothesis that this prevention is due to the Ca^{2+}-entry action.

Acknowledgement

I sincerely thank my colleagues and co-workers which made the described experiments possible: D. Ashton, G. Clincke, J. Fransen, W. Melis, C.J.E. Niemegeers, J. Van Reempts. I also thank D. Ashton for his help in the preparation of the manuscript.

References

Agnew, W.F., Yuen, T.G.H., Bullara, L.A., Jacques, D. and Punolenz, R.H. Intracellular calcium deposition in brain following electrical stimulation. *Neurol. Res.*, **1**, 187-202 (1979).

Amery, W., Wauquier, A., Van Nueten, J., De Clerck, F., Van Reempts, J. and Janssen, P.A.J. The anti-migrainous pharmacology of flunarizine (R 14 950), a calcium antagonist. *Drug Exp. Clin. Res.*, **7**, 1-10 (1981).

Ashton, D., Van Reempts, J. and Wauquier, A. Behavioural electroencephalographic and histological study of the protective effect of etomidate against histotoxic dysoxia produced by cyanide. *Arch. Int. Pharmacodyn. Ther.*, **254**, 196-213 (1981).

Blaustein, M.P., Ratzlaff, R.W. and Kendrick, N.K. The regulation of intracellular calcium in presynaptic nerve terminals. *Ann. N.Y. Acad. Sci.*, **307**, 195-211 (1978).

Bleyaert, A.L., Nemoto, E.M., Safar, P., Stezoski, W., Mickell, J.J., Moossy, J. and Rao, G.R. Thiopental amelioration of brain damage after global ischemia in monkeys. *Anesthesiology*, **49**, 390 (1978).

Borgers, M., De Brabander, M., Van Reempts, J., Awouters, F. and Jacob, W.A. Intranuclear microtubules in lung mast cells of guinea pigs in anaphylactic shock. *Lab. Invest.*, **37**, 1-8 (1977).

Borgers, M. The action of the calcium entry blockers flunarizine and cinnarizine in cells and tissues. In: Proceedings of the Hearing on Vasoactive Drugs (Ricci, G., Ed.), Raven Press, New York, (1981).

Brown, A.W. Structural abnormalities in neurones. *J. Clin. Pathol.*, **30** (Suppl. 11), 155-169 (1977).

De Clerck, F., Beerens, M., Thoné, F. and Borgers, M. The effects of flunarizine on the human RBC shape change and calcium deposition induced by ionophore A 23187. *Biorheologie*, **16**, 513 (1980).

Emery, A.E.H. and Burt, D. Intracellular calcium and pathogenesis and antenatal diagnosis of Duchenne muscular dystrophy. *Brit. Med. J.*, **280**, 355-357 (1980).

Farber, J.L. The role of calcium in cell death. *Life Sci.*, **29**, 1289-1295 (1981).

Flameng, W., Daenen, W., Xhonneux, R., Van de Water, A., Thoné, F. and Borgers, M. Lidoflazine protection in normothermic myocardial ischemia in the dog. *RCM Int. Congress and Symposium Series*, **29**, 89-95 (1980).

Graham, D.J. Pathology of hypoxic brain damage in man. *J. Clin. Pathol.*, **30** (Suppl. 11), 170-180 (1977).

Hackel, D.B., Mikat, E.M., Whalen, G., Reimer, K. and Rochlani, S.P. Treatment of hemorrhagic shock in dogs with verapamil. Effects on survival and on cardiovascular lesions. *Lab. Invest.*, **41**, 356-359 (1979).

Hansen, A.J. and Zeuthen, T. Extracellular ion concentrations during spreading depression and ischemia in the rat brain cortex. *Acta Physiol. Scand.*, **113**, 437-445 (1981).

Henkart, M. Identification and function of intracellular calcium stores in neurons. Introduction. *Fed. Proc.*, **39**, 2776-2777 (1980).

Hermans, C., De Reese, R., Van Loon, J., Loots, W. and Jageneau, A.H.M. A cardiac arrest model in rats for the evaluation of the antihypoxic action of flunarizine. *Eur. J. Pharmacol.* **81**, 137-140 (1982).

Hladovec, J. and De Clerck, F. Protection by flunarizine against endothelial cell injury *in vivo*. *Angiology*, **32**, 448-462 (1981).

Hoffmeister, F., Kazda, S. and Krause, H.P. Influence of nimodipine on the postischemic changes of brain function. *Acta Neurol. Scand.*, **60** (Suppl. 72), 358-359 (1979).

Joó, R., Ponduez, Á., Fóth, I., Kamushina, I. and Barca-Barca, M.A. Attempts at localizing calcium in relation to synaptic transmission: an X-ray microanalytical study. *J. Physiol.*, **76**, 403-411 (1980).

Katz, B. Release of neural transmitter substances. Charles C. Thomas - Springfield III (1964).

Katz, B. and Miledi, R. The effects of calcium on acetylcholine release from motor terminals. *Proc. R. Soc. B.*, **161**, 496-503 (1965).

Katz, B. and Miledi, R. Tedrodoxin-resistant electrical activity in presynaptic terminals. *J. Physiol.* (Lond.), **203**, 459-487 (1969).

Katz, B. and Miledi, R. Further study of the role of calcium in synaptic transmission. *J. Physiol.* (Lond.), **207**, 789-801 (1970).

Kraig, R.P. and Nicholson, C. Extracellular ionic variation during spreading depression. *Neuroscience*, **3**, 1045-1059 (1978).

Levine, S. Anoxic-ischemic encephalopathy in rats. *Am. J. Pathol.*, **36**, 1-17 (1960).

Llinàs, R. and Hess, R. Tetrodoxin-resistant dendritic spikes in avian Purkinje cells. *Proc. Natl. Acad. Sci.*, **73**, 2520-2523 (1976).

Meldrum, B.S. Metabolic effects of prolonged epileptic seizures and the causation of epileptic brain damage. In: Metabolic Disorders of the Nervous System (Clifford Rose, Ed.), Pitman Publ. Co., London, pp. 175-187 (1981).

Miledi, R. Transmitter release induced by injection of calcium into nerve terminals. *Proc. R. Soc. Lond. B.*, **183**, 421-425 (1973).

Mullie, A., Hermans, C., Van de Velde, K., Wauquier, A. and Jageneau, A. Resuscitability with brain protective drugs during cardiopulmonary resuscitation in dogs. *Crit. Care Med.*, **9**, 183 (1981).

Nugent, M., Artue, A.A. and Michenfelder, J.D. Cerebral metabolic vascular and protective effect of midazolam maleate. *Anaesthesiology*, **56**, 172-176 (1982).

Phillis, J.W. The role of calcium in the central effects of biogenic amines. *Life Sci.*, **14**, 1189-1201 (1974).

Rahwan, R.G., Piascik, M.F. and Witiak, D.T. The role of calcium antagonism in the therapeutic action of drugs. *Can. J. Physiol. Pharmacol.*, **57**, 443-460 (1979).

Siesjö, B.K. Cell damage in the brain: a speculative synthesis. *J. Cerebral Blood Flow and Metabolism*, **1**, 155-185 (1981).

Schanne, F.A.X., Kane, A.B., Young, E.E. and Farber, J.L. Calcium dependence of toxic cell death: a final common pathway. *Science*, **206**, 700-702 (1981).

Schwartzkroin, P.H. and Slawsky, M. Probable calcium spikes in hippocampal neurons. *Brain Res.*, **135**, 157-161 (1977).

Traub, R.D. Neocortical pyramidal cells: a model with dendritic calcium conductance reproduces repetitive firing and epileptic behavior. *Brain Res.*, **173**, 243-257 (1979).

Van Nueten, J.M. Vasodilatation or inhibition of peripheral vasoconstriction? In: Mechanisms of Vasodilatation (Vanhoutte, P., Leusen, I., Eds.), Karger, Basel, pp. 137-143 (1978).

Van Nueten, J.M. and Vanhoutte, P.M. Improvement of tissue perfusion with inhibitors of calcium ion influx. *Biochem. Pharmacol.*, **29**, 479-481 (1980).

Van Nueten, J.M., Van Beek, J. and Janssen, P.A.J. Effect of flunarizine on calcium-induced responses of peripheral vascular smooth muscle. *Arch. Int. Pharmacodyn. Ther.*, **232**, 42-52(1978).

Van Reempts, J., Borgers, M., Van Eyndhoven, J. and Hermans, C. The protective effects of etomidate in hypoxic-ischemic brain damage in the rat. Morphologic assessment. *Exp. Neurol.*, **76**, 181-195 (1982).

Van Reempts, J., Borgers, M., Van Dael, L., Van Eyndhoven, J. and de Ven, M. Protection with flunarizine against hypoxic-ischemic damage of the rat cerebral cortex. A quantitative morphologic approach. Arch. Int. Pharmacodyn. Ther., **262** 76-88 (1983)

Wauquier, A., Ashton, D., Clincke, G., Niemegeers, C.J.E. and Janssen, P.A.J. Etomidat: ein barbituratfreies Hypnotikum, antikonvulsive, antianoxische, und hirnprotektive Wirkung in Tierexperiment. In: Anaesthesia bei Zerebralen Krampfanfällen und Intensivtherapie des Status Epileptics, (Opitz, A., Degen, R., Eds.), Verlagsgesellschaft mbH, Erlangen, pp. 183-203 (1980a).

Wauquier, A., Van den Broeck, W.A.E., Hermans, C., Jageneau, A. and François, P. Electroencephalography in etomidate, thiopental and pentobarbital treated hemorrhagic dogs. 7th World Congress of Anaesthesiologists, Abstracts, p. 433 (1980b).

Wauquier, A., Ashton, D., Clincke, G. and Niemegeers, C.J.E. Anti-hypoxic effects of etomidate, thiopental and methohexital. *Arch. Int. Pharmacodyn. Ther.*, **249**, 330-334 (1981a).

Wauquier, A., Clincke, G., Ashton, D. and Van Reempts, J. Considerations on models and treatment of brain hypoxia. In: Functional Recovery from Brain Damage, (Van Hof, M., Mohn, J., Eds.), Elsevier/North-Holland Biomedical Press, Amsterdam, pp. 95-114 (1981b).

Wauquier, A., Ashton, D., Clincke, G. and Van Reempts, J. Pharmacological protection against brain hypoxia: the efficacy of flunarizine, a calcium entry blocker. In: Cerebral Hypoxia in the Pathogenesis of Migraine Attacks, (Amery, W., Clifford-Rose, Eds.), Pittman Publish. Co., 139-154 (1982).

White, B.C., Gadzinski, D.S., Hoehner, P.J., Krome, P.J., Krome, C., Hochner, T., White, J.D. and Trombley, J.H. Correction of canine cerebral cortical blood flow and vascular resistance after cardiac arrest using flunarizine, a calcium antagonist. *Ann. Emerg. Med.*, **11**, 118 (1982).

Wong, R.K.S., Prince, D.A. and Basbaun, A.I. Intradendritic recordings from hippocampal neurons. *Proc. Natl. Acad. Sci.*, **76**, 986-990 (1979).

Calcium entry blockers in the therapy of vertebrobasilar insufficiency

B.Hofferberth

Summary

Today, the so-called calcium antagonists have not found wide use yet in the treatment of vertebrobasilar insufficiency. The aim of the present study was restricted to discuss the effect of these substances on vestibular nystagmus. As to their effects on clinicial symptoms in particular, many questions are still unsolved.

Partly in acute trials and partly in studies during which they were applied during various weeks, three substances were evaluated both in animals and in man. Each of these had been shown to be a calcium entry blocker. Bencyclane produced a disinhibition of the nystagmus parameters along with rhythmicity of the curve pattern. With flunarizine and nimodipine, a disinhibition of the nystagmus frequency was obtained. The pathologically disinhibited electronystagmogram , a feature of brain flow disorders, is normalized with these substances. The correlation of subjective symptoms — dizziness and all its associated autonomic symptoms — and of the normalized nystagmus parameters should be investigated in larger studies.

Whether a vasodilatory effect can be assumed to be the working mechanism for the substances mentioned, or whether a direct effect on the vestibular system in the sense of an inhibited transmission of impulses is involved is not yet clear.

Because of the clear-cut effect on experimentally induced nystagmus, further comparative studies which also give attention to clinical symptoms seem to make sense.

Résumé

Aujourd'hui, ce qu'on appelle les antagonistes de calcium sont largement utilisés déjà dans le traitement de l'insuffisance vertébro-basilaire. L'objectif de la présente étude se limite à la discussion de l'effet de ces substances sur le nystagmus vestibulaire. De nombreuses questions demeurent encore sans réponse quant à leurs effets sur les symptômes cliniques en particulier. Trois substances ont été évaluées tant chez l'animal que chez l'homme, en partie dans des tests aigus et en partie dans des études pendant lesquelles elles étaient administrées plusieurs semaines durant. Chacune d'elles s'était avérée être un bloqueur de l'entrée de calcium. Le bencyclane produisait une désinhibition des paramètres du nystagmus tout en rendant l'allure de la courbe plus rhythmique. Avec la flunarizine et la nimodipine, une désinhibition de la fréquence du nystagmus a été obtenue. L'électronystagmogramme pathologiquement désinhibé, l'un des traits des troubles circulatoires cérébraux, est normalisé par ces substances. La corrélation des symptômes subjectifs — étourdissements et tous les symptômes autonomes y associés — et les paramètres du nystagmus normalisé devraient être explorés dans le cadre d'études plus amples. On ne peut encore préciser si un effet vasodilatateur est susceptible d'être le mécanisme d'action des substances mentionnées ou s'il y a un effet direct sur le système vestibulaire dans le sens d'une transmission inhibée d'impulsions. Compte tenu de l'effet tranché obtenu sur le nystagmus induit de façon expérimentale, des études comparatives nouvelles qui accordent également de l'importance aux symptômes cliniques semblent nécessaires et indiquées.

Resumen

Hasta hoy en día, los llamados antagonistas del calcio aún no han encontrado gran uso en el tratamiento de la insuficiencia vertebrobasilar. El objetivo de este estudio se limita a discutir el efecto de estas sustancias en el nistagma vestibular. En lo que se refiere a sus efectos en síntomas clínicos en particular, muchas preguntas quedan sin resolver.
Parcialmente en experimentos agudos, y parcialmente en estudios aplicados, durante varias semanas, se evaluaron tres sustancias, tanto en animales como en el hombre. Cada una había demostrado ser un inhibidor de la penetración intracelular del calcio. Benciclano produjo una desinhibición de los parámetros del nistagma junto con una ritmicidad de la curva. Con flunarizina y nimodipino se obtuvo una desinhibición de la frecuencia del nistagma. El electronistagmograma, desinhibido patológicamente — una característica de los trastornos del flujo cerebral — se normaliza con estas sustancias. La correlación entre la mejoría de los síntomas subjetivos — el vértigo y todos sus autonómicos síntomas asociados — y la de los parámetros del nistagma, necesitan más estudios.
Hasta ahora, no está claro si un efecto vasodilatador puede ser considerado como el mecanismo de acción de las sustancias mencionadas, o si se trata de un efecto directo en el sistema vestibular, es decir, una inhibición de la transmisión de impulsos.
A causa del importante efecto en el nistagma, provocado experimentalmente, se requieren más estudios comparativos, que también presten atención a síntomas clínicos.

Zusammenfassung

Die Anwendung der sogenannten Kalziumantagonisten in der Therapie der vertebrobasilären Insuffizienz ist bis heute noch nicht sehr verbreitet. In der vorliegenden Arbeit wurde bewusst nur der Einfluss dieser Substanzen auf den vestibulären Nystagmus referiert. Für eine endgültige Aussage über die Wirksamkeit dieser Substanzen, insbesondere auch auf die klinische Symptomatik, bleiben noch viele Fragen offen. Teilweise im Akutversuch, teilweise mit Hilfe einer oralen Applikation über mehrere Wochen, wurden drei verschiedene Substanzen sowohl tierexperimentell als auch bei Patienten eingesetzt, deren kalziumantagonistische Eigenschaften als gesichert gelten können. Für Bencyclan ergab sich eine Enthemmung der Nystagmusparameter bei gleichzeitiger Rhythmisierung des Kurvenbildes. Für Flunarizin und Nimodipin ergab sich eine Hemmung der Nystagmusfrequenz. Das bei Hirnduchblutungsstörungen pathologisch enthemmte Elektronystagmogramm wird mit Hilfe dieser Substanzen normalisiert. Eine Korrelation der subjektiven Beschwerden — des Schwindels und all seiner vegetativen Begleitsymptome — mit der Normalisierung der Nystagmusparameter muss noch in grösseren Studien durchgeführt werden.
Ob als Wirkmechanismus bei den genannten Substanzen ein vasodilatatorischer Effekt angenommen werden muss, oder ob eine direkte Wirkung im vestibulären System im Sinne einer Hemmung der Erregungsübertragung vorliegt, kann derzeit nicht entschieden werden.
Wegen des deutlichen Effekts auf den experimentell erzeugten Nystagmus erscheinen weitere vergleichende Studien, die auch die klinische Symptomatik mit einbeziehen, notwendig und sinnvoll.

1. Introduction

The notion "vertebrobasilar insufficiency" (VBI) covers nearly the same area as "cerebrovascular insufficiency", except that the first delimits the area that is insufficiently supplied with blood to the vertebral arteries and the basilar artery. Symptoms typical of VBI are dizziness (particularly on reclination of the head), drop attacks, transitory affection of the cranial nerves, transitory bulbar disorders, affections of the long routes through the brain stem and occipital headache which often is of longer standing (Gänshirt, 1978). To conclude to a diagnosis of VBI, at least two of the above symptoms are required.

The most important neurophysiological examination in disorders of the brain stem can be considered to be electronystagmography (ENG) (Jung, 1953). By means of the experimental induction of brain stem reflexes and the deviation from eye movements involved with these reflex paths, also statements regarding the functional diagnosis of the brain stem can be made.

Calcium entry blockers represent a new type of drug, which, particularly under hypoxic conditions block the influx of calcium into the cell. Whereas this therapeutic principle at the level of the myocardium has been known and applied for a few years, only recently substances have been developed which exert their calcium-antagonizing effect primarily on the cerebral vessels. Their major activity probably consists in an antivasoconstrictive effect on the cerebral vessels under hypoxic conditions (Edvinsson et al., 1979).

In this report, the calcium entry blockers bencyclane, flunarizine and nimodipine are examined. It gives results of animal experiments and clinical trials, both in healthy volunteers and in patients with VBI.

2. Material and method

2.1. VBI in an animal experiment model

In animals, the blood supply to the brain stem was reduced so as to simulate the pathological conditions under VBI. It was assessed whether this would result in reproducible changes of the nystagmus parameter. In two test series of 12 shepherd dogs each (both male and female, average weight 28.7 kg), the femoral artery was punctured according to SELDINGER's technique. Through the puncture cannula, a catheter was inserted into the aorta and the left vertebral artery was probed. The diameter of the vertebral artery was defined radiologically. Using a balloon, which could be filled via the double-way catheter, the diameter of the vessel was narrowed by half. In a second step, the vessel was closed by further filling the balloon. The arterial pressure at the catheter tip was measured by means of a Statham element. Blood flow in the vertebral artery was recorded at the atlas loop, using Doppler sonography.
EEG and ENG were recorded with needle electrodes. As an 8-channel recording apparatus, a mingograph of the Siemens Elema company was used. Amplification was 100 μV/cm for the EEG and 200 μV/cm for the ENG. For the filters 70 and 15 Hz were used, respectively. The time constant was 0.3 and 1.5 s, respectively.

In order to keep the sedative effect on the eye movements as low as possible, neuro-leptanalgesia was chosen for narcosis following various previous testings. Initially, De-hydrobenzperidol in a dosage of 0.1 mg/kg was administered. Narcosis was maintained with fentanyl hydrogen citrate in doses of 0.1 mg, seeing to it that the corneal reflex of the animals was not affected.

Rotatory nystagmus was used as a measuring value, with automatic recording by means of a laboratory computer of the following parameters: frequency, angular velocity of the slow phase and total amplitude (Hofferberth, 1981). The animals were rotated in a construction of our own design with a motor-driven revolving chair of the Tönnies company. Angular acceleration during rotation was 1.5, 3 and 6°/s^2. During the rotation tests a lying balloon catheter was used. The balloon was subsequently filled and rotatory nystagmus again induced. Thereafter, 12 dogs were given 5 mg flunarizine while the other 12 received 10 mg nimodipine I.V. and the rotation tests were again performed.

2.2. Clinical trials

Nothing has been published on the use of bencyclane in vertebrobasilar insufficiency. In a study from Hoeft (1972), only a slightly positive effect was observed as compared with placebo in 64 patients with dizziness. Whether this substance exerts a vestibular effect was investigated by us in 10 healthy volunteers (both male and female, average age 31.4 years). A continuous caloric stimulation was thereby exerted for 45 minutes, consisting in flushing the right external auditory meatus with water at a temperature of 30°C. Ten minutes after flushing was started, 50 mg bencyclane was slowly applied by intravenous route. The nystagmus parameters were analysed at three 10-second intervals before and at 5-minute intervals after the administration of bencyclane.

During the trials with flunarizine and nimodipine, a complete electronystagmographic examination was each time carried out, as described elsewhere (Hofferberth and Dessauer, 1980). The basic tests thereby comprised the recording of saccade speed and the consecutive movements of the eye, as well as searches for spontaneous nystagmus. Subsequently, opticokinetic, thermic and rotatory nystagmus were investigated. The investigations with flunarizine were performed in 40 patients with VBI. They were compared with a reference substance according to a double-blind procedure. The criteria for inclusion were: 1/ clinical evidence of at least 2 or more symptoms of VBI; 2/presence of a high-frequency, low-amplitude nystagmus writing, the so-called "petite écriture" on the electronystagmogram at assessment of the vestibulo-ocular reflex. The patient material comprised 13 females and 27 males, their average age being 62.5 years. The dosage amounted to 21 mg flunarizine in 3 single doses per day during 18 weeks. Electronystagmographic controls were performed before treatment, as well as within 4, 8, 10, 14 and 18 weeks of the treatment period. Apart from anamnesis and clinical examination, the ENG, the EEG and the acoustically induced brain stem potentials (BERA) were recorded.

The effect of nimodipine on ENG parameters in patients with VBI was assessed in an open pilot study involving 10 patients who received one oral dose of 40 mg. These patients, with an average age of 54 years (3 females, 7 males), also had to exhibit at least 2 clinical symptoms of VBI. Moreover, their ENG had to contain a low-amplitude, high-frequency nystagmus writing.

Before they had to take 2 nimodipine tablets of 20 mg, their pulse rate and blood pressure were controlled. Furthermore, the carotid arteries, the supratrochlear artery and the radial artery were examined bilaterally by Doppler sonography. One hour after intake, the electronystagmogram and the Doppler sonogram were repeated, whereas pulse rate and blood pressure as well as the possible occurrence of undesired effects were recorded continuously.

Although in the above-mentioned experimental series not only electro-nystagmographic examinations, but also other objective parameters were recorded such as EEG, BERA or Doppler sonography, and although, as a matter of fact, also the subjective symptoms and anamnestic data were noted, only the results on nystagmus recording will be presented and discussed.

3. Results

3.1. Results from the animal experiments

In the animal experiments, the reduction of the blood supply of the brain stem through a vertebral artery resulted in an increased frequency and a decreased amplitude of nystagmus. These findings became more pronounced after full obstruction of the vessel by means of the balloon catheter. However, after the I.V. administration of flunarizine (Table 1) as well as of nimodipine (Table 2), values returned to normal despite the occlusion of the vertebral artery. Both tables show the measuring values obtained at an angular acceleration of $3°/s^2$ and relate to the data obtained in 12 dogs. Their first column lists the initial values with a lying catheter, the second the values obtained with the artery occluded by half, and the third with the artery occluded fully. In the last column, the parameters recorded after the I.V. administration of either substance are represented. The values measured were the frequency and amplitude of the ENG, arterial pressure at the catheter tip proximally to the balloon, the amplitude of the systolic Doppler signal, and EEG frequency.

Table 1: Rotatory deviation at an angular acceleration of $3°/s^2$ in 12 shepherd dogs, with lying catheter in the left vertebral artery (normal), after reduction of the vascular volume by half by means of a balloon (1/2), after complete occlusion (1/1), and after I.V. administration of 5 mg flunarizine.

	normal	1/2	1/1	5 mg flunarizine I.V.
ENG frequency (Hz)	1.4	1.9	2.7	1.6
ENG nystagmus amplitude (°)	29	16	8	25
blood pressure (mmHg)	117	53	0	0
Doppler amplitude (%)	100	38	0	0
EEG frequency (Hz)	16	18	14	16

Table 2: Rotatory deviation at an angular acceleration of 3°/s² in 12 shepherd dogs, with lying catheter in the left vertebral artery (normal), after reduction of the vascular volume by half by means of a balloon (1/2), after complete occlusion (1/1), and after I.V. administration of 10 mg nimodipine.

	normal	1/2	1/1	10 mg nimodipine I.V.
ENG frequency (Hz)	1.2	1.6	2.9	1.3
ENG nystagmus amplitude (°)	26	21	5	22
blood pressure (mmHg)	134	76	0	0
Doppler amplitude (%)	100	44	0	0
EEG frequency (Hz)	14	14	12	15

3.2. Results from the clinical trials

During acute studies, the parameters of continuous ENG recordings before and 10 minutes after I.V. injection of bencyclane were evaluated. The results of two representative 30-second intervals are given in Table 3, which comprises the following criteria: frequency, average angular velocity of the slow phases and total amplitudes of the rapid phases.

Table 3: Electronystagmographic findings in 10 healthy volunteers during continuous caloric stimulation with water at 30 °C at the right ear. Evaluation of 30-second intervals before and 10 minutes after I.V. injection of 50 mg bencyclane.

	before	10 min. after I.V. injection
frequency (30 s)	36	38
angular velocity (°/s)	22	38
total amplitude (°)	242	436

Whereas the nystagmus frequency during the acute trials was barely affected, the angular velocity of the slow phases as well as the total amplitude of the nystagmus beats clearly increased.

The 40 patients with vertebrobasilar insufficiency and with resulting changes in their electronystagmograms showed a clear effect after administration of 21 mg flunarizine per day during 18 weeks (Table 4). All showed evidence of pathologically disinhibited vestibulo-ocular reflexes. During preliminary examinations, an average frequency of 78.5 nystagmus beats over 30 s was recorded on caloric heat flushing at the right.

Table 4: Electronystagmographic results of a long-term trial implying 40 patients with vertebrobasilar insufficiency who received an oral daily dose of 21 mg flunarizine. Evaluation of right-sided nystagmus after heat flushing of the right auditory meatus with water at 44 °C.

	before	4 weeks	10 weeks	18 weeks
frequency (30 s)	78.5	53	49	55
angular velocity (°/s)	19	17	14	16
total amplitude (°)	296	312	284	306

The decrease of frequency during treatment was not accompanied by a change in total amplitude, which means that the separate nystagmus beats again increased in amplitude during treatment. Already after 4 weeks the normalization of the electronystagmograms took place. This effect lasted during the total observation period.

Also an investigation with nimodipine was performed in 10 patients with vertebrobasilar insufficiency. The criterion for inclusion in the study was evidence of a high-frequency, low-amplitude nystagmus writing. In the acute trial, the effect of nimodipine on the parameters of the pathologically disinhibited nystagmus was evaluated. Eight of the 10 patients thereby showed a normalization of the curves (Table 5). Whereas the nystagmus frequency, on average, was 86 beats in 30 s before intake of nimodipine, this was 51 beats in 30 s one hour after intake of this drug. Apart from the frequency decrease, the amplitudes of the separate nystagmus beats increased, so that the total amplitudes showed no essential changes.

Tabel 5: Electronystagmographic results in 10 patients with vertebrobasilar insufficiency who received 40 mg nimodipine. Evaluation of right-sided nystagmus beats after heat flushing of the right auditory meatus with water at 44°C.

	before	after 1 hour
frequency (30 s)	86	51
angular velocity (°/s)	15	16
total amplitude (°)	334	326

References

Edvinsson, L., Brand, L., Anderson, K. and Bengtson, B. Effect of a calcium antagonist on experimental construction of human brain vessels. *Surg. Neurol.*, **11**, 327-330 (1979).

Gänshirt, H. Die Vertebralisinsuffizienz. In: Lechner, H., Ladurner, G., Ott, E. (ed.), Die zerebralen transitorisch-ischämischen Attacken, Verlag H. Huber, Bern-Stuttgart-Wien, 21-28 (1979).

Hoeft, H. Fludilat im Doppelblindversuch. *Therapiewoche*, **22**, 905-908 (1972).

Hofferberth, B. and Dessauer, M. Fluctuations of electronystagmogram parameters. In: Lechner, H., Aranibar, A. (ed.), EEG and clinical neurophysiology, Excerpta Medica, Amsterdam, 662-665 (1980).

Hofferberth, B. The use of the computer in the equilibrium laboratory. *Royal Society of Medicine Series*, **33**, 13-21 (1980).

Jung, R. Nystagmographie. In: Bergmann, G. und Mitarb. (ed.), Hdb.inn.Med., 4. Aufl., Bd. V/1, Springer, Berlin-Göttingen-Heidelberg (1953).

Calcium entry blockers and pharmacological aspects of migraine

R. Towart

Summary

Accumulating evidence suggests that, despite an unknown and probably heterogeneous aetiology, classical migraine attacks are preceded by a prodromal phase of localised cerebral ischaemia. The cerebral anti-vasoconstrictor and anti-ischaemic effects of calcium entry blockers are reviewed with special reference to nimodipine, which acts predilectively on the cerebral vasculature. Calcium entry blockers with this pharmacological profile represent a novel and rational pharmacological prophylaxis against the cerebral vasoconstriction which precipitates classical migraine. Initial clinical trials in man are proving promising.

Résumé

Un grand nombre de preuves suggèrent que, malgré une étiologie inconnue et probablement hétérogène, les accès de migraine classique sont précédés par une phase prodromique d'ischémie cérébrale localisée. Les effets cérébraux anti-vasoconstricteurs et anti-ischémiques des agents bloqueurs de l'entrée de calcium sont étudiés avec une attention toute spéciale pour la nimodipine, qui agit avec prédilection sur le système vasculaire cérébral. Les agents bloqueurs de l'entrée de calcium possédant ce profil pharmacologique représentent une nouvelle prophylaxie pharmacologique rationnelle contre la vasoconstriction cérébrale qui précipite la migraine classique. Les premières expériences cliniques chez l'homme semblent fort prometteuses.

Resumen

Más y más evidencia va sugeriendo que, a pesar de una estología desconocida y probablemente heterogénea, clásicos ataques de jaqueca son precedidos por una fase prodrómica de isquemia cerebral localizada. Los efectos antivasoconstrictores y antiisquémicos cerebrales de los inhibidores de la penetración intracelular de Ca^{2+} se examinan con especial referencia a nimodipino, que actúa preferentemente en el sistema vascular cerebral. Los inhibidores de la penetración intracelular de Ca^{2+}, con este perfil farmacológico, representan una original y racional profilaxis farmacológica contra la vasoconstricción cerebral que precede a la jaqueca clásica. Las pruebas clínicas iniciales en el hombre son prometedoras.

Zusammenfassung

Zunehmendes Beweismaterial deutet darauf hin, dass, ungeachtet einer unbekannten und heterogenen Ätiologie, klassischen Migräneanfällen eine Prodromalphase örtlicher Hirnischämie vorangeht. Die antivasokonstriktions- und anti-ischämischen Wirkungen der Kalzium-Einstromhemmer werden kurz beschrieben, wobei dem Nimodipin, welches eine Prädilektion für Hirngefässe zeigt, besondere Aufmerksamkeit geschenkt wird. Kalzium-Einstromhemmer mit diesem pharmakologischen Profil bedeuten eine neue und rationale Prophylaxe gegen zerebrale Vasokonstriktion, die zu klassischer Migräne führen kann. Erste klinische Versuche beim Menschen sind erfolgversprechend.

Introduction

The aetiology of the debilitating condition migraine is still unknown. The wide range of drugs used either prophylactically or symptomatically (see Raskin, 1981 and Friedman, 1982, for reviews) emphasises the uncertainty as to either the cause of the disease or to reliable and rational therapy. Interested readers are referred to recent reviews for an overview of the fascinating multiplicity of factors which may contribute to the pathophysiology of migraine (see Burnstock, 1981; Crook, 1981; Hanington et al., 1981).

Migraine — the triggering role of vasoconstriction

Nearly 50 years ago Wolff and his colleagues proposed that an initial cerebral vasoconstriction was an important triggering factor in migraine (Graham and Wolff, 1938). Recent direct measurements of regional blood flow have produced convincing evidence that in at least one form, "classical" migraine, constriction of cerebral blood vessels occurs during the prodromal or "aura" phase (Skinhoj, 1973; Edmeads, 1977; Olesen, 1982). The reflex vasodilation which follows is believed to be responsible for the consequent headache phase, as the pain receptors on the dilated vessels are stimulated (Caviness and O'Brien, 1980; Amery, 1982). Thus it has been suggested that a suitable strategy for migraine prophylaxis might be the prevention of the initial vasoconstriction and its associated hypoxia. Some early support for this view comes from the report that the cerebral vasodilator drug papaverine could be an effective prophylactic drug (Poser, 1974). However, until recently few drugs termed as "cerebral vasodilators" have been considered to have any significant effects on cerebral hypoxia, partly because of "steal" effects (see e.g. Vanhoutte, 1982).

A recent more promising approach to cerebral hypoxia has been the development of certain "second generation" calcium entry blockers, which, while still not completely selective as cerebral vasodilators, certainly increase cerebral blood flow in doses which have little or no effects on systemic blood pressure (Kazda et al., 1982a; Haws et al., 1983).

Calcium entry blockers and cerebral vessels

As has been discussed in depth in the other chapters of this volume, the calcium entry blockers, or "calcium antagonists" are drugs which, by nature of their pharmacological properties, are potent anti-vasoconstrictor agents. The importance of calcium ions in the excitation-contraction coupling of vascular smooth muscle (Casteels, 1984) ensures that block of calcium influx into isolated blood vessels leads to an inhibition of vasoconstrictor reactions. However, as has also been pointed out (Van Nueten, 1984), the in vivo response of any particular vascular bed to calcium entry blockers is influenced by many factors.

The comparative pharmacology of the group of drugs known as calcium antagonists has been much reviewed (e.g. Henry, 1980; Kazda et al., 1983b), and is complex. It has been found empirically that a certain degree of tissue selectivity exists. Tissue selectivity may be demonstrated by comparative studies in which a particular agent is more potent at relaxing certain tissues in vitro under comparable conditions (e.g. Van Nueten and Vanhoutte, 1981; Bevan, 1983; Kazda et al., 1980). An additional effect may be due to the pharmacokinetics of the agents involved, i.e. on administration to the whole animal, a predilective dilatation of a particular vascular bed is observed. For example the calcium antagonists nitrendipine or felodipine are reported to be potent **peripheral** vasodilators (Kazda et al., 1983a; Johnsson et al., 1983) whereas nimodipine increases **cerebral** blood flow in doses that have little or no effect on systemic blood pressure (Kazda et al., 1982a; Haws et al., 1983). Thus at least some of the second generation calcium antagonists at present undergoing clinical trials show predilective effects on the cerebral circulation.

Effects of nimodipine on cerebral vessels

Several distinct chemical structures possess calcium antagonistic properties, but the 1,4-dihydropyridine derivatives were early found to be the most potent and specific agents (see Fleckenstein, 1977). The prototype compound is nifedipine, which is widely used as an antianginal and antihypertensive agent. Kazda and Meyer developed the "second generation" dihydropyridine derivative nimodipine, which has predilective effects on the cerebral vasculature (Kazda et al., 1982a). Many independent studies have now confirmed that nimodipine increases cerebral blood flow in animals and in man with little effect on arterial blood pressure (Tanaka et al., 1980; Auer, 1981; Harper et al., 1981; Gelmers, 1982; Steen et al., 1983; Haws et al., 1983). Several studies from my laboratory have demonstrated that nimodipine potently relaxes isolated cerebral blood vessels stimulated by a variety of contractile stimuli: potassium depolarisation, serotonin, catecholamines, histamine, thromboxane, and even whole blood (Towart and Kazda, 1980; Towart, 1981a; Towart and Perzborn, 1981; Towart et al., 1982). In addition nimodipine, like some other calcium entry blockers (see Bevan, 1983) selectively inhibits the effects of contractile agonists on cerebral vessels; the effects on peripheral vessels such as aorta or saphenous artery are little affected (Towart, 1981a).

Nimodipine's pharmacological profile of anti-vasoconstrictor effects against a variety of contractile stimuli which may be released in ischaemic areas of the brain (see Siesjo, 1981 for review) emphasises the pathological role of calcium ions in cerebral hypoxia (Hass, 1981). Thus calcium antagonists such as nimodipine, by inhibiting the increase in intracellular calcium concentration, which constitutes the final common pathway for vasoconstriction, constitute a rational prophylaxis against cerebral vasoconstriction.

Other effects of nimodipine

A much-discussed possibility is that platelets are in some way involved in the pathogenesis of migraine (see e.g. Hanington et al., 1981). Calcium entry blockers have been reported by many groups to possess anti-aggregatory properties, but the concentrations required are high in comparison to those which relax blood vessels. Even in concentrations of around $1.5 \times 10^{-4}M$ nimodipine had no effect on arachidonic acid- or ADP-induced platelet aggregation (Schmunck and Lefer, 1982).

Despite its lack of action on platelets, nimodipine possesses a variety of anti-ischaemic effects, which may or may not be directly related to its calcium-antagonistic actions. Both circulatory (Kazda et al., 1982a) and behavioural effects (Hoffmeister et al., 1982) have been reported after ischaemic or hypoxic insult in several species. Nimodipine improves neurologic recovery in dogs after complete cerebral ischaemia (Steen et al., 1983). Chronic nimodipine treatment of stroke-prone spontaneously hypertensive rats reduces mortality and the incidence of histological cerebrovascular lesions (Kazda et al., 1982b). In addition nimodipine in low concentrations has been reported to stimulate Na+-, K+-activated ATPase activity of vascular smooth muscle microsomes (Pan and Janis, 1982). Whether this action contributes to its vasodilator effects in vivo is at present unknown.

Although the models of cerebral ischaemia or insult used in the studies above are obviously more severe than would be found in the prodromal phase of human migraine, the results clearly demonstrate that nimodipine possesses protective effects against cerebral ischaemia or hypoxia. Similar protective actions have been demonstrated for other calcium antagonists (e.g. flunarizine, see Amery, 1982).

Effects of calcium entry blockers in migraine

In the light of the foregoing discussion, certain calcium antagonists could have a prophylactic effect at least in classical migraine, in which an initial vasoconstriction is observed during the aura phase (see e.g. Olesen, 1982). The calcium entry blockers, both by their inhibitory effects on cerebral vasoconstriction, and by their other, less well explained cerebral anti-ischaemic effects (see above) would prevent or abort the initial vasoconstriction, and prevent or lessen any ischaemic effects leading to reflex cerebral vasodilatation and stimulation of pain receptors.

Several small scale trials, all with some degree of success, have taken place using diltiazem (Riopelle and McCans, 1982), verapamil (Solomon, 1982), cinnarizine or flunarizine (Drillisch and Girke, 1980, Louis, 1981; Amery, 1982; Rose, 1982; Amery et al., 1981), nifedipine (Kahan et al., 1983) or nimodipine (Gelmers, 1983; Havanka-Kannianen et al., 1982) (see also Blau, 1983). The interested reader is referred to the individual reports for details. As all of these preliminary investigations showed superiority of the calcium entry blocker over placebo, a larger scale controlled trials of a calcium entry blocker for migraine prophylaxis would seem to be indicated to determine the therapeutic potential of these drugs in the prophylaxis of migraine.

Acknowledgement

The author wishes to thank Dr. S. Kazda and Dr. D. Tettenborn (Bayer AG) for many helpful discussions, and Mrs. K.B. Crocker for preparing the manuscript.

References

Amery, W.K. Brain hypoxia in migraine: pathophysiologic and therapeutic implications. *J. Cereb. Blood Flow Met.*, **2**, Suppl. 1, S62-65. (1982)

Amery, W.K., Wauquier, A., Van Nueten, J.M., De Clerck, F., Van Reempts, J.V., Janssen, P.A.J. The anti-migrainous pharmacology of flunarizine (R 14 950), a calcium antagonist. *Drugs Exptl. Clin. Res.*, **7**, 1-10. (1981)

Auer, L.M. Pial arterial vasodilatation by intravenous nimodipine in cats. *Arzneimittel-Forsch. (Drug Res.)*, **31**, 1423-1425. (1981)

Bevan, J.A. Diltiazem selectively inhibits cerebrovascular extrinsic but not intrinsic myogenic tone. *Circ. Res.*, **52** (Suppl.1), 104-109. (1983)

Blau, J.N. News on headache (editorial). *Brit. Med. J.*, **287**, 166. (1983)

Burnstock, G. Pathophysiology of migraine. *Lancet*, **I**, 1397-1399. (1981)

Casteels, R. Calcium ions and excitation-contraction coupling in vascular smooth muscle cells. In: Calcium entry blockers in cardiovascular and cerebral dysfunctions. Editors: T. Godfraind, A. Herman, D. Wellens. *Martinus Nijhoff Publishers*, pp 45-52. (1984)

Caviness, V.S. and O'Brien, P. Current Concepts: headache. *N. Engl. J. Med.*, **302**, 446-450. (1980)

Crook, M. Migraine: a biochemical headache. *Biochem. Soc. Trans.*, **9**, 351-357. (1981)

Edmeads, J. Cerebral blood flow in migraine. *Headache*, **17**, 148-152. (1977)

Fleckenstein, A. Specific pharmacology of calcium in myocardium, cardiac pacemakers, and vascular smooth muscle. *Ann. Rev. Pharmacol. Toxicol.*, **17**, 149-166. (1977)

Friedman, A.P. Overview of migraine. In: Advances in Neurology, vol. 33 (Critchley, M. et al., eds.). Raven Press, New York, 1982, pp 1-17. (1982)

Gelmers, H.J. Effect of nimodipine (BAY e9736) on postischemic cerebrovascular reactivity as revealed by measuring regional cerebral blood flow (rCBF). *Acta-Neurochir.* (Wien), **63**, 283-290. (1982)

Gelmers, H.J. Nimodipine, a new calcium antagonist in the prophylactic treatment of migraine. *Headache*, **23**, 106-109. (1983)

Graham, J.R. and Wolff, H.G. Mechanism of migraine headache and action of ergotamine tartrate. *Arch. Neurol. Psychiatry*, **39**, 737-763. (1938)

Hanington, E., Jones, R.J., Agmess, J.A.L. and Wachowicz, B. Migraine: a platelet disorder. *Lancet*, **ii**, 720-723. (1981)

Harper, A.M., Craigen, L. and Kazda, S. Effect of the calcium antagonist nimodipine on cerebral blood flow and metabolism in the primate. *J. Cereb. Blood Flow Metab.*, **1**, 349-356. (1981)

Hass, W.K. Beyond cerebral blood flow, metabolism and ischaemic thresholds: Examination of the role of calcium in initiation of cerebral infarction. In: Cerebral Vascular Disease Vol. 3 (Meyer, J.S. et al., eds.). Excerpta Medica, Amsterdam, pp3-17. (1981)

Havanka-Kanniainen, H., Myllyla, V.V. and Hokkanen, E. Nimodipine in the prophylaxis of migraine, a double blind study. *Acta Neurol. Scand.*, **65**, Suppl. 90, 77-78. (1982)

Haws, C.W., Gourley, J.K. and Heistad, D.D. Effects of nimodipine on cerebral blood flow. *J. Pharmac. Exp. Ther.*, **225**, 24-28. (1983)

Henry, P.D. Comparative pharmacology of Ca^{2+}-antagonists. *Am. J. Cardiol.*, **46**, 1047-1058. (1980)

Hoffmeister, F., Benz, U., Heise, A., Krause, H.-P. and Neuser, V. Behavioural effects of nimodipine in animals. *Arzneim.-Forsch. (Drug Res.)*, **32**, 347-360. (1982)

Johnsson, G., Murray, G., Tweddel, A. and Hutton, I. Haemodynamic effects of a new vasodilator drug, felodipine, in healthy subjects. *Eur. J. Clin. Pharmacol.*, **24**, 49-53. (1983)

Kahan, A., Weber, S., Amor, B., Guerin, F. and Degeorges, M. Nifedipine in the treatment of migraine in patients with Raynaud's phenomenon. *N. Engl. J. Med.*, **308**, 1102-1103. (1983)

Kazda, S., Garthoff, B., Krause, H.P. and Schlossmann, K. Cerebrovascular effects of the calcium antagonistic dihydropyridine derivative nimodipine in experimental animals. *Arzneim.-Forsch. (Drug Res.)*, **32**, 331-338. (1982a)

Kazda, S., Garthoff, B., Luckhaus, G. and Nash, G. Prevention of cerebrovascular lesions and mortality in stroke-prone spontaneously hypertensive rats by the calcium antagonist nimodipine. In: Calcium Modulators, Godfraind, T. et al., eds. Elsevier, Amsterdam, pp. 155-167. (1982b)

Kazda, S., Garthoff, B., Meyer, H., Schlossmann, K., Stoepel, K., Towart, R., Vater, W. and Wehinger, E. Pharmacology of a new calcium antagonistic compound, isobutyl methyl 1,4-dihydro-2,6-dimethyl-4-(2-nitrophenyl)-3,5-pyridinedicarboxylate (nisoldipine, BAY K 5552). *Arzneim.-Forsch. (Drug Res.)*, **30** (II), 2144-2162. (1980)

Kazda, S., Garthoff, B. and Knorr, A. Nitrendipine and other calcium entry blockers (calcium antagonists) in hypertension. *Fed. Proc.*, **42**, 196-200. (1983a)

Kazda, S., Knorr, A. and Towart, R. Common properties, and differences between, various calcium antagonists. *Progress in Pharmacology*, **5**, 83-116. (1983b)

Louis, P. A double-blind placebo-controlled prophylactic study of flunarizine in migraine. *Headache*, **21**, 235-239. (1981)

Olesen, J. Is ischaemia involved in the pathogenesis of migraine? *Path. Biologie*, **30**, 318-324. (1982)

Pan, M. and Janis, R.A. Nimodipine, a new cerebral vasodilator, stimulates Na^+, K^+-activated ATPase of smooth muscle microsomes. *Fed. Proc.*, **42**, 1483. (1982)

Poser, C.M. Papaverine in prophylactic treatment of migraine. *Lancet*, **i**, 1290. (1974)

Raskin, N.H. Pharmacology of migraine. *Ann. Rev. Pharmacol. Toxicol.*, **21**, 463-478. (1981)

Riopelle, R.J. and McCans, J.L. A pilot study of the calcium antagonist diltiazem in migraine syndrome prophylaxis. *Le Journal Can. d. Sciences Neurol.*, **9**, 269 (abst.). (1982)

Rose, F.C. Possible role for flunarizine in the prophylaxis of migraine. In: Cerebral Hypoxia in the Pathogenesis of Migraine. Rose, F.C. and Amery, W.K., eds., Pitman, London, pp. 185-194. (1982)

Schmunck, G.A. and Lefer, A.M. Anti-aggregatory actions of calcium channel blockers in cat platelets. *Res. Commun. Chem. Path. Pharmacol.*, **35**, 179-187. (1982)

Siesjo, B.K. Cell damage in the brain: A speculative synthesis. *J. Cerebral Blood Flow Met.*, **1**, 155-185. (1981)

Skinhoj, E. Haemodynamic studies within the brain during migraine. *Arch. Neurol.*, **29**, 95-98. (1973)

Solomon, G.D. Calcium channel blockers in migraine. *Lancet*, **II**, 1982, 162. (1982)

Steen, P.A., Newberg, L.A., Milde, J.H. and Michenfelder, J.D. Nimodipine improves cerebral blood flow and neurologic recovery after complete cerebral ischaemia in the dog. *J. Cereb. Blood Flow Metab.*, **3**, 38-43. (1983)

Tanaka, K., Gotoh, F., Muramatsu, F., Fukuuchi, Y., Amano, T., Okayasu, H. and Suzuki, N. Effects of nimodipine (BAY e9736) on cerebral circulation in cats. *Arzneim.-Forsch. (Drug Res.)*, **30**, 1494-1497. (1980)

Towart, R. The selective inhibition of serotonin-induced contractions of rabbit cerebral vascular smooth muscle by calcium antagonistic dihydropyridines. An investigation of the mechanism of action of nimodipine. *Circ. Res.*, **48**, 650-657. (1981a)

Towart, R. Predilective relaxation by the calcium antagonist nimodipine (BAY e9736) of isolated cerebral blood vessels contracted with autalogous blood. *Brit. J. Pharmacol.*, **74**, 268P-269P. (1981b)

Towart, R. and Kazda, S. The effect of nimodipine (BAY e9736), a calcium antagonist dihydropyridine, on cerebral and peripheral vessels. In: Pathophysiology and Pharmacotherapy of Cerebrovascular Disorders, Betz, E., Grote, J., Heuser, D. and Wullenweber, R., eds., Baden-Baden: Verlag Gerhard Witzstrock, pp. 64-67. (1980)

Towart, R. and Perzborn, E. Nimodipine inhibits carbocyclic thromboxane-A_2-induced contractions of cerebral arteries. *Eur. J. Pharmacol.*, **69**, 213-215. (1981)

Towart, R., Wehinger, E., Meyer, H. and Kazda, S. The effects of nimodipine, its optical isomers and metabolites on isolated vascular smooth muscle. *Arzneim.-Forsch. (Drug Res.)*, **32**, 338-346. (1982)

Vanhoutte, P.M. Hypoxia and tissue perfusion. In: Cerebral Hypoxia in the Pathogenesis of Migraine. Rose, F.C. and Amery, W.K., eds., Pitman, London, pp. 3-11. (1982)

Van Nueten, J.M. and Vanhoutte, P.M. Selectivity of calcium-antagonism and serotonin-antagonism with respect to venous and arterial tissues. *Angiology*, **32**, 476-484. (1981)

Van Nueten, J.M. Vascular pharmacology of calcium entry blockers. In: Calcium entry blockers in cardiovascular and cerebral dysfunctions. Editors: T. Godfraind, A. Herman, D. Wellens. *Martinus Nijhoff Publishers*, 59-72. (1984)

270

Clinical evaluation of calcium entry blockers in migraine

E.L.H. Spierings

Summary

In this paper the clinical studies are reviewed on the efficacy of the calcium entry blockers, flunarizine, nimodipine, nifedipine and verapamil, in the prophylactic treatment of migraine. Of these four drugs the prophylactic antimigraine activity of flunarizine is best documented and has been demonstrated to be roughly equal to that of the well established antimigraine drug, pizotifen. However, more and in general better designed and longer studies are needed before this class of drugs can be fully considered a new generation of prophylactic antimigraine drugs.

Résumé

Des études cliniques sont passées en revue, qui portent sur l'efficacité des bloqueurs d'entrée de calcium tels que la flunarizine, la nimodipine, la nifédipine et le vérapamil dans le traitement prophylactique de la migraine. Parmi les activités antimigraineuses de ces quatre substances, celle de la flunarizine est la mieux connue. Il a été démontré à son sujet que son activité était à peu près identique à celle d'une autre substance antimigraineuse bien établie, le pizotifene. Toutefois, il faudra que des études plus nombreuses et en général mieux bâties viennent étayer ces constatations avant que cette catégorie de substances soit pleinement reconnue comme constituant une nouvelle génération de substances antimigraineuses prophylactiques.

Resumen

Este papel reseña los ensayos clínicos de la eficacia de los inhibidores de la penetración intracelular de calcio, flunarizina, nimodipino, nifedipino y verapamilo, en el tratamiento profiláctico de la jaqueca. De estas cuatro drogas la actividad profiláctica antijaqueca de flunarizina está mejor documentada y ha demostrado ser aproximadamente igual a la de la droga antijaqueca de probada eficacia, pizotifeno. Sin embargo, se necesitan más estudios, y en general mejor concebidos y más largos, antes de que esta clase de drogas se pueda considerar verdaderamente como una nueva generación de drogas profilácticas antijaqueca.

Zusammenfassung

In diesem Beitrag wird eine Übersicht über klinische Studien gegeben, die sich mit der Wirksamkeit der Kalziumantagonisten Flunarizin, Nimodipin, Nifedipin und Verapamil in der Migräneprophylaxe befassen. Bei diesen vier Arzneimitteln ist die prophylaktische Antimigränewirkung von Flunarizin am besten belegt und hat sich als ähnlich der des bewährten Antimigränemittels Pizotifen erwiesen. Dennoch sind weitere, besser kontrollierte und längerdauernde Versuche durchzuführen, bevor diese Arzneimittelgruppe als eine vollwertige neue Generation prophylaktischer Antimigränemittel betrachtet werden kann.

Introduction

The calcium entry blockers, formerly called calcium antagonists, are gradually secur-
ing themselves a place of importance in various fields of medicine, including the treatment of migraine. Double-blind studies to evaluate their efficacy as prophylactic
antimigraine drugs have been published for flunarizine, nimodipine, nifedipine and
verapamil. These studies will be reviewed here, preceded by some general remarks
on the methodology of prophylactic drug trials in migraine.

Prophylactic drug trials in migraine

Migraine is a chronic paroxysmal headache disorder which often seems to occur on
the basis of a clear hereditary predisposition. However, the first appearance of the attacks may be marked by events like prolonged psychological stress, a head or neck
injury, menarche, the use of oral contraceptives, etc.

The frequency with which migraine attacks occur varies greatly, both in the same patient as well as between patients, and is particularly sensitive to stress. Stress is also a
common precipitating factor of individual attacks, and then migraine attacks
characteristically occur after the stress rather than during it, a feature which may even
be considered diagnostic for the condition.

In contrast to stress, reassurance, which may emanate from the attention of a
thoughtful physician, is able to decrease the attack frequency. When a patient agrees
to participate in a drug study he is likely to receive, apart from a tablet or a capsule, also
increased medical attention. The "spontaneous" decrease in attack frequency which
may result from it, is in this context usually referred to as "placebo effect".

Another effect that also has to be corrected for in drug studies in migraine is the so-
called time effect, which is the "spontaneous" decrease in attack frequency which may
occur with time. The explanation of this effect is that a patient usually consults his physician when the attack frequency is high. Then the most likely course for the condition
to take is to decrease, even without medical interference.

Both the "placebo" and the "time effect" make the use of a placebo in prophylactic
drug studies in migraine mandatory. If it concerns a crossover study, i.e. when each
patient receives both the drug and the placebo, the order in which the two treatments
are given should be determined by chance to occur randomly, with the same number
of patients starting with the drug and with the placebo. In a non-crossover study, i.e.
when each patient receives either the drug or the placebo, it also necessitates inclusion
in the study of a base-line observation period which should last at least one month. A
base-line observation period is then also necessary to ensure comparability in
headache suffering between the two treatment groups.

A major advantage of the crossover method over the non-crossover one is that in the
former each patient serves as his own control, thus eliminating inter-patient variability
and reducing the number of patients required.

However, because every patient is treated with both the drug and the placebo the duration of the study is considerably longer than when the non-crossover method is used, which, in turn, increases the risk of drop-outs.

Whatever the nature of the study is, i.e. crossover or non-crossover, the treatment period should always be of sufficient duration and should preferably last at least three months. In addition, in a crossover study, a wash-out period should be interposed between the two treatment periods. The wash-out period should last from two to four weeks and should prevent a carry-over effect of the first treatment on the state of the condition during the second treatment.

In a crossover study with its already longer duration a base-line observation period is not as absolutely necessary as in a non-crossover one. In the latter a base-line observation period is indispensable because without it it is impossible to determine whether the drug is at all able to influence the condition. It also allows to observe whether the patient's attack frequency is indeed high enough, i.e. more than two per month, to participate in a prophylactic drug trial. Furthermore, from the base-line observation period an indication can be obtained of the patient's compliance. This could decrease the drop-out rate and drop-outs are especially deleterious in a non-crossover study.

A base-line observation period also provides an opportunity to recognize and to deal with patients in whom the high attack frequency is due to a high intake of ergotamine. Because this presents a situation intractable to treatment with a prophylactic antimigraine drug, these patients should be requested to entirely discontinue the use of ergotamine before entering the study proper. Of course, alternative attack treatment should then be provided, e.g. in the form of metoclopramide in combination with an analgesic like aspirin or paracetamol (acetominophen), or indomethacin suppositories.

The advantage of the non-crossover method over the crossover one is that in the former the duration of the study is relatively short. However, the non-crossover method needs more patients which makes both methods in terms of economy of resources about equal. Nevertheless, in view of what has been stated above, the crossover method can generally be regarded as preferable.

Flunarizine (Sibelium®)

Flunarizine is a derivative of cinnarizine. Cinnarizine, in turn, is a histamine H_1-receptor blocking agent widely employed in the treatment of vertigo. Flunarizine also has antihistamine properties and, in addition, both drugs have been shown to inhibit the influx of calcium into vascular smooth muscle cells.

With regard to the prophylactic antimigraine action of flunarizine, three double-blind studies have been published, all employing the non-crossover method. One of them concerns a placebo-controlled study while in the other two the prophylactic antimigraine activity of the drug was compared with that of cinnarizine and pizotifen, respectively.

Pizotifen is a serotonin-antagonist and a prophylactic antimigraine drug of good reputation. Cinnarizine, on the other hand, has never entered the realm of migraine treatment probably because its major action has always been considered to be on histamine-receptors, and histamine has never been regarded to play a major role in the pathogenesis of the migraine attack.

The placebo-controlled study with flunarizine was conducted by Louis (1981) and involved 58 patients (40 with common and 18 with classical migraine) of whom half received the placebo and the other half the drug. A base-line observation period was not included in the study but each patient was questioned about the number of attacks experienced during the six months preceding the trial. The duration of treatment was three months and the dose of flunarizine was 5 mg twice daily.

The conclusion of the study was that flunarizine lowered the attack frequency but that the drug did not affect the duration and severity of the attacks. With regard to the attack frequency the conclusion was drawn on the observation that during the treatment period the number of attacks was significantly lower in the flunarizine group, as compared with the placebo group (Table 1). The average number of attacks suffered by the patients in the six months preceding the trial was the same in both groups and amounted to 1.2 per month. However, if a base-line observation period had been included in the study, the above conclusion could have been drawn on more solid grounds.

Table 1: Results of a randomized double-blind non-crossover study comparing flunarizine (5 mg b.i.d.) with placebo in 2 x 29 patients with migraine[1]

	placebo (3 months)	flunarizine (3 months)
number of attacks per month	1.0	0.6
	$p < 0.001$	

[1] data obtained from Louis, (1981)

Of the two studies in which the efficacy of flunarizine was compared with that of another drug, a base-line observation period was included in the cinnarizine study but not in the pizotifen one. However, in a study in which two drugs with "proven" prophylactic antimigraine activity are compared, a base-line observation period is not as necessary as it is in a placebo-controlled one, except to ensure comparability in migraine suffering between the two groups. In the flunarizine-pizotifen study conducted by Louis and myself (1982) the latter was established on the basis of the information obtained from the patients about their migraine suffering during the six months preceding the trial.

The flunarizine-cinnarizine study was conducted by Drillisch and Girke (1980) and was the first to suggest a prophylactic antimigraine action for flunarizine. It involved 27 patients of whom 14 received flunarizine and 13 cinnarizine.

The patients suffered either from classical or ophthalmoplegic migraine and patients with common migraine were not included in the study. The dose of flunarizine was 3 mg t.i.d. and that of cinnarizine 75 mg t.i.d. The base-line observation period lasted six weeks and the treatment periods three months. The results of the study with regard to the attack frequency and the duration of the attacks are shown in Figure 1. However, not only these two variables but also the severity of the attacks decreased significantly in both treatment groups.

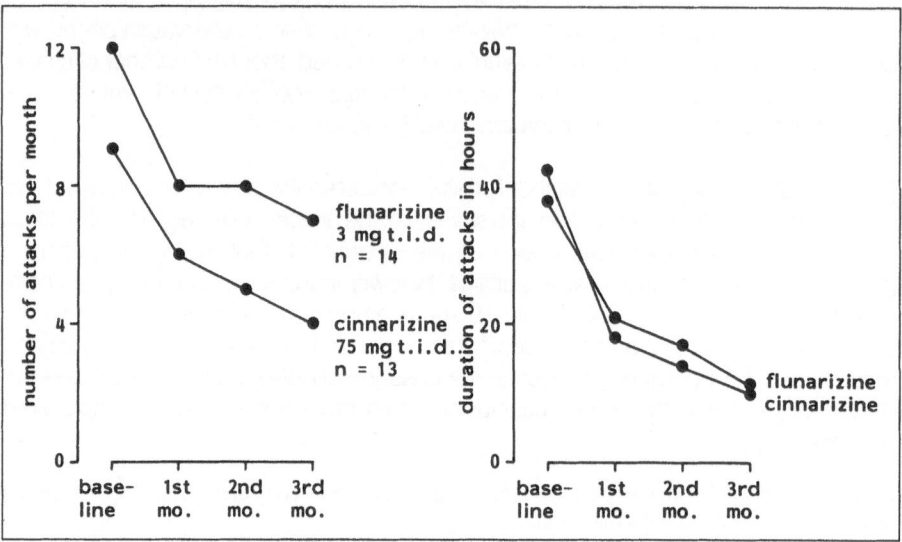

Figure 1: The effects of flunarizine and cinnarizine on attack frequency (left hand diagram) and duration (right hand diagram) as observed by Drillisch and Girke (1980) in a double-blind non-crossover study in migraine.

The effect of flunarizine on the attack duration and severity as observed in the flunarizine-cinnarizine study contrasts with Louis's finding in the placebo-controlled study where the drug had no effect on these variables. In the flunarizine-pizotifen study conducted by Louis and myself (1982) an effect of flunarizine was observed on attack severity but not on the duration of the attacks.

The flunarizine-pizotifen study involved 72 patients (28 with classical and 44 with common migraine) of whom 38 received flunarizine and 34 pizotifen. The dose of flunarizine was 10 mg, taken every evening before retiring, and that of pizotifen 2 - 3 mg per day in three intakes. The duration of treatment was four months. The results of the study with regard to the attack frequency are shown in Figure 2. Judging from the course the attack frequency takes from the first to the fourth month, it can be concluded that as far as this variable goes, both drugs are equally potent. As in Louis's placebo controlled study, in this study no differences in response to flunarizine were observed between patients with classical and common migraine.

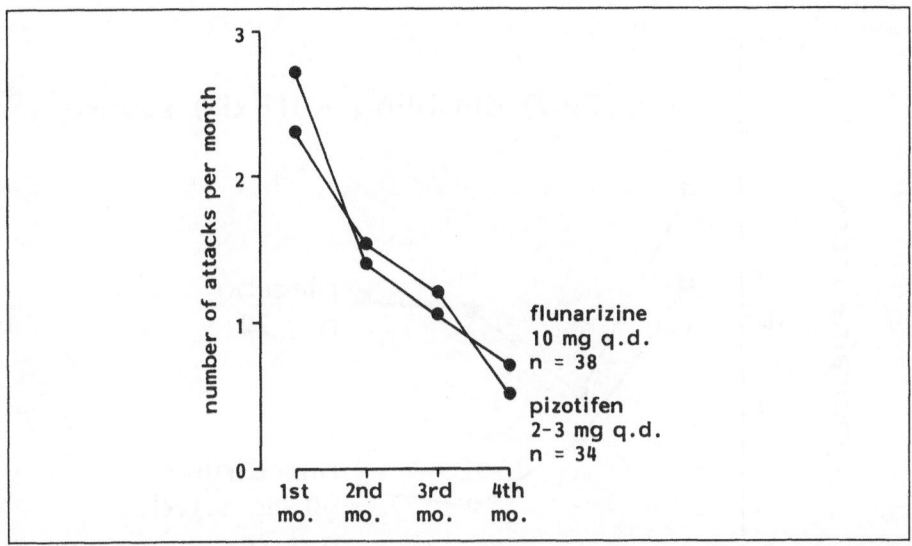

Figure 2: The effects of flunarizine and pizotifen on attack frequency as observed by Louis and Spierings (1982) in a randomized double-blind non-crossover study in migraine.

Nimodipine (Nimotop®)

Nimodipine as a prophylactic antimigraine drug has been the subject of study in two double-blind placebo-controlled trials of which one has only been published in abstract form. In both studies the drug was administered in the dose of 120 mg per day in three or four intakes. One of the studies (Gelmers, 1983) applied the non-crossover method with the treatment being preceded by a two-week base-line observation period. The duration of treatment was in this study three months and the results, as presented in Figure 3, showed a decrease in "migraine index", which over the whole three months period amounted to 62% for nimodipine and 35% for placebo. A difference between the drug and the placebo was, however, not noted until after the first month of treatment.

The other study (Havanka-Kanniainen *et al.*, 1982) was set up in a crossover design which, however, was not clear from the abstract itself; the information was obtained from the pharmaceutical company. The study involved 20 patients and the duration of treatment was two months. Presumably 10 patients were treated first with placebo and then with nimodipine whereas the other 10 *vice versa*, and the allocation of the patients occurred randomly. The number of attacks per month amounted to 3.2 during treatment with placebo and to 2.5 during treatment with the drug. The decrease in attack frequency was 22% and was reported to be statistically significant at the 0.025 level. Both studies involved patients with classical as well as common migraine.

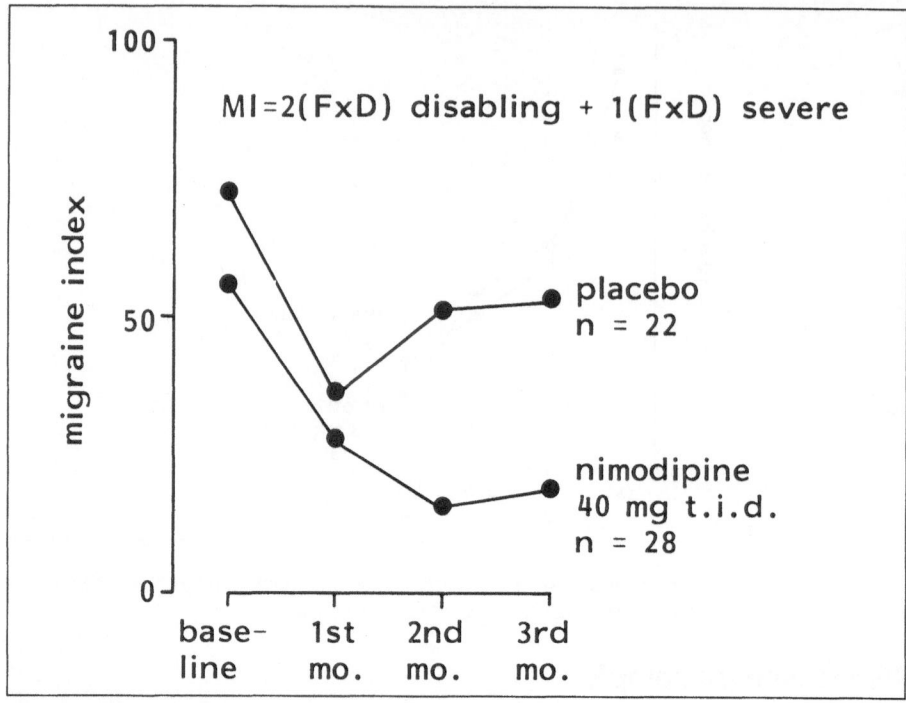

$$MI = 2(FxD) \text{ disabling} + 1(FxD) \text{ severe}$$

placebo
n = 22

nimodipine
40 mg t.i.d.
n = 28

base-line · 1st mo. · 2nd mo. · 3rd mo.

migraine index

Figure 3: The effects of nimodipine and placebo on the migraine index as observed by Gelmers (1983) in a randomized double-blind non-crossover study.

Nifedipine (Adalat®/Procardia®)

Two double-blind studies have been performed with nifedipine as a prophylactic an-timigraine drug. One of them is published by Kahan et al. (1983) and the other one is known to me from a personal communication with Selmaj, Poland. Both studies employed the crossover method with randomized allocation of the patients, were placebo-controlled and used the drug in the dose of 10 mg t.i.d. The published study concerned eight patients with migraine and Raynaud's phenomenon. It included a base-line observation period of the same duration as the treatment periods, i.e. one month. The results of the study are summarized in Table 2 and show a highly signifi-cant reduction in the frequency of the attacks as well as in their severity, both when compared to base-line and to placebo treatment.

In sharp contrast to the observations by Kahan et al. are those of Selmaj et al. (1983) which are summarized in Table 3. In Selmaj's study which involved 10 patients and which did not include a base-line observation period but where the treatment periods were twice as long as in Kahan's study, no significant differences, when compared with placebo treatment, were observed.

Table 2: Results of a randomized double-blind crossover study comparing nifedipine (10 mg t.i.d.) with placebo in 8 patients with migraine and Raynaud's phenomenon[1]

	base-line (1 month)	placebo (1 month)	nifedipine (1 month)
number of attacks per month	8.0 ± 1.5	7.6 ± 1.3 (-74%) p < 0.001	2.0 ± 3.3
	(-75%) p < 0.001		
	p < 0.001		
severity of attacks[2]	5.6 ± 1.6	5.2 ± 1.5 (-71%) p < 0.001	1.5 ± 1.6
	(-73%) p < 0.001		
	p < 0.001		

[1] data obtained from Kahan *et al.*, (1983)
[2] assessed by patients on a 10-cm visual analogue scale

Table 3: Results of a randomized double-blind crossover study comparing nifedipine (10 mg t.i.d.) with placebo in 10 patients with migraine[1]

	placebo (2 months)	nifedipine (2 months)
number of attacks per month	5.8 (-12%) p < 0.2	5.1
weekly headache index[2]	28.7 (-8%) p < 0.2	26.3

[1] data obtained from Selmaj et al., personal communication, 1983
[2] number of attacks per week x intensity

Verapamil (Isoptin®)

The double-blind placebo-controlled study of verapamil in the prophylactic treatment of migraine has also only been published in abstract form (Solomon et al., 1983). It concerns a randomized crossover study in five patients and the drug was given in the dose of 80 mg q.i.d. No base-line observation period was included in the study. The results of the study are presented in Table 4 and show a significant reduction in attack frequency and "headache unit index", when compared with placebo treatment. Two patients in this study suffered from classical migraine and they were reported to have responded considerably better to the drug than the other three patients with common migraine (93.5% versus 45% reduction in attack frequency).

Table 4: Results of a randomized double-blind crossover study comparing verapamil (80 mg q.i.d.) with placebo in 5 patients with migraine[1]

	placebo (3 months)	verapamil (3 months)
number of attacks per month	9.3 ± 1.7 (-52%) $p < 0.01$	4.5 ± 0.9
headache unit index[2]	0.83 (-37%) $p < 0.05$	0.52

[1] data obtained from Solomon et al., (1983)
[2] total score of headache severity/total number of days observed

Acknowledgement

I would like to thank my wife, Malina, for valuable assistance in the preparation of this manuscript.

280

References

Drillisch, C., Girke, W. Ergebnisse der Behandlung von Migräne-Patienten mit Cinnarizin and Flunarizin. *Med. Welt*, **31**, 1870-1872. (1980)

Gelmers, H.J. Nimodipine, a new calcium antagonist, in the prophylactic treatment of migraine. *Headache*, **23**, 106-109. (1983)

Havanka-Kanniainen, H., Myllylä, V.V., Hokkanen, E. Nimodipine in the prophylaxis of migraine, a double-blind study. *Acta Neurol. Scand.*, **65** (Suppl. 90), 77-78. (1982)

Kahan, A., Weber, S., Amor, B., Guerin, F., Degeorges, M. Nifedipine in the treatment of migraine in patients with Raynaud's phenomenon. *N. Engl. J. Med.*, **308**, 1102-1103. (1983)

Louis, P. A double-blind placebo-controlled prophylactic study of flunarizine (**Sibelium**) in migraine. *Headache*, **21**, 235-239. (1981)

Louis, P., Spierings, E.L.H. Comparison of flunarizine (**Sibelium**) and pizotifen (**Sandomigran**) in migraine treatment: a double-blind study. *Cephalalgia*, **2**, 197-203. (1982)

Selmaj, K., Durko, A., Guszcz-Zielinska, A., Szymanska, R., Sykulski, J. Failure of nifedipine in migraine prophylaxis. Personal communication. (1983)

Solomon, G.D., Steel, J.G., Spaccavento, L.J. Migraine prophylaxis with verapamil - a preliminary report. *Headache*, **23**, 139. (1983)

Chapter V:

Calcium entry blockers
in hypertension treatment

Double-blind comparison of the antihypertensive effects of verapamil and nifedipine

K. Midtbø, O. Hals, J. van der Meer,
L. Storstein and K.-D. Rämsch

Summary

It may be concluded that both verapamil and nifedipine are efficient antihypertensive drugs in mild to moderate essential hypertension. The effect is maintained, possibly increased, for at least up to 6 weeks of treatment. Heart rate is reduced by verapamil and insignificantly increased by nifedipine. On the actual doses, side effects are mainly moderate and transient and decrease with time. Determination of plasma concentration of verapamil and nifedipine may be valuable when poor patient compliance, interaction with other drugs or accumulation are suspected. In the case of poor therapeutic response drug plasma concentration values may be important before increasing the dose.

Résumé

On peut conclure que tant le vérapamil que la nifédipine sont des substances antihypertensives efficaces dans l'hypertension essentielle faible à modérée. L'effet est maintenu, éventuellement accru, pendant au moins 6 semaines de traitement. La fréquence cardiaque diminue sous l'effet du vérapamil et augmente de façon non significative sous l'effet de la nifédipine. Aux doses utilisées, les effets secondaires sont principalement modérés et passagers et diminuent avec le temps. La détermination de la concentration plasmatique du vérapamil et de la nifédipine peut être utile lorsqu'on suspecte une faible compléance de la part du patient, une interaction avec d'autres substances ou une accumulation. Dans le cas d'une réaction thérapeutique faible, il peut être important de connaître les valeurs de la concentration plasmatique de la substance avant d'augmenter la dose.

Resumen

Se puede concluir que ambos verapamilo y nifedipino son eficaces en el tratamiento de la hipertensión esencial ligera a moderada. El efecto sigue mantenido, posiblemente aumentado, durante, por lo menos, seis semanas de tratamiento. La frecuencia cardíaca se reduce con verapamilo y se aumenta de manera insignificante con nifedipino. Con las dosis actuales, los efectos secundarios son sobre todo moderados y pasajeros y disminuyen con el tiempo. La determinación de la concentración plasmática de verapamilo y nifedipino puede ser valiosa cuando se sospechan una toma del medicamento irregular por parte del patiente, interacción con otras drogas o acumulación. En el caso de poca respuesta terapéutica el control de la concentración plasmática de la droga puede ser importante antes de aumentar la dosis.

Zusammenfassung

Sowohl Verapamil als auch Nifedipin sind bei leichter bis mäßiger Hypertonie wirkungsvolle Antihypertonika. Die Wirkung bleibt während sechswöchiger Behandlung erhalten bzw. steigt an. Die Herzfrequenz wird durch Verapamil verringert, während sie nach Nifedipin nichtsignifikant ansteigt. Bei den üblichen Dosen sind die Nebenwirkungen meist mäßiger und vorübergehender Art und nehmen allmählich ab. Bei ungenügender Patientenzuverlässigkeit, Wechselwirkung mit anderen Arzneimitteln oder Akkumulation kann die Bestimmung der Konzentration von Verapamil und Nifedipin im Plasma nützlich sein. Auch im Falle eines mangelhaften Therapieresultates können Plasmakonzentrationswerte vor einer Steigerung der Dosis nützlich sein.

Introduction

The calcium ions play a central role in the regulation of blood pressure (Lederballe Pedersen, 1981, Aoki et al., 1976), and perhaps a causal role in high blood pressure (Aoki et al., 1976, Postnov et al., 1979).

The hypothesis that pathological cellular handling of calcium may be a mechanism underlying essential hypertension has by now considerable experimental support (Aoki et al., 1976, Noon et al., 1978).

If this is the case the calcium blockers may be a specific approach to the treatment of . high blood pressure.

The hypotensive action of the calcium blockers verapamil and nifedipine is well documented (de Leeuw et al., 1981; Lederballe Pedersen and Mikkelsen, 1978).

However, direct comparisons of the two drugs in the treatment of hypertension have been done in small groups of patients only and for short periods (Lewis et al., 1981, Muiesan et al., 1981). In these studies the agents had an equipotent hypotensive effect, but side effects were much more pronounced in patients taking nifedipine.

The present controlled study compares verapamil and nifedipine in a group of patients with essential hypertension treated for periods of 6 weeks with special attention to side effects.

Patients and methods

We studied 28 patients — aged 30-64 years, mean age 53 — with mild to moderate essential hypertension, having secondary hypertension excluded.

Twenty-one patients had been treated medicamentally prior to the study and previous drugs were mainly beta-blockers. Except for 2 the patients had been satisfactorily controlled on existing medication.

The selection criterion was diastolic blood pressure $\geqq$ 100 mg Hg at the end of the pretreatment period. The usual exclusion criteria for verapamil and nifedipine were used (Opie, 1980).

All antihypertensive medication was stopped, — beta-blockers gradually over one week — and after a pretreatment period of at least 2 weeks with no medication the patients were selected for the study. They were now randomized and allocated to a double-blind cross-over trial including 2 periods of 6 weeks each during which they were given verapamil 160 mg (Isoptin "Knoll", tablets of 80 mg) three times daily or nifedipine 20 mg (Adalat "Bayer", slow release tablets of 20 mg) twice daily in a fixed-dose regimen. A double dummy method was used. In order to enhance patients compliance, the tablets were dispensed into boxes (dosettes) divided in daily doses and containing medication for one week each.

Blood pressure and heart rate were measured after 3 minutes in supine, sitting and standing positions by the same observer and at the same time of day, at the end of the pretreatment period and every second week throughout the trial. The mean values of 3 measurements were recorded in each position.

At the end of the pretreatment period and at the end of both treatment periods a 12-lead ECG was recorded, body weight registered and the following lab-tests determined: serum electrolytes (Na, Cl and K), liver function tests, serum creatinine and serum lipoproteins (HDL-cholesterol, total cholesterol and triglycerides).

During both treatment periods plasma concentrations of verapamil, the active metabolite nor-verapamil and nifedipine were determined. For verapamil a high-pressure liquid chromatographic method (Harapat and Kates, 1979) was used. Nifedipine was analysed with a gaschromatographic method (Rämsch, 1979). Side effects were asked for and registered at fortnightly intervals. Immediately after the study was finished the patients were asked to make a global evaluation of which treatment period they preferred. The data were statistically analysed with the paired t-test and in addition a computerized procedure was used for a multivariate linear modelling of the blood pressure data.

Results shown in tables and figures are mean values ± standard deviations.

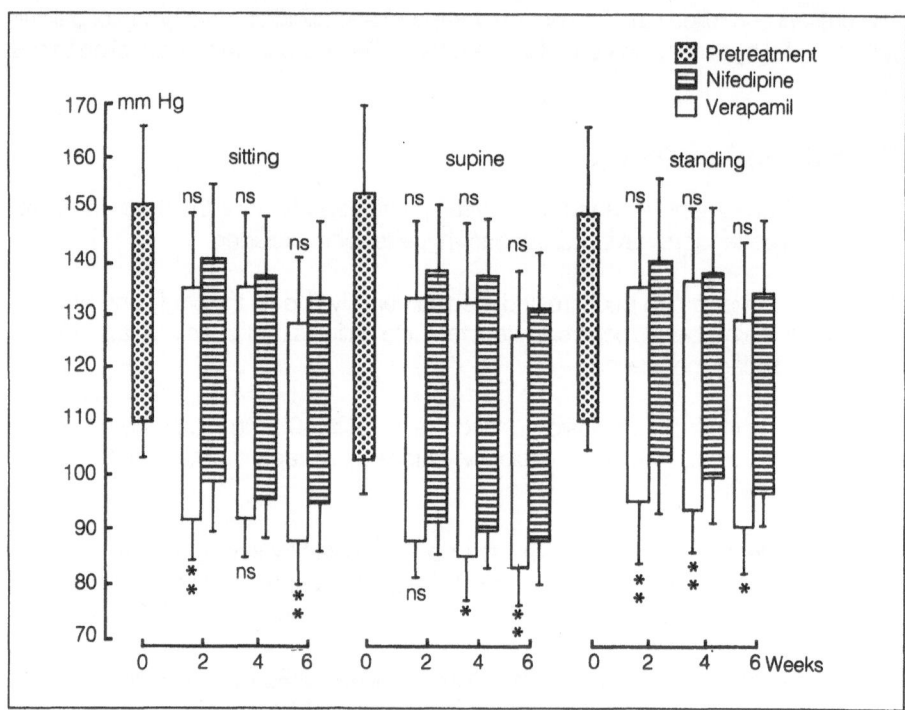

Figure 1: Mean systolic and diastolic blood pressure in patients in the sitting, supine and standing positions before treatment and after 2, 4 and 6 weeks of treatment with verapamil and with nifedipine. The indication of significance (ns = not significant; * = p ≤ 0,05; * = p ≤ 0,01) refers to the mean differences between verapamil and nifedipine.

Results

Two patients, one in each group of drug, were withdrawn because of serious side effects, i.e. 26 patients completed the trial. The results of the blood pressure part of the study is shown in figure 1 and table 1. Treatment with verapamil resulted in a highly significant reduction of mean systolic and diastolic blood pressure in all positions after 2, 4 and 6 weeks (all p-values < 0.001 with both statistical methods). Nifedipine reduced diastolic blood pressure significantly in all positions (all p-values < 0.001) after 2 weeks and increased this effect from 2 to 6 weeks. Standing systolic pressure was not significantly reduced by nifedipine after 2 weeks, but in the other positions, and after 4 and 6 weeks standing, all systolic pressures were significantly lowered by nifedipine.

Table 1: Mean values of supine, sitting, and standing blood pressure (mm Hg) together before treatment, after 6 weeks of treatment with nifedipine, and after 6 weeks of treatment with verapamil.

	Pretreatment	Nifedipine	Verapamil
Systolic blood pressure	149 ± 13	133 ± 12	128 ± 13
Diastolic blood pressure	107 ± 5	93 ± 8	87 ± 8

(n = 26)

Neither drug produced any rebound rise or carry over effect on blood pressure. For both drugs the hypotensive action increased throughout the periods.

However, none of the observed mean differences between blood pressure after 2 weeks and 6 weeks was statistically significant, except for standing blood pressure during nifedipine.

Mean diastolic blood pressure was significantly more reduced by verapamil than by nifedipine in all positions ($p < 0.05$ and < 0.01, see fig. 1. For mean of the whole treatment period $p < 0.001$ for all positions).

In 5 patients (19%) nifedipine had no significant effect on either systolic or diastolic pressure, 4 of these having favourable effect from verapamil. During verapamil 2 patients (= 8%) had hardly any reduction of systolic blood pressure and one had no diastolic lowering.

After 6 weeks of treatment diastolic blood pressure was still greater than 95 mm in 12 patients (= 43%) in the nifedipine group and in 5 patients (= 19%) treated with verapamil. These patients would probably have benefited from a higher dose or an additional drug.

There was no significant correlation between pretreatment blood pressure levels and pressure reduction by any of the agents.

The lesser hypotensive effect achieved with nifedipine than with verapamil in the present study, may partly be due to the slow-release nifedipine preparation tested in this trial, probably resulting in dose intervals that were too long and/or the total daily quantity of 40 mg nifedipine may have been inadequate in some patients.

Mean heart rate was significantly decreased by verapamil compared with pretreatment values (see table 2).

Table 2: Mean heart rates (min $^{-1}$) in the different positions before treatment and during the treatment periods with nifedipine and with verapamil.

		Nifedipine			Verapamil		
	Pretreatment	2 weeks	4 weeks	6 weeks	2 weeks	4 weeks	6 weeks
Supine	67 ± 6	70 ± 9	69 ± 8	68 ± 9	63 ± 8	61 ± 6	61 ± 7
Sitting	69 ± 6	74 ± 9	70 ± 8	71 ± 8	66 ± 8	63 ± 6	65 ± 7
Standing	74 ± 7	78 ± 9	77 ± 8	77 ± 9	70 ± 8	68 ± 8	71 ± 8

(n = 26)

Nifedipine produced no significant effect on heart rate compared with pretreatment, but increased heart rate significantly compared with verapamil ($p < 0.001$ for mean of the whole treatment period). This difference in heart rate was less pronounced at the end of the treatment periods. The demonstrated heart rate response may support the hypothesis of gradually decreasing sympathetic tone during long-term nifedipine treatment (Lederballe Pedersen, 1981).

Neither verapamil nor nifedipine changed the levels of serum lipoproteins. A slight rise of HDL-cholesterol during verapamil was observed. Liver function tests, serum electrolytes and serum creatinine were not significantly affected by either drug.

Fluid retention has been reported to be a problem in long-term treatment with nifedipine (Lederballe Pedersen, 1981). None of our patients had significant increase in body weight.

Nifedipine did not affect AV-conduction significantly, but mean PQ-time was significantly prolonged by verapamil compared with both pretreatment and nifedipine, although the maximum PQ-time measured was only 0,22 seconds. It should be noted that in one of our nifedipine patients PQ-time increased from 0.18 to 0.22 sec. with unchanged heart rate.

The pharmacokinetic/-dynamic part of the study will be detailed in a separate report (Storstein et al.). A wide scatter of maximum plasma concentrations was observed, probably owing to considerable interindividual first pass metabolism of the drugs (Opie, 1980).

We found mean maximum plasma concentration of verapamil after one hour and for nifedipine after two hours, following the morning dose during chronic treatment. Blood pressure was significantly reduced with both drugs one hour after the morning dose compared with pre-dose pressure.

There was no significant correlation between blood pressure reduction and plasma concentration of either drug.

One patient developed SA-block after 7 days on verapamil but was unaffected by nifedipine. After withdrawal of verapamil he recovered promptly. This patient turned out to have a moderate renal failure and should have been excluded from the trial.

Another patient had to be withdrawn because of increasing intolerable tiredness and dizziness during 3 weeks on nifedipine, but had no discomfort during verapamil treatment.

This list of side effects (see table 3) may seem impressive, but, except for the withdrawn patients, the side effects were, however, mainly mild and temporary and decreasing during treatment. The dominating adverse reactions were light to moderate constipation with verapamil and initial headache during nifedipine treatment. It is noteworthy that altogether 8 patients (V: 3, N: 5) reported increased urination (diuresis?) during the first days of treatment. This could have been caused by increased natriuresis as reported previously (Zanchetti, 1981), but unfortunately this was not studied in detail. Having finished the trial, the majority of the patients had no period preference, while 6 against one preferred verapamil.

Table 3: Side effects.

	Nifedipine	Verapamil
Headache	11	2
Constipation	4	9
Increased urination	5	3
Flushing	3	2
Fatigue	3	2
alpitations	2	2
Dizziness	3	0
Urticaria	0	1
Sinoatrial block	0	1

Acknowledgement

The authors wish to acknowledge Vera Haakenstad for her valuable help in the preparation of this manuscript.

References

Aoki, K., Yamashita, K., Suzuki, A. et al. Uptake of calcium ions by sarcoplasmic reticulum from heart and arterial smooth muscle in the spontaneously hypertensive rat (SHR). *Clin. Exp. Pharmacol. Physiol.*, **Suppl. 3**, 27 (1976).

de Leeuw, P.W., Smout, A.J.P.M., Willemse, P.J., Birkenhäger, W.H. Effects of verapamil in hypertensive patients. In: Zanchetti, A., Krikler, D.M., eds. Calcium antagonism in cardiovascular therapy. Experience with verapamil 1980. Amsterdam, Oxford, Princeton: Excerpta Medica, 222 (1981).

Doyle, A.E., Anavekar, S.N., Oliver, L.E. A clinical trial of verapamil in the treatment of hypertension. In: Zanchetti, A., Krikler, D.M., eds. Calcium antagonism in cardiovascular therapy. Experience with verapamil 1980. Amsterdam, Oxford, Princeton: Excerpta Medica, 252 (1981).

Guazzi, M.D., Fiorintini, C., Olivari, M.T. Short- and long-term efficacy of a calcium-antagonistic agent (nifedipine) combined with methyldopa in the treatment of severe hypertension. *Circulation*, **61**, 913 (1980).

Harapat, S.R., Kates, R.E. Rapid high-pressure liquid chromatographic analysis of verapamil in blood and plasma. *J. Chromatog.*, **170**, 385 (1979).

Lederballe Pedersen, O., Mikkelsen, E. Acute and chronic effects of nifedipine in arterial hypertension. *Europ. J. Clin. Pharmacol.*, **14**, 375 (1978).

Lederballe Pedersen, O. Calcium blockade as a therapeutic principle in arterial hypertension. *Acta Pharmacol. Toxicol.*, **49** (Suppl. II), 1 (1981).

Lewis, G.R.J., Morley, K.D., Lewis, B.M., Bones, P.J. The treatment of hypertension with verapamil. *N. Zeal. J. Med.*, **87**, 351 (1978).

Lewis, G.R.J., Stewart, D.J., Lewis, B.M., Bones, P.J., Morley, K.D., Janus, E.D. The antihypertensive effect of oral verapamil — acute and long-term administrations and its effects on the high-density lipoprotein values in plasma. In: Zanchetti, A., Krikler, D.M., eds. Calcium antagonism in cardiovascular therapy. Experience with verapamil 1980. Amsterdam, Oxford, Princeton: Excerpta Medica, 270 (1981).

Midtbø, K., Hals, O. Verapamil in the treatment of hypertension. *Curr. Therap. Res.*, **27**, 830 (1980).

Muiesan, G., Agabiti-Rosei, E., Alicandri, C. et al. Influence of verapamil on catecholamines, renin and aldosterone in essential hypertensive patients. In: Zanchetti, A., Krikler, D.M., eds. Calcium antagonism in cardiovascular therapy. Experience with verapamil 1980. Amsterdam, Oxford, Princeton: Excerpta Medica, 238 (1981).

Noon, J.P., Rice, P.J., Baldessarini, R.J. Calcium leakage as a cause of the high resting tension in vascular smooth muscle from the spontaneously hypertensive rat. *Proc. Natl. Acad. Sci. U.S.A.*, **75**, 1605 (1978).

Olivari, M.T., Bartorelli, C., Polese, A. Treatment of hypertension with nifedipine, a calcium antagonistic agent. *Circulation*, **59**, 1056 (1979).

Opie, L.H. Drugs and the heart III: Calcium antagonists. *Lancet*, **1**, 806 (1980).

Postnov, Y.V., Orlov, S.N., Pokudin, N.I. Decrease of calcium binding by the red blood cell membrane in spontaneously hypertensive rat and in essential hypertension. *Pflügers Arch.*, **379**, 191 (1979).

Rämsch, K.D. Nifedipine: detection in blood plasma by gas chromatography following administration of therapeutic doses. Pharma Report no. 8773 and methodological appendix HP/Rä, Bayer AG, Wupperthal (1979).

Storstein, L., Midtbø, K., Hals, O., van der Meer, J., Rämsch, K. A comparative study of the antihypertensive effects of verapamil and nifedipine in relation to plasma concentrations of the drugs. In preparation for publication.

Zanchetti, A. Perspectives in antihypertensive treatment. In: Zanchetti, A., Krikler, D.M., eds. Calcium antagonism in cardiovascular therapy. Experience with verapamil 1980. Amsterdam, Oxford, Princeton: Excerpta Medica, 292 (1981).

Treatment of hypertension emergencies and chronic arterial hypertension with calcium entry blockers

W. Klein

Summary

Vasodilators may lead to reflex activation of the sympathetic nervous system and the renin-angiotensin-aldosteron system and fluid retention when used as a monotherapy. Calcium antagonists do have some significant advantages over other vasodilators justifying their use in hypertension treatment and add another group of drugs to all those already available on the market.

Résumé

Les vasodilatateurs peuvent conduire à une activation réflexe du système nerveux sympathique et du système rénine-angiotensine ainsi que de la rétention de liquide, lorsqu'utilisés en monothérapie. Les antagonistes de calcium présentent certains avantages significatifs par rapport à d'autres vasodilatateurs, ce qui justifie leur utilisation dans le traitement de l'hypertension et apportent un nouveau groupe de substances venant s'ajouter à toutes celles déjà existantes sur le marche.

Resumen

Vasodilatadores pueden conducir a la activación refleja del sistema nervioso simpático y del sistema renina-angiotensina-aldosterona y de la retención fluida, cuando se usan como una monoterapia. Antagonistas de calcio tienen sin duda importantes ventajas comparados con otros vasodilatadores, y esto justifica su uso en el tratamiento de la hipertensión. Añaden otro grupo de drogas a todos los otros que ya están disponibles en el mercado.

Zusammenfassung

Vasodilatatoren können als Monotherapie zur Aktivierung der Reflexe des sympathischen Nervensystems und des Renin-Angiotensin-Aldosteron-Systems, ebenso wie zu Flüssigkeitsretention führen. Kalziumantagonisten haben im Vergleich zu anderen Vasodilatatoren bedeutende Vorteile, die ihren Gebrauch bei Hypertonie rechtfertigen. Sie bedeuten eine Bereicherung der schon bestehenden Palette um eine weitere Arzneimittelgruppe.

Calcium antagonists have been extensively used in the treatment of supraventricular arrhythmias and vasospastic as well as stable effort angina.

By impairing calcium ion entry into the cell during depolarization calcium blockers decrease the strength of contraction of cardiac and smooth muscle, the latter producing peripheral vasodilatation.

Since the principal hemodynamic abnormality in hypertension is an increase in peripheral resistance, use of drugs which lower peripheral vascular resistance by a direct action on arteriolar smooth muscle is rational. Calcium blockers therefore should be effective in the treatment of high blood pressure.

Hemodynamic studies in 6 patients with hypertensive emergencies show a significant reduction of systolic (- 26%) and diastolic (- 47%) blood pressure after 20 mg nifedipine sublingually due to a vigorous drop of peripheral resistance (- 45%), while cardiac output is increased (+ 15%). Pulmonary vascular resistance is also reduced (- 20%), heart rate and stroke volume reveal a different behavior depending of the functional status of the myocardium.

Nifedipine has some advantages over other calcium antagonists in the treatment of hypertensive crises: it can be administered sublingually with a very rapid onset of action, the effect lasting for several hours and it may be also used in hypertensive emergencies complicated by acute left heart failure.

A double-blind, placebo-controlled comparison between diltiazem and nifedipine in mild to moderate chronic essential hypertension reveals a responder-rate of 80% for both drugs. Diastolic blood pressure is lowered at rest and during exercise by 10-15%, systolic blood pressure is only reduced at rest. Heart rate is not changed significantly after nifedipine, but is decreased with diltiazem.

As a part of the study, in 20 consecutive patients hemodynamics were measured during rest and bicycle ergometry by means of a Swan-Ganz-Thermodilution catheter and blood samples were taken for analysis of adrenaline, noradrenaline and dopamine. Catecholamine concentrations were measured radioenzymatically.

Both drugs lead to a decrease of peripheral resistance by 20% at rest and 30% during work; as a consequence of afterload reduction, cardiac output, stroke index and stroke work index increase by 17%, 21% and 7% with nifedipine and by 34%, 26% and 20% with diltiazem. During exercise these changes are even more pronounced. Pulmonary artery pressures, however, and pulmonary vascular resistance are reduced only by nifedipine, not by diltiazem.

Adrenaline and dopamine changes during therapy were not significant, plasma noradrenaline increased more under nifedipine (+ 41%) than under diltiazem (+ 23%). Statistically, only the increase after nifedipine at rest was significant ($P < 0.05$).

In the nifedipine-group 6/24 patients experienced side effects (headache, sweating, tremor, giddiness, peripheral edema). In 2 patients the dosage had to be reduced for relief of symptoms.

In the diltiazem-group 4/23 patients had symptoms (headache, palpitations, drowsiness, gastric pain), but in no instance the medication had to be stopped or reduced. There were no side effects on the electrocardiogram.

Nifedipine therapy usually is associated with a reflex activation of the sympathetic nervous system with increase of plasma norepinephrine concentration and sometimes tachycardia. With diltiazem, side effects due to vasodilatation like tachycardia, increase of plasma norepinephrine and fluid retention are less.

In the treatment of chronic arterial hypertension therefore diltiazem seems to be superior to nifedipine because of lesser side effects.

At present, the usual approach to the treatment of hypertension includes diuretics and/or betablockers and/or vasodilators. The hemodynamic pattern characteristic of established essential hypertension is represented by an unchanged cardiac output with augmented vascular resistance, this derangement being present at rest and during exercise. It is interesting that the two classes of drugs that, because of the paucity of their side effects, are generally classified as first choice in antihypertensive treatment, namely diuretics and betablockers, reduce blood pressure acutely by lowering cardiac output rather than peripheral resistance.

Despite the physiological rationale of their use in a disease like hypertension, which is characterized by vasoconstriction, peripheral vasodilators are still relegated to the upper steps of the antihypertensive staircase, and for good reasons. Vasodilators may lead to reflex activation of the sympathetic nervous system and the renin-angiotensin-aldosteron system and fluid retention when used as a monotherapy.

Calcium antagonists do have some significant advantages over other vasodilators justifying their use in hypertension treatment and add another group of drugs to all those already available on the market. 1. They have obviously less side effects than other hypotensive drugs, 2. they reduce only the elevated, but not the normal blood pressure avoiding overdosage-effects and hypotension, 3. they treat hypertension associated heart failure by increasing cardiac output, 4. they are effective also in coronary heart disease and peripheral vascular disease which are often combined with hypertension and 5. there are preliminary observations that calcium blockers cause a regression of left ventricular hypertrophy in this condition.

The effect of nifedipine on arterial pressure and reflex cardiac control

W. A. Littler

Summary

Nine patients with untreated, essential hypertension (mean casual BP 173/109 ± 14/7 mmHg) were studied in the control state and then following 16 weeks treatment with nifedipine 10 mg orally 8 hourly. Direct arterial blood pressure, monitored continuously over 24 hours, demonstrated that nifedipine significantly reduced systolic and diastolic blood pressure throughout the day and the night. The variability of blood pressure was not altered by nifedipine therapy. There was no significant change in heart rate after nifedipine therapy.

Chronic nifedipine therapy was associated with an increase in forearm blood flow and a decrease in forearm vascular resistance consistent with its action as a vasodilator. There was a reduction in the absolute blood pressure responses to tilt, handgrip and cold but the percentage increase in pressure was not altered by therapy. Plasma renin activity was unaltered by chronic nifedipine therapy.

The sensitivity and setting of the baroreflex response to intravenous phenylephrine was measured. Following chronic nifedipine therapy there was re-setting of the sino-aortic baroreflex and an increase in its sensitivity.

Finally, successful control of blood pressure with nifedipine led to a significant reduction in the left ventricular mass index of these patients.

Résumé

Neuf patients présentant une hypertension essentielle non traitée (173/109 ± 14/7 mm Hg) ont été étudiés lors de la phase de contrôle et après 16 semaines de traitement par la nifédipine à raison d'une dose de 10 mg administrée par voie orale toutes les 8 heures. La tension artérielle directe, contrôlée de façon continue pendant 24 heures, a démontré que la nifédipine réduisait significativement la tension artérielle systolique et diastolique pendant le jour et la nuit. La variabilité de la tension artérielle n'était pas modifiée suite au traitement par la nifédipine. On n'a pas relevé de changement significatif de la fréquence cardiaque après le traitement par la nifédipine.

Le traitement chronique par la nifédipine était associé à une augmentation de la circulation sanguine dans l'avant-bras et une diminution de la résistance vasculaire dans l'avant-bras conformément à son action en tant que vasodilatateur. Il y avait diminution des réactions absolues de la tension artérielle au changement de position, à la poignée de main et au froid mais le pourcentage d'augmentation de la tension n'était pas modifié suite au traitement. L'activité de la rénine plasmatique était inchangée suite au traitement chronique par la nifédipine.

La sensibilité et l'ajustage de la réaction baroréflexe à la phényléphrine ont été mesurés. Après le traitement chronique par la nifédipine, il y avait un réajustement du baroréflexe sino-aortique et une augmentation de sa sensibilité.

Enfin, un contrôle satisfaisant de la tension artérielle par la nifédipine a conduit à une réduction significative de l'indice de masse ventriculaire gauche chez ces patients.

Resumen

Se ha estudiado a nueve pacientes sin tratamiento previo con hipertensión esencial durante el estado de control (promedio de 173/109 ± 14/7 mm Hg) y después durante un tratamiento de 16 semanas con nifedipino 10 mg por vía oral cada 8 horas. Se controlaba continuamente la presión arterial directa de la sangre durante 24 horas y se comprobó que nifedipino reducía de manera significativa la presión sanguínea sistólica y diastólica, tanto de día como de noche. La variabilidad de la presión sanguínea no sufrió alteración por el tratamiento con nifedipino. Tampoco se dio cambio significativo del ritmo cardíaco después del tratamiento con nifedipino.

El tratamiento crónico iba acompañado de un incremento del flujo sanguíneo en el antebrazo mostrando su acción vasodilatadora. Hubo una reducción en la amplitud de las reacciones de la presión sanguínea provocadas por inclinación, apretón de manos y frío, pero la modificación proporcional de la presión no cambió. La actividad renina del plasma no fue alterada por la terapia crónica con nifedipino.

Mediante inyecciones intravenosas de fenilefrina se midió el nivel de la presión arterial que causó una respuesta baroreflexiva y la sensibilidad de esta respuesta. La terapia crónica con nifedipino cambió el nivel de reacción del baroreflejo sino-aórtico y aumentó su sensibilidad.

Finalmente, el control adecuado de la presión sanguínea con nifedipino condujo a una reducción significativa en el índice de la masa ventricular en estos pacientes.

Zusammenfassung

Neun Patienten mit unbehandeltem essentiellem Hochdruck bei einem mittleren Blutdruck von 173/109 ± 14/7 mmHg wurden vor und nach einer 16wöchigen Behandlung mit 10 mg Nifedipin, das aller acht Stunden oral verabreicht wurde, untersucht. Direkte Messungen des arteriellen Blutdrucks, die laufend über 24 Stunden durchgeführt wurden, zeigten, daß Nifedipin den systolischen sowie den diastolischen Blutdruck Tag und Nacht bedeutend herabsetzt. Die Variabilität des Blutdrucks wurde durch die Nifedipinbehandlung nicht bedeutend beeinflußt. Auch die Herzfrequenz zeigte nach Nifedipin keine erhebliche Veränderung.

Bei chronischer Behandlung mit Nifedipin wurde, seiner Wirkung als Vasodilatator entsprechend, eine erhöhte Durchblutung bei erniedrigtem Gefäßwiderstand im Unterarm beobachtet. Die absoluten Blutdruckwerte bei geneigter Lage, Handgriffübung und Kälte sanken ab, jedoch wurde der prozentuale Blutdruckanstieg durch die Behandlung nicht beeinflusst. Die Plasma-Renin-Aktivität blieb unverändert. Die Empfindlichkeit und Regulierung des Baroreflexes bei intravenöser Gabe von Phenylephrin wurden gemessen. Chronische Nifedipingabe resultierte in einer veränderten Regulation und einer erhöhten Empfindlichkeit des sinoaortischen Baroreflexes.

Schließlich ergab eine erfolgreiche Blutdruckregulierung mit Nifedipin eine bedeutende Erniedrigung des linksventrikulären Massenindex.

Nifedipine belongs to the group of drugs known as calcium antagonists. These drugs are vasodilators and have proved useful agents in the short-term treatment of both moderate and severe hypertension. However, the evidence for the hypotensive activity of nifedipine is limited and the mechanism and mode of action of blood pressure reduction remains uncertain.

We have measured the effect of nifedipine therapy alone on direct arterial pressure and its variability in hypertensive patients and have examined the effect of the drug on forearm blood flow and resistance, sino-aortic baroreflex activity, the responses to tilt, isometric exercise and cold and the renin-angiotensin system.

Patients and methods

Nine patients (7 male, 2 female) with an average casual blood pressure greater than 160 mmHg systolic and 95 mmHg diastolic on at least three separate occasions over a period of one month or more were studied. The mean casual blood pressure ± 1 SD for the group was 173 ± 14/109 ± 7 mmHg. The mean age was 40 years (range 33 to 53 years). No patient had evidence of target organ damage, and none had previously received treatment for their hypertension.

The following investigations were carried out:

1. Ambulatory intra-arterial blood pressure measurement.

2. Forearm blood flow measurement.

3. Plasma renin activity.

4. Upright tilt.

5. Handgrip.

6. Cold pressor.

7. Sino-aortic baroreflex sensitivity.

8. Left ventricular mass.

Protocol

At the completion of the first intra-arterial blood pressure study, each patient was started on nifedipine 10 mg 8 hourly orally and was followed up at two week intervals and then monthly intervals for a period of 16 weeks. The visits were at the same time of day on each occasion. Within these clinic visits symptoms and side-effects were recorded. Compliance was checked by capsule counts. At the end of the treatment period patients were re-studied under identical conditions whilst taking their medication.

Results

1. Casual blood pressure

Casual blood pressure was reduced from 173 ± 14/109 ± 7 mmHg to 138 ± 7/86 ± 6 mmHg after 16 weeks treatment (p < 0.001). Over the same 16 week period the heart rate did not significantly change. Control: 77 ± 13 beats/minute; 16 weeks: 80 ± 19 beats/minute.

2. Intra-arterial pressure

For the whole 24 hour period there was a significant fall in both systolic and diastolic blood pressure (153/98 ± 19/11 mmHg to 133/85 ± 13/8 mmHg, p < 0.001).

3. Heart rate

There was no significant difference in heart rate following nifedipine therapy over a 24 hour period. Control: 80 ± 9 beats/minute; nifedipine: 77 ± 9 beats/minute.

4. Forearm blood flow measurement

There was a significant increase in forearm blood flow coupled with a decrease in arterial pressure leading to a significant reduction in calculated vascular resistance.

5. Response to tilting

In both treated and untreated states there was an increase in diastolic blood pressure on tilting and insignificant rise in systolic pressure. The heart rate also rose after tilting. When the changes in systolic blood pressure, diastolic blood pressure and heart rate from supine control to the tilt-up position at 15 minutes before and after treatment were compared, no significance was found in these responses.

6. Plasma renin activity

Resting and stimulated plasma renin activity was not significantly altered by nifedipine therapy.

7. Sino-aortic baroreflex sensitivity

Mean baroreflex sensitivity was 6.3 ± 3.7 msec/mmHg before treatment and significantly increased to 8.8 ± 4.0 msec/mmHg after treatment (p < 0.05).

8. Left ventricular mass

The left ventricular mass fell significantly from 126.1 ± 31.3 g/m^2 before treatment to 117 ± 27.3 g/m^2 after nifedipine (p < 0.05).

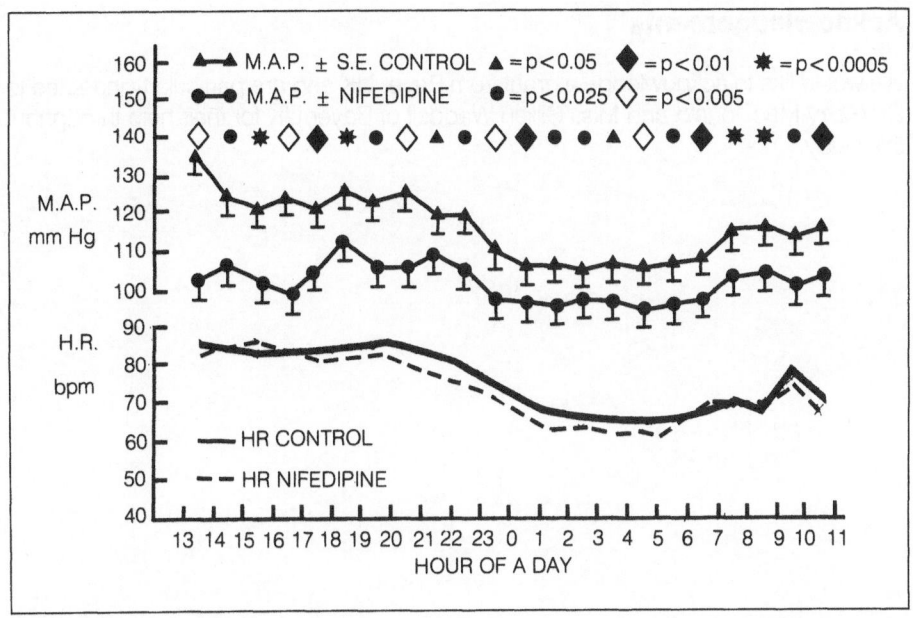

Figure 1: The effect of chronic nifedipine therapy on ambulatory mean arterial pressure (MAP) and heart rate (HR) over 24 hours.

Discussion

Our results have confirmed the hypotensive action of nifedipine when used alone to treat essential hypertension. Our study demonstrates that nifedipine given in a daily dose of 10 mg three times a day significantly reduces blood pressure throughout the day and night. Heart rate did not change significantly after 16 weeks treatment of nifedipine therapy. An understanding of these heart rate changes may come from examination of our baroreflex data. We found that there was a significant change in the set point of the reflex, in that the regression line of systolic blood pressure on R-R interval had shifted to the left. The lowered blood pressure combined with an unchanged heart rate reflects re-setting of the baroreflex so that the regulating mechanism has been re-set to buffer arterial pressure at a lower level. In addition, we have demonstrated an increased sensitivity of the baroreflex heart rate control which means that for any increase in blood pressure there is an increase in reflex cardiac slowing. We suggest that these effects of nifedipine on the baroreflex arc may be due to a direct effect of the drug on the pressor receptors in the carotid sinus and aortic arch. It is likely that relaxation of the smooth muscle elements at these sites could alter the distensibility of the vessel and thus alter the characteristics of the reflex response.

We have observed that there is a reduction in peripheral resistance and increase in forearm blood flow following chronic nifedipine therapy in keeping with the drugs action on vascular smooth muscle with consequent vasodilatation. Finally, our findings with regard to left ventricular mass are compatible with a sustained lowering of blood pressure over the period of study.

303

Acknowledgements

We would like to acknowledge a grant from Bayer UK and are particularly indebted to Dr. Garry MacDonald and Miss Gillian Waddell of Bayer UK for their help throughout this study.

Concluding remarks

Why are Ca²⁺ entry blockers effective in the treatment of hypertension and tissue hypoxia?

P.M. Vanhoutte, M.D.

Summary

The beneficial effects of Ca²⁺ entry blockers in hypertension can be attributed to the prevention of abnormal vasoconstriction and inhibition of myogenic vascular activity in precapillary vessels. The beneficial effects on tissue hypoxia can be attributed to a multiplicity of actions including: antagonism of vasospasms, increase in deformability of red blood cells, and inhibition of intracellular Ca²⁺ accumulation. A potential prophylactic effect on atherosclerosis through reduced endothelium desquamation has to be further investigated.

Résumé

L'effet bénéfique antihypertenseur de certains inhibiteurs de l'entrée de calcium peut être attribué à la prévention d'une vasoconstriction anormale et à l'inhibition de l'activité myogène vasculaire dans les vaisseaux précapillaires. Les effets bénéfiques dans l'hypoxie tissulaire peuvent être attribués à une multiplicité d'actions telles que: antagonisme des vasospasmes, augmentation de la déformabilité des érythrocytes et inhibition de l'accumulation intracellulaire de Ca^{2+}. Un effet prophylactique potentiel dans l'athérosclérose par une diminution de la desquamation endothéliale requiert une étude plus approfondie.

Resumen

La acción benéfica de ciertos inhibidores de la penetración intracelular de Ca^{2+} en la hipertensión puede atribuirse a la prevención de vasoconstricciones anormales y la inhibición de la actividad vascular miogénica en vasos precapilares. Los efectos benéficos en la hipoxia del tejido pueden atribuirse a varias acciones, tales como: antagonismo de vasoespasmos, mejoramiento de la deformabilidad de los eritrocitos e inhibición de la acumulación intracelular de Ca^{2+}. Un potencial efecto profiláctico en la arteriosclerosis basado por la reducción de la descamación endotelial tiene que estudiarse a fondo.

Zusammenfassung

Der günstige Effekt von Ca^{2+}-Blockern bei Hypertonie kann auf die Verhütung abnormer Vasokonstriktion und Hemmung der myogenen Gefässaktivität im präkapillären Bereich zurückgeführt werden. Der günstige Einfluss auf die Gewebehypoxie hängt von einer Vielzahl von Wirkungen ab: Antagonisierung des Vasospasmus, Steigerung der Deformabilität der Erythrozyten und Hemmung der intrazellulären Ca^{2+}-Akkumulation. Der potentielle prophylaktische Effekt bei Arteriosklerose durch Verminderung der Endothelschädigung muss weiter untersucht werden.

The beneficial effect of certain Ca^{2+} entry blockers in the treatment of arterial hypertension is easy to explain, as these substances not only reduce the constriction of precapillary vessels to most naturally occurring neurohumoral mediators but also prevent myogenic activity of vascular smooth muscle. Actually, the latter probably is the most important as calcium entry blockers which are most potent in inhibiting this myogenic activity are also better antihypertensive drugs (see chapters by Casteels, by Godfraind and Miller, by Klein, by Littler, by Midtbo et al., by Van Nueten).

It is more difficult to understand the beneficial effects of the Ca^{2+} entry blockers under hypoxic conditions. In the intact organism, ischemia of peripheral and cerebral tissues occurs mainly when the blood supply becomes inadequate. Except for an inability of the heart to maintain its output resulting in generalized symptoms, ischemia usually is localized and results from a reduction in the diameter of a large artery, under conditions where the collateral circulation is insufficient to meet the demands of the active cells. The beneficial effects of Ca^{2+} entry blockers in the treatment of hypoxic conditions can be explained by the multiplicity of their effects (Fig. 1). If the restriction of blood flow is due only to mechanical factors (atherosclerosis, embolism, external compression), one may predict little therapeutical effect of Ca^{2+} entry blockers; indeed, the vasodilatation they can cause may steal the blood away from underperfused tissues to normally oxygenated vascular beds.

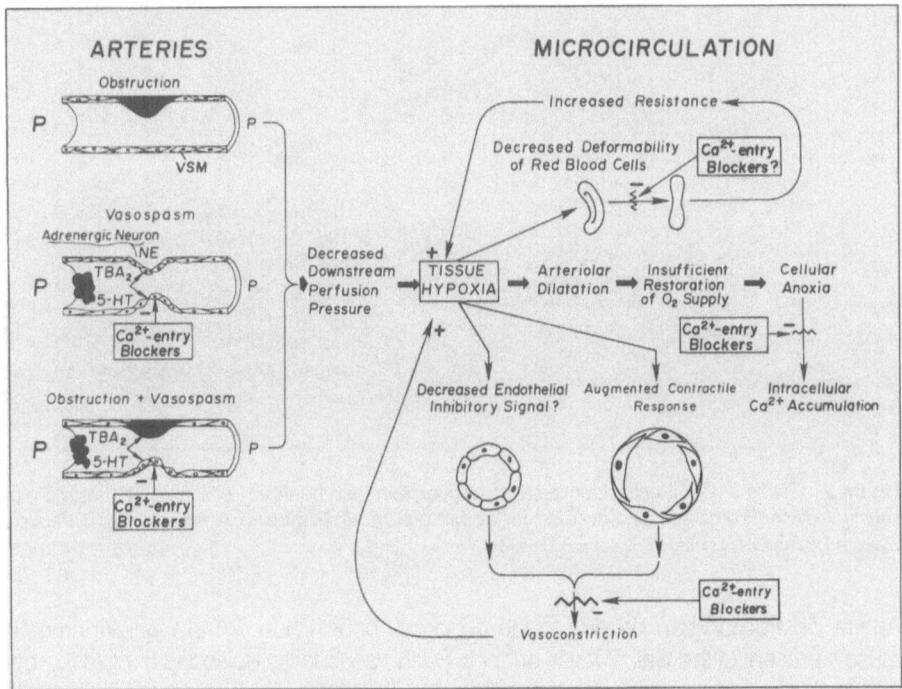

Figure 1: Events leading to and maintaining tissue hypoxia, with indication of the possible sites of action of calcium entry blockers with vasodilator and other properties. P = blood pressure; VSM = vascular smooth muscle; 5-HT = 5-hydroxytryptamine; TBA_2 = thromboxane A_2. (From Vanhoutte, Am. Coll. Clin. Pharmacol., in press, 1983).

However, these compounds may have a potential prophylactic effect on atherosclerosis or reduce its progression as they reduce endothelium-desquamation and can inhibit platelet aggregation, which is known to play a primary role in the genesis of the disease (see chapter by De Clerck and Hladovec). In addition, in the case of patients with angina pectoris the reduction in afterload, due to arteriolar dilatation, and possibly the reduction in preload, due to a selective effect on the splanchnic veins, will reduce the work of the myocardium and thus restore the balance between oxygen demand and supply (Fig. 2; see chapters by Bourassa, by Cohn, by Lichtlen *et al.*, by Van Nueten).

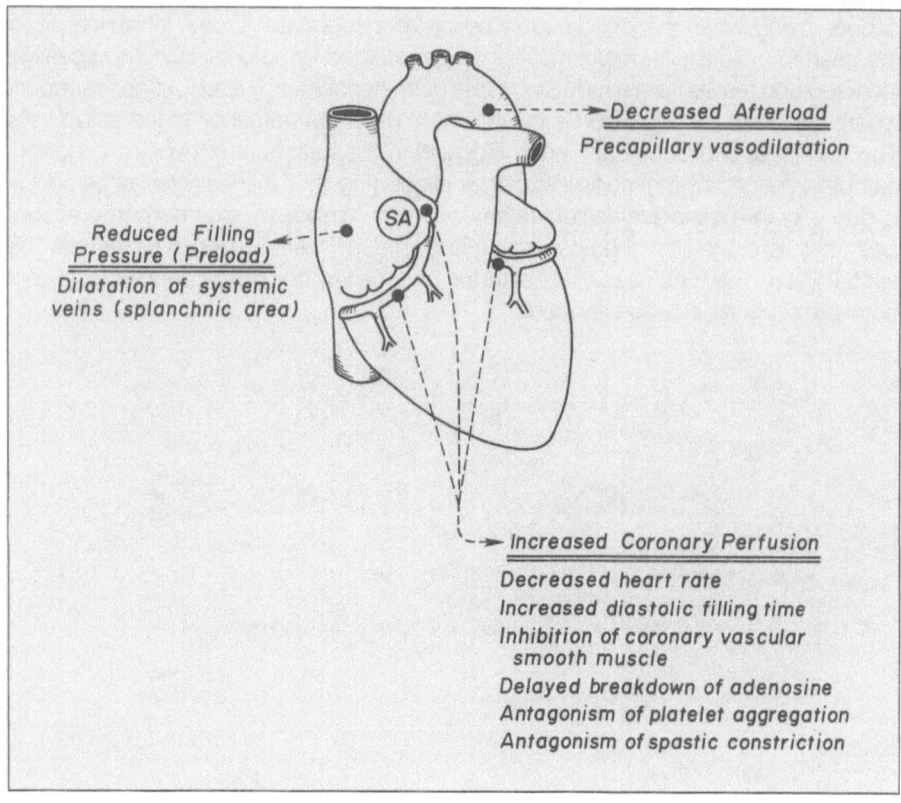

Figure 2: Effects of Ca^{2+} entry blockers that help explain their beneficial effects in the treatment of angina pectoris. (From Vanhoutte, in "Calcium Modulators", ed. T. Godfraind, A. Albertini and R. Paoletti, Elsevier Biomedical Press, 1982, pp. 351-362).

Arterial obstruction can be due to the abnormal constriction of the vascular smooth muscle present in the wall of large arteries. Such vasospastic episodes explain the occurrence of variant angina (see chapters by Bourassa, by Kidner), of Raynaud's disease, of peripheral obliterative arterial disease (see chapter by Di Perri *et al.*) and possibly also of migraine (see chapters by Spierings, by Towart). The exact etiology of vasospasm is unknown and may involve abnormal responsiveness of vascular smooth muscle, exaggerated release of norepinephrine and subsequent activation of postjunctional alpha-adrenoceptors, production of vasoconstrictor autocoids by the tissues or release of substances such as serotonin or thromboxane A_2 from aggregating platelets at sites of endothelial lesions. Whatever the cause of vasospasm may be, it appears that the contraction of smooth muscle cells of large arteries depends mainly on the entry of Ca^{2+} through specific channels in their cell membranes (see chapters by Casteels, by Godfraind and Miller, by Van Nueten). Hence, the beneficial effect of Ca^{2+} entry blockers is easy to understand. If the vasospasm is due to substances released from aggregating platelets, an inhibitory effect on platelet aggregation would contribute (see chapter by De Clerck and Hladovec).

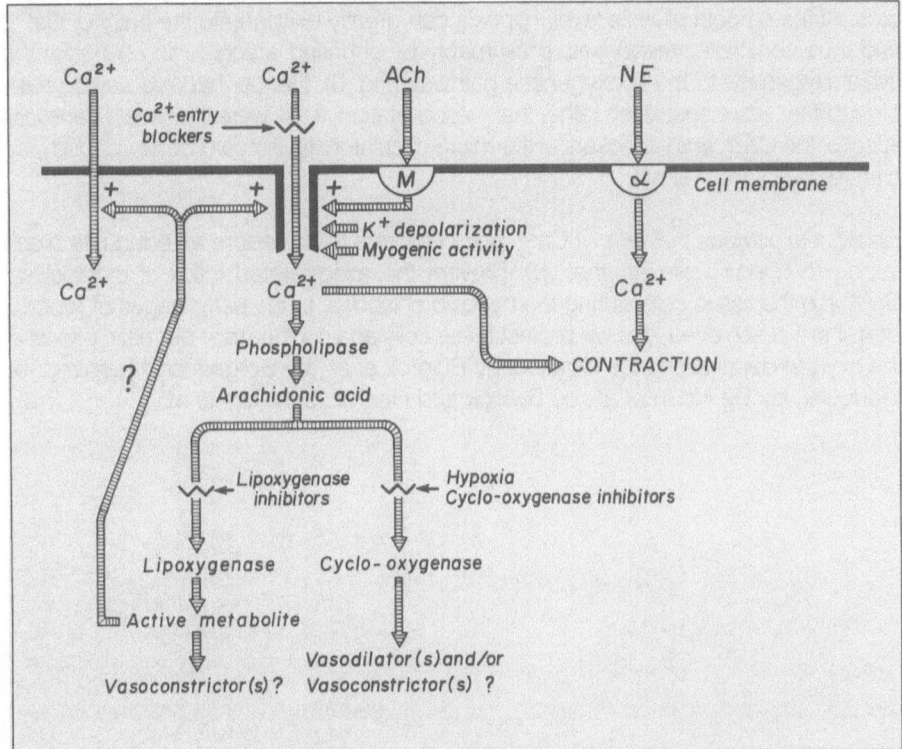

Figure 3: Proposed interaction between calcium entry and arachidonic acid metabolism in canine vascular smooth muscle. In the saphenous vein, contractions induced by acetylcholine (ACh) and potassium (K^+) are inhibited by the calcium entry blockers, but potentiated by inhibitors of cyclo-oxygenase. Contractions induced by norepinephrine (NE) are only moderately reduced by calcium entry blockers and not augmented by inhibitors of cyclo-oxygenase. In the coronary artery, hypoxia inhibits cyclo-oxygenase and induces a contraction that can be inhibited by the calcium entry blockers. Augmentation of the entry of calcium by ACh, K^+ and hypoxia results in activation of phospholipase. The produced arachidonic acid is diverted into the lipoxygenase pathway (when cyclo-oxygenase is inhibited by indomethacin or hypoxia), the products of which in an unknown fashion enhance the entry of calcium through the calcium channel or possibly by acting as a calcium ionophore. M = muscarinic receptor; a = alpha-adrenoceptor; Ca^{2+} = calcium; + = augmentation; ? = unknown. (From Vanhoutte, in "Calcium Modulators", ed. T. Godfraind, A. Albertini and R. Paoletti, Elsevier Biomedical Press, 1982, pp. 351-362).

It is generally admitted that tissue hypoxia causes arteriolar dilatation, an attempt to restore the oxygen supply. However, hypoxia can have several consequences which do not necessarily favor tissue perfusion. Thus, metabolic deprivation reduces red blood cell deformability, which in turn increases the viscosity of the blood, which may increase the local resistance to flow and impair the transport of oxygen at the capillary level; an effect of Ca^{2+} entry blockers to increase red blood cell deformability of hypoxic blood hence would be beneficial (see chapters by De Clerck and Hladovec, by Schatzmann, by Stoltz). Hypoxia may also perturb considerably normal local regulatory mechanisms. For example, it reduces or prevents certain inhibitory signals generated by the endothelial cells, or even triggers vasoconstrictor signals from these cells. At the smooth muscle level, hypoxia can greatly exaggerate the entry of Ca^{2+}, and thus constrictor responses, presumably by shunting arachidonic acid from the cyclo-oxygenase to the lipoxygenase pathway (Fig. 3). Hence, hypoxia could cause precapillary vasoconstriction rather than vasodilatation. If this were the case a beneficial effect of the Ca^{2+} entry blockers at the micro-circulatory level could be envisaged (see chapter by Di Perri et al.).

Finally, it is obvious that even if Ca^{2+} entry blockers fail to restore an adequate blood supply to hypoxic tissues, they will prevent the exaggerated influx of extracellular Ca^{2+} into the tissue cells during the hypoxic episodes. In the early stages of reperfusion, if this is achieved, this will protect these cells against the most dramatic effects of the oxygen deprivation (see chapters by Ruigrok et al., by Borgers and Flameng, by Wauquier, by De Nollin et al., by Bullock and Hearse, by White et al.).

List of authors and co-authors

This list provides the names, academic degrees and addresses of all authors and co-authors. If available, photos are given for the first author of each article as well as for the second author if there are only two of them.

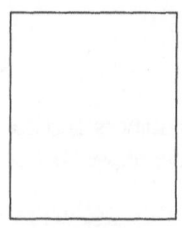

Amende, Ivo,
Division of Cardiology, Hannover Medical School, Hannover, West-Germany.

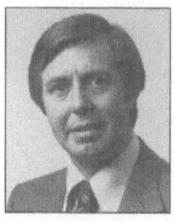

Borgers, Marcel, Dr.
Laboratory of Cell Biology
Janssen Pharmaceutica Research Laboratories
B-2340 Beerse, Belgium

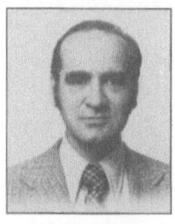

Bourassa, Martial G.,
Montreal Heart Institute,
Montreal, Quebec, Canada.

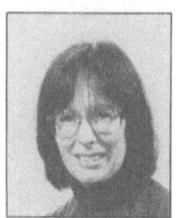

Bullock, Gillian R.,
Research Centre
Ciba-Geigy Pharmaceuticals Division
RH12 4AB Horsham, England

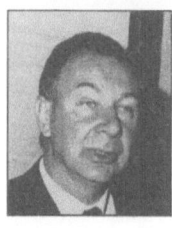

Casteels, Rik,
Professor of Physiology, K.U. Leuven,
Laboratorium voor Fysiologie, Academisch Ziekenhuis Gasthuisberg,
Herestraat 49, B-3000 Leuven, Belgium.

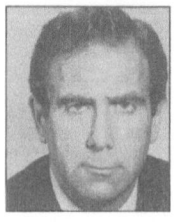

Cohn, Peter F.,
Professor of Medicine and Chief, Cardiology Division
State University of New York
Health Sciences Center
Stony Brook, New York, U.S.A.

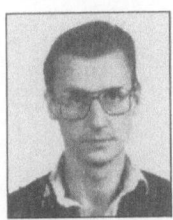

De Clerck, Fred, M. Sc.
Laboratory of Haematology,
Janssen Pharmaceutica Research Laboratories,
B-2340 Beerse, Belgium

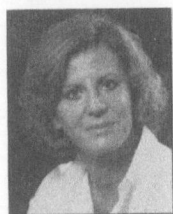

De Nollin, Sonja, Ph. D.
University of Antwerp, UIA, Dept. of Medicine,
Universiteitsplein 1, B-2610 Wilrijk, Belgium.

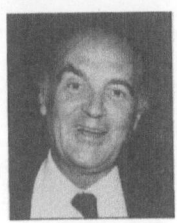

Di Perri, Tullio, M.D.
Istituto di Patologia Medica
e Metodologia Clinica
University of Siena
53100 Siena, Italy

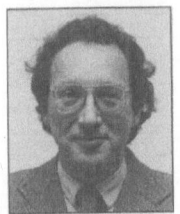

Flameng, Willem, M.D.
Professor, K.U. Leuven
Department of Cardiovascular Surgery
Academisch Ziekenhuis Gasthuisberg,
Herestraat 49,
B-3000 Leuven, Belgium

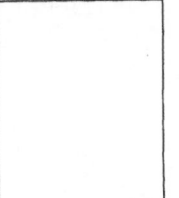

Gadzinski Daniel S., M.D.
Section of Emergency Medicine, Department of Surgery,
Wayne State University School of Medicine,
Detroit, Michigan, U.S.A.

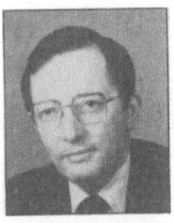

Godfraind, Théophile, M.D.
Professor of Pharmacology, Université Catholique de Louvain,
Labo de Pharmacodynamie Générale et de Pharmacologie,
U.C.L. 7350, Avenue Emmanuel Mounier, 73, B-1200 Bruxelles,
Belgium

Guerrini, Maurizio
Istituto di Patologia Medica
e Metodologia Clinica
University of Siena
53100 Siena, Italy

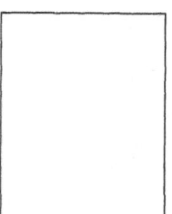

Hals, Ottar, M.D.
Medical Department 8, Ullevaal Hospital, University of Oslo,
Kirkevn. 166, Oslo 1, Norway.

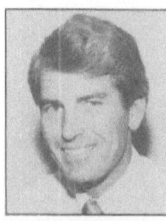

Hearse, David J., Ph.D.
St. Thomas Hospital
London, England

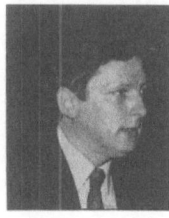

Herman, Arnold G., M.D.
Professor of Pharmacology,
University of Antwerp, UIA, Dept. of Medicine
Universiteitsplein 1, B-2610 Wilrijk, Belgium.

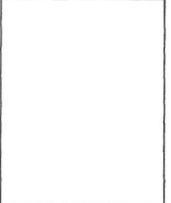

Hertsens, Robert C., M. Sc.
University of Antwerp, UIA, Dept. of Medicine,
Universiteitsplein 1, B-2610 Wilrijk, Belgium.

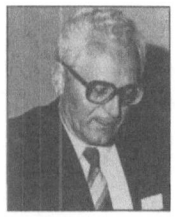

Hladovec, Josef, M.D.
Institute of Clinical and Experimental Medicine, Praha,
Czechoslovakia.

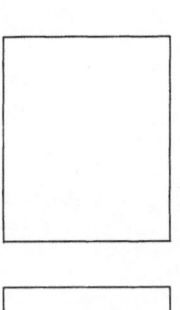

Hoehner Paul J.
Section of Emergency Medicine, Department of Surgery,
Wayne State University School of Medicine,
Detroit, Michigan, U.S.A.

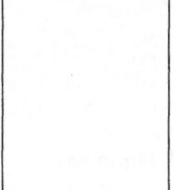

Hoehner Thomas
Section of Emergency Medicine, Department of Surgery,
Wayne State University School of Medicine,
Detroit, Michigan, U.S.A.

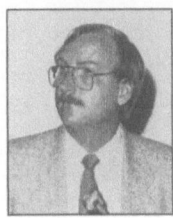

Hofferberth, Bernhard, M.D.
Neurological University Hospital (Dir. Prof. G.G.Brune)
Münster, West-Germany.

Jacob, Willem A., Ph. D.
University of Antwerp, UIA, Dept. of Medicine,
Universiteitsplein 1, B-2610 Wilrijk, Belgium.

Kidner, Peter H., M.A., B.M., B.Ch., F.R.C.P.
Physician,
Waller Cardiopulmonary Unit,
St. Mary's Hospital,
Praed Street,
London W.2, U.K.

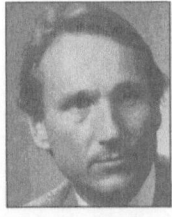

Klein, Werner, M.D.
Professor,
Department of Cardiology,
University hospital, A-8036 Graz, Austria.

Laghi Pasini, Franco
Istituto di Patologia Medica
e Metodologia Clinica
University of Siena
53100 Siena, Italy

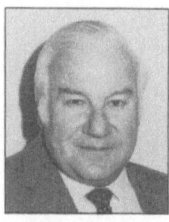

Lichtlen, Paul R., M.D.
Professor,
Division of Cardiology, Hannover Medical School, Hannover,
West-Germany.

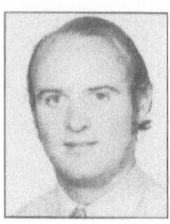

Littler, William A., M.D.
Professor of Cardiovascular Medicine,
University of Birmingham and East Birmingham Hospital,
Bordesley Green East, Birmingham B9 5ST, England.

Meijler, Frits L., M.D.
Professor of Cardiology, University Hospital, Utrecht,
The Netherlands

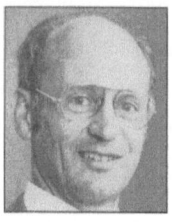

Meldrum, Brian S., M.B., B. Chir., Ph. D.
Senior Lecturer,
Department of Neurology, Institute of Psychiatry,
De Crespigny Park, London SE5 8AF, U.K.

Midtbø, Kjell, M.D.
Medical Department 8, Ullevaal Hospital, University of Oslo,
Kirkevn. 166, Oslo 1, Norway.

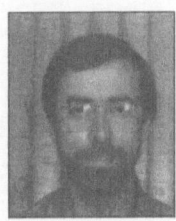

Miller, Robert C., M.D.
Université Louis Pasteur,
Laboratoire de Pharmacodynamie,
B.P. 10, F-67048 Strasbourg Cedex, France

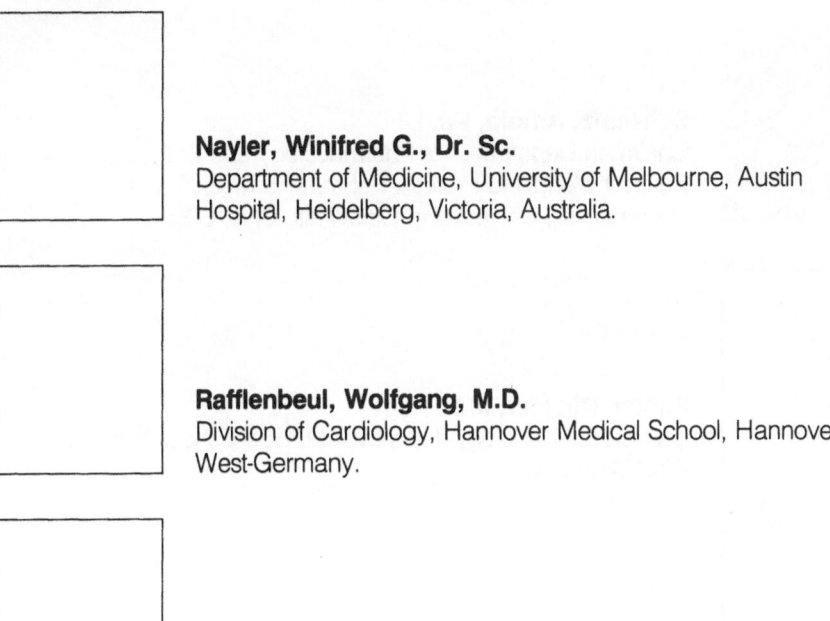

Nayler, Winifred G., Dr. Sc.
Department of Medicine, University of Melbourne, Austin
Hospital, Heidelberg, Victoria, Australia.

Rafflenbeul, Wolfgang, M.D.
Division of Cardiology, Hannover Medical School, Hannover,
West-Germany.

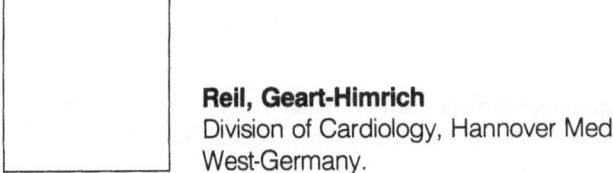

Rämsch, Klaus-Dieter, Ph. D.
Bayer AG, Wupperthal, West Germany.

Reil, Geart-Himrich
Division of Cardiology, Hannover Medical School, Hannover,
West-Germany.

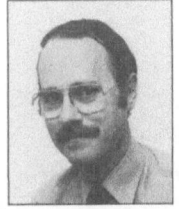

Ruigrok, Tom J.C., Ph.D.
Department of Cardiology, University Hospital, Utrecht, The
Netherlands

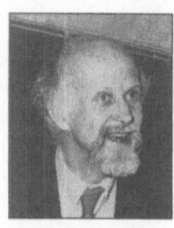

Schatzmann, Hans Jürg, M.D.
Department of Veterinary Pharmacology,
University of Bern,
Bern, Switzerland.

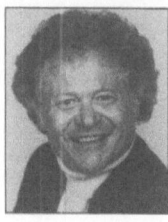

Schwartz, Arnold, Ph. D.
Chairman Department of Pharmacology and Cell Biophysics,
Edward Wendland Professor of Materia Medica and
Therapeutics, University of Cincinnati, Ohio, U.S.A.

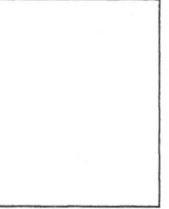

Simon, Rüdiger, M.D.
Division of Cardiology, Hannover Medical School, Hannover,
West-Germany.

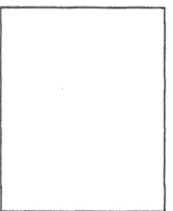

Slade, Anthony M., Ph. D.
Cardiothoracic Institute, University of London,
London, England.

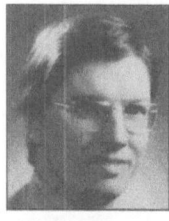

Spierings, Egilius L.H., M.D., Ph.D.
Department of Neurology, University Hospital "Dijkzigt"
3015 GD Rotterdam, The Netherlands

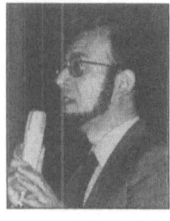

Stoltz, Jean-François
Research Director, Groupe d'Hémorhéologie, Centre de
Transfusion Sanguine, Brabois, 54500 Vandoeuvre les Nancy,
France

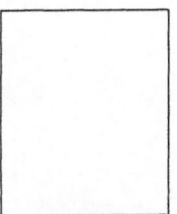

Storstein, Liv, M.D.
Medical Department 8, Ullevaal Hospital, University of Oslo,
Kirkevn. 166, Oslo 1, Norway.

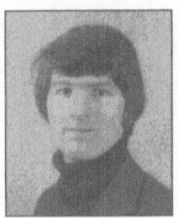

Towart, Robbie, B.Sc., Ph. D.
Head of Biochemical Pharmacology
Miles Laboratories Ltd.
Stoke Poges, Slough SL24LY
U.K.

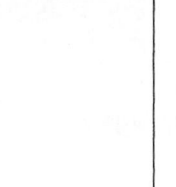

Trombley John Jr., R. Ph.
Section of Emergency Medicine, Department of Surgery,
Wayne State University School of Medicine,
Detroit, Michigan, U.S.A.

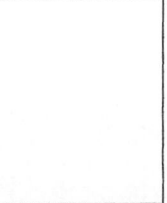

van der Meer, Joop, M. Ph. Sci.
Granliveien 33, N-3440 Royken, Norway.

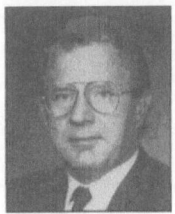

Vanhoutte, Paul M., M.D.,
Professor of Physiology and Pharmacology
Department of Physiology and Biophysics
Mayo Clinic and Mayo Foundation
Rochester, Minnesota 55905, U.S.A.

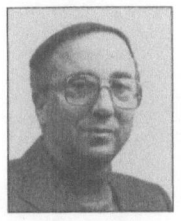

Van Nueten, Jan M., Dr. Sc.
Department of Pharmacology,
Janssen Pharmaceutica Research Laboratories
B-2340 Beerse, Belgium.

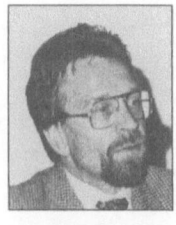

Wauquier, Albert, Ph. D.
Department of Neuropharmacology,
Janssen Pharmaceutica Research Laboratories,
B-2340 Beerse, Belgium

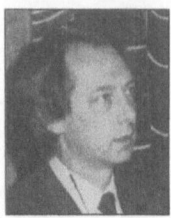

Wellens, Donald, Dr. Sc.
Janssen Pharmaceutica,
B-2340 Beerse, Belgium.

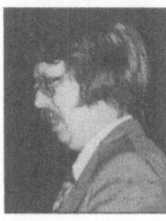

White, Blaine C., M.D.
Section of Emergency Medicine, Department of Surgery,
Wayne State University School of Medicine,
Detroit, Michigan, U.S.A.

Winegar Carl D., M.D.
Section of Emergency Medicine, Department of Surgery,
Wayne State University School of Medicine,
Detroit, Michigan, U.S.A.